Head and Neck Cancer

Editor

GLENN J. HANNA

HEMATOLOGY/ONCOLOGY CLINICS OF NORTH AMERICA

www.hemonc.theclinics.com

Consulting Editors
GEORGE P. CANELLOS
EDWARD J. BENZ Jr

October 2021 • Volume 35 • Number 5

ELSEVIER

1600 John F. Kennedy Boulevard • Suite 1800 • Philadelphia, Pennsylvania, 19103-2899

http://www.theclinics.com

**HEMATOLOGY/ONCOLOGY CLINICS OF NORTH AMERICA Volume 35, Number 5
October 2021 ISSN 0889-8588, ISBN 13: 978-0-323-80930-6**

Editor: Stacy Eastman
Developmental Editor: Ann Gielou M. Posedio

Hematology/Oncology Clinics (ISSN 0889-8588) is published bimonthly by Elsevier Inc., 360 Park Avenue South, New York, NY 10010-1710. Months of issue are February, April, June, August, October, and December. Business and Editorial Offices: 1600 John F. Kennedy Blvd., Ste. 1800, Philadelphia, PA 19103–2899. Customer Service Office: 3251 Riverport Lane, Maryland Heights, MO 63043. Periodicals postage paid at New York, NY and at additional mailing offices. Subscription prices are $456.00 per year (domestic individuals), $1150.00 per year (domestic institutions), $100.00 per year (domestic students/residents), $480.00 per year (Canadian individuals), $100.00 per year (Canadian students/residents), $1213.00 per year (Canadian institutions) $547.00 per year (international individuals), $1213.00 per year (international institutions), and $255.00 per year (international students/residents). International air speed delivery is included in all *Clinics* subscription prices. All prices are subject to change without notice. **POSTMASTER:** Send address changes to *Hematology/Oncology Clinics of North America*, Elsevier Health Sciences Division, Subscription Customer Service, 3251 Riverport Lane, Maryland Heights, MO 63043. Customer Service (orders, claims, online, change of address): Elsevier Health Sciences Division, Subscription **Customer Service, 3251 Riverport Lane, Maryland Heights, MO 63043. Tel: 1-800-654-2452 (U.S. and Canada); 314-447-8871 (outside U.S. and Canada). Fax: 314-447-8029. E-mail: journalscustomerservice-usa@elsevier.com (for print support); journalsonlinesupport-usa@elsevier.com (for online support).**

Reprints. For copies of 100 or more, of articles in this publication, please contact the Commercial Reprints Department, Elsevier Inc., 360 Park Avenue South, New York, New York 10010-1710; Tel.: 212-633-3874, Fax: 212-633-3820, E-mail: reprints@elsevier.com.

Hematology/Oncology Clinics of North America is covered in *MEDLINE/PubMed (Index Medicus), EMBASE/ Excerpta Medica, and BIOSIS.*

Contributors

CONSULTING EDITORS

GEORGE P. CANELLOS, MD
William Rosenberg Professor of Medicine, Department of Medical Oncology, Dana-Farber
Cancer Institute, Boston, Massachusetts

EDWARD J. BENZ Jr, MD
Professor, Pediatrics, Richard and Susan Smith Professor, Medicine, Professor, Genetics,
Harvard Medical School, President and CEO Emeritus, Office of the President, Dana-
Farber Cancer Institute, Boston, Massachusetts

EDITOR

GLENN J. HANNA, MD
Medical Oncologist, Center for Head and Neck Oncology, Director, Center for Salivary and
Rare Head and Neck Cancers, Dana-Farber Cancer Institute, Assistant Professor of
Medicine, Harvard Medical School, Boston, Massachusetts

AUTHORS

CHARU AGGARWAL, MD, MPH
Department of Medicine, Division of Hematology-Oncology, University of Pennsylvania,
Perelman Center for Advanced Medicine, Philadelphia, Pennsylvania

NISHANT AGRAWAL, MD
University of Chicago, Chicago, Illinois

DINESH K. CHHETRI, MD
Vice-Chair of the UCLA, Department of Head and Neck Surgery, David Geffen School of
Medicine at UCLA, UCLA Head and Neck Cancer Program, Los Angeles, California

KRISTEN A. ECHANIQUE, MD
Department of Head and Neck Surgery, David Geffen School of Medicine at UCLA, Los
Angeles, California

LAURAN K. EVANS, MD, MPH
Department of Head and Neck Surgery, David Geffen School of Medicine at UCLA, Los
Angeles, California

ZHEN GOOI, MBBS
University of Chicago, Chicago, Illinois

JEFFREY P. GUENETTE, MD
Assistant Professor of Radiology, Director of Head and Neck Imaging and Interventions,
Division of Neuroradiology, Brigham and Women's Hospital, Dana-Farber Cancer
Institute, Harvard Medical School, Boston, Massachusetts

ALBERT Y. HAN, MD, PhD
Department of Head and Neck Surgery, David Geffen School of Medicine at UCLA, Los Angeles, California

ANDREW J. HOLCOMB, MD
Assistant Professor of Otolaryngology–Head and Neck Surgery, Creighton Medical School, Nebraska Methodist Hospital, Omaha, Nebraska

ADAM HOWARD, MD
University of Chicago, Chicago, Illinois

GINO K. IN, MD, MPH
Assistant Professor of Medicine and Dermatology, Norris Comprehensive Cancer Center, University of Southern California Keck School of Medicine, Los Angeles, California

VIDHYA KARIVEDU, MD
Division of Medical Oncology, The Ohio State University, Columbus, Ohio

ELENI M. RETTIG, MD
Head and Neck Surgeon, Division of Otolaryngology–Head and Neck Surgery, Department of Surgery, Brigham and Women's Hospital, Center for Head and Neck Oncology, Dana-Farber Cancer Institute, Department of Otolaryngology–Head and Neck Surgery, Harvard Medical School, Boston, Massachusetts

JEREMY D. RICHMON, MD
Associate Professor of Otolaryngology–Head and Neck Surgery, Mass Eye and Ear, Harvard Medical School, Boston, Massachusetts

NABIL F. SABA, MD, FACP
Professor, Hematology, Medical Oncology and Otolaryngology, Director, Head and Neck Oncology Program, Winship Cancer Institute, Emory University, Atlanta, Georgia

ROSH K.V. SETHI, MD, MPH
Head and Neck Surgeon, Division of Otolaryngology–Head and Neck Surgery, Department of Surgery, Brigham and Women's Hospital, Center for Head and Neck Oncology, Dana-Farber Cancer Institute, Department of Otolaryngology Head and Neck Surgery, Harvard Medical School, Boston, Massachusetts

HIRA SHAIKH, MD
Division of Hematology/Oncology, University of Cincinnati, Cincinnati, Ohio

ANN W. SILK, MD, MS
Dana-Farber Cancer Institute, Harvard Medical School, Boston, Massachusetts

MAIE A. ST. JOHN, MD, PhD
Chair of the UCLA, Department of Head and Neck Surgery, David Geffen School of Medicine at UCLA, UCLA Head and Neck Cancer Program, Los Angeles, California

LOVA SUN, MD
Department of Medicine, Division of Hematology-Oncology, University of Pennsylvania, Perelman Center for Advanced Medicine, Philadelphia, Pennsylvania

MELISSA A. TAYLOR, MD, MPH
Department of Internal Medicine, Emory University, Atlanta, Georgia

VATCHE TCHEKMEDYIAN, MD, MEd
Assistant Professor of Medicine, Tufts University School of Medicine, MaineHealth
Cancer Care, South Portland, Maine

JACOB S. THOMAS, MD
Assistant Professor of Clinical Medicine, Norris Comprehensive Cancer Center, University
of Southern California Keck School of Medicine, Los Angeles, California

SUMITA TRIVEDI, MD
Department of Medicine, Division of Hematology-Oncology, University of Pennsylvania,
Perelman Center for Advanced Medicine, Philadelphia, Pennsylvania

HARISH N. VASUDEVAN, MD, PhD
Department of Radiation Oncology, University of California, San Francisco, San
Francisco, California

TRISHA M. WISE-DRAPER, MD, PhD
Division of Hematology/Oncology, University of Cincinnati, Cincinnati, Ohio

SUE S. YOM, MD, PhD, MAS
Department of Radiation Oncology, University of California, San Francisco, San
Francisco, California

Contents

CT, PET, ultrasound, and MRI examinations all have roles in the staging and surveillance of cancers in the head and neck. Contrast-enhanced CT is generally the primary examination because of availability, cost, reproducibility, and good overall quality regardless of where performed. PET, ultrasound, and MRI have more specific and nuanced applications. Good interdisciplinary interactions with radiologist consultation can streamline the examination process and reduce the examination burden on patients by limiting the number and maximizing the quality of the examinations and image-guided interventions performed.

Technological developments have disrupted the practice of medicine throughout history. Endoscopic and robotic techniques in head and neck surgery have emerged over the past half-century and have been incrementally adapted to expanding indications within otolaryngology. Robotic and endoscopic surgery have an established role in treatment of oropharyngeal and laryngeal cancers, reducing surgical morbidity and improving survival relative to traditional open approaches. Surgical treatment of human papillomavirus-mediated oropharyngeal cancer via transoral robotic surgery offers equivalent oncologic and functional outcomes relative to radiotherapy. Newer iterations of single-port robotic systems continue to expand the scope of robotics in head and neck surgery.

Lip and oral cavity squamous cell carcinoma (SCC) develop from progressive dysplasia of these mucosal structures. The cancers are often preceded by premalignant lesions, and any nonhealing ulcers of the lip or oral cavity should be biopsied. Some risk factors for these 2 subsites overlap and include tobacco use, alcohol use, and an immunocompromised state. Lip and oral cavity SCC are clinically staged based on physical examination and imaging. The 5-year overall survival for early-stage lip and oral cavity SCC is around 70% to 90% but decreases to about 50% for late-stage disease.

> Squamous cell carcinoma of the oropharynx (OPC) consists of human papillomavirus (HPV)-negative disease caused by tobacco and alcohol use, and HPV-positive disease caused by the sexually transmitted infection HPV. These entities have unique but overlapping risk factors, epidemiologic trends, staging systems, and survival outcomes. HPV-positive tumor status confers a significant survival benefit compared with HPV-negative disease. OPC treatment entails a combination of surgery, radiation, and chemotherapy. Ongoing trials will determine whether treatment of HPV-related disease may be safely deintensified to decrease morbidity. Emerging HPV-related biomarkers are under study as tools to inform screening, diagnosis, treatment, and surveillance for HPV-positive OPC.

> The Radiation Therapy Oncology Group 91-11 trial and US Veterans Affairs trial revolutionized the way locally advanced laryngeal cancers are treated. Adjuvant therapies exist aimed toward laryngeal preservation using docetaxel, cisplatin, and fluorouracil. Cetuximab is a cornerstone of treatment due to the large role of epidermal growth factor receptor in laryngeal and hypopharyngeal carcinomas. In addition, the immune system is vital in the prevention of recurrence, and various immunomodulators against programmed cell death receptor 1 are being investigated. Multidisciplinary management of the patient with laryngeal and hypopharyngeal is key, as many vital functions are affected by this devastating disease.

> Sinonasal malignancies rare and pathologically diverse and make up <1% of all malignancies. Due to their anatomical location, they can cause significant morbidity with involvement of surrounding critical structures. They often present at a late stage with insidious onset of symptoms. Treatment of sinonasal malignancies is challenging and they often require a multimodality approach with surgery, radiation, and chemotherapy. Outcomes are poor with 5-year overall survival around 32%, but this varies greatly depending on histologic subtype. There is an urgent need for more randomized controlled trials to better define the appropriate therapeutic regimens and to improve clinical outcomes.

> Nasopharyngeal carcinoma (NPC) is caused by Epstein-Barr virus (EBV) infection, yet incorporating measurement of EBV DNA levels into clinical practice remains a challenge. Here, we summarize the relationship between NPC and EBV infection before describing the use of cell-free DNA as a plasma biomarker in cancer. We then compare conventional polymerase chain reaction methods and emerging next-generation sequencing

approaches for EBV viral load detection emphasizing their prognostic and predictive utility. We conclude by considering how assay standardization, novel molecular approaches, and alternative clinical specimens may be leveraged to bring EBV testing into the routine care of patients with NPC.

Vatche Tchekmedyian

Salivary gland carcinomas are a rare and heterogenous group of cancers with varying underlying biology and clinical behavior. A quickly evolving body of data has advanced the understanding of these tumors, leading to effective therapeutics for several histologic subtypes. Biologically rational clinical trials have developed from an understanding of MYB and NOTCH signaling in adenoid cystic carcinoma. The recognition of androgen receptor signaling and HER2-targeted therapy has offered therapeutic options in non-ACC salivary cancers. The use of TRK inhibitors in salivary secretory carcinoma has led to exceptional responses. Immunotherapy is an exciting new therapeutic avenue that requires further exploration.

Gino K. In, Jacob S. Thomas, and Ann W. Silk

Cutaneous malignancies (CMs), or skin cancers, are the most common cancer worldwide, with a quarter million cases diagnosed annually in the United States alone. The best described risk factor for CM is ultraviolet radiation from sunlight, and therefore most of these cancers develop in sun-exposed skin, including the head and neck. Beginning with melanoma, immunotherapy has increasingly been used over the past decade for treatment of unresectable CM, and immune checkpoint inhibitors are now Food and Drug Administration–approved for first-line treatment of unresectable melanoma, Merkel cell carcinoma, and cutaneous squamous cell carcinoma, and second-line for basal cell carcinoma.

Hira Shaikh, Vidhya Karivedu, and Trisha M. Wise-Draper

Head and neck squamous cell carcinoma (HNSCC) treatment is often associated with high morbidity especially in the recurrent and/or metastatic (R/M) setting, limiting effective treatment options. Local disease control is important. Therefore, local therapies including reirradiation and salvage surgery, either alone or in combination with systemic treatment, may be used for selected patients with R/M HNSCC. Although chemotherapy and targeted agents have modest efficacy in HNSCC, the advent of immunotherapy has revolutionized the treatment paradigm of R/M HNSCC. Multiple trials have resulted in the past 5 years advocating for its use alone or in combination with chemotherapy.

Sumita Trivedi, Lova Sun, and Charu Aggarwal

Head and neck squamous cell carcinomas (HNSCC) remain an important cause of global cancer morbidity and mortality. Historically, outcomes for patients with recurrent or metastatic disease were poor with limited treatment options. In recent decades, the demographic profile of this disease has evolved with an increase in human papilloma virus–associated oropharyngeal carcinoma and a decrease in tobacco-related disease. The treatment paradigm for HNSCC has rapidly evolved with identification of novel, immune-directed, therapeutic strategies that take advantage of immune dysregulation commonly seen in HNSCC. This review summarizes recent developments in this field and discusses emerging strategies for future therapies.

HEMATOLOGY/ONCOLOGY
CLINICS OF NORTH AMERICA

FORTHCOMING ISSUES

December 2021
Inherited Bleeding Disorders
Nathan T. Connell, *Editor*

February 2022
Central Nervous System Malignancies
David A. Reardon, *Editor*

April 2022
**New Developments in the Understanding
and Treatment of Autoimmune Hemolytic
Anemia**
Alexandra P. Wolanskyj-Spinner and
Ronald S. Go, *Editors*

RECENT ISSUES

August 2021
Chronic Lymphocytic Leukemia
Jennifer R. Brown, *Editor*

June 2021
Bladder Cancer
Guru P. Sonpavde, *Editor*

April 2021
Myeloproliferative Neoplasms
Ronald Hoffman, Ross Levine, John
Mascarenhas, and Raajit Rampal, *Editors*

SERIES OF RELATED INTEREST

Surgical Oncology Clinics of North America
https://www.surgonc.theclinics.com/

Preface

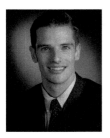

Glenn J. Hanna, MD
Editor

Head and neck cancers comprise a unique set of distinct disease entities, from carcinogen-related and viral-mediated mucosal cancers to the rare salivary gland malignancies, all of which necessitate multidisciplinary expert collaboration to diagnose and treat. In the last few years, there have been important advances made within the head and neck oncology community. This often underrecognized and highly specialized area of cancer medicine has been revolutionized by the established benefits of immunotherapy in the advanced disease setting, and we have made further strides toward treatment deintensification while preserving favorable outcomes in human papillomavirus (HPV)-associated disease. But despite these improvements, there remains a continued need to push our understanding of head and neck cancer biology and immunology to improve patient outcomes.

In this issue of *Hematology/Oncology Clinics of North America*, we review the current landscape of head and neck cancer diagnosis and treatment while providing insights on where the field may be headed: dividing the issue into eleven subtopics worthy of individual attention. We start by reviewing optimal radiologic evaluation of the complex head and neck anatomy and focus on technological advances permitting minimally invasive techniques to access delicate aerodigestive structures, both of which have improved our diagnostic accuracy and reshaped our approach to surgically manage these cancers. The middle articles cover the principles of treating mucosal head and neck malignancies, dominated by squamous cell carcinomas, focusing on definitive surgical and nonsurgical concurrent chemoradiotherapy paradigms. These articles also highlight advances toward treatment deescalation for favorable risk HPV oropharyngeal cancers and biomarker utility like that of circulating Epstein-Barr virus DNA monitoring. The later articles in the issue start by featuring a review of the rare salivary gland cancers and the molecularly targeted approaches being adopted to personalize therapy for this constellation of histologic entities when disease becomes advanced or incurable. Finally, we turn to cutaneous and recurrent metastatic head and neck disease, where immunotherapy has redefined treatment algorithms and improved survival

Hematol Oncol Clin N Am 35 (2021) xiii–xiv
https://doi.org/10.1016/j.hoc.2021.07.013
0889-8588/21/© 2021 Published by Elsevier Inc.

outcomes for the first time in decades. This immuno-oncology revolution has welcomed newer trials investigating immunotherapy in all disease settings: neoadjuvant or preoperatively, in the definitive setting with concurrent chemoradiation, and in the adjuvant setting to prevent recurrence among high-risk disease.

I hope the issue provides a means to understanding our current diagnostic and treatment approaches in this collection of diseases and sheds light on areas for improvement and opportunities for cancer therapeutic research development to benefit our patients now, and in the future.

Glenn J. Hanna, MD
Center for Head & Neck Oncology
Center for Salivary and Rare Head and Neck Cancers
Dana-Farber Cancer Institute
Harvard Medical School
Boston, MA 02215, USA

E-mail address:
glenn_hanna@dfci.harvard.edu

Radiologic Evaluation of the Head and Neck Cancer Patient

Jeffrey P. Guenette, MD

KEYWORDS

- Head and neck neoplasms • Spiral computed tomography
- Positron-emission tomography • Diagnostic ultrasound
- Magnetic resonance imaging

KEY POINTS

- Contrast-enhanced CT is generally the primary examination for staging and surveillance of head and neck cancers because of availability, cost, reproducibility, and good overall quality regardless of where performed.
- Ultrasound is the primary examination for thyroid and superficial salivary gland lesions.
- PET has a variable role based on availability and provider preference but can help improve detection of some primary cancers and small metastases with a good negative predictive value for surveillance imaging.
- MRI is the examination of choice for deep salivary gland lesions and when there is concern for a fixed or infiltrative mass, bone involvement, or perineural tumor spread.

INTRODUCTION

The complexity of head and neck anatomy, with many small structures, can make diagnostic medical imaging of this region quite challenging. This article is written for medical oncologists, radiation oncologists, and surgeons who manage patients with cancers of the head and neck. The focus of the article is on outlining the advantages and disadvantages of the different imaging examination choices for the most common scenarios. The article is meant to serve as a practical guide to ordering the highest-yield imaging examinations. Advanced imaging techniques are beyond the scope of this article. While prior review articles on this topic tend to focus on imaging by disease process, this article focuses on imaging examination type so that readers can ulti-mately make informed—as opposed to algorithmic—decisions, thereby facilitating decision-making in nonroutine and challenging cases.

Division of Neuroradiology, Brigham and Women's Hospital, Dana-Farber Cancer Institute, Harvard Medical School, 75 Francis Street, Boston, MA 02115, USA
E-mail address: jpguenette@bwh.harvard.edu

Hematol Oncol Clin N Am 35 (2021) 863–873
https://doi.org/10.1016/j.hoc.2021.05.001
0889-8588/21/© 2021 Elsevier Inc. All rights reserved.

hemonc.theclinics.com

APPROACH
Computed tomography

Computed tomography (CT) is available throughout the United States, including in most remote areas, and in major health centers and cities in most parts of the world. For imaging of head and neck cancer, intravenous iodine-based contrast material improves visibility of tumor margins and abnormal lymph nodes. An advantage over ultrasound, CT examinations yield images of the entire evaluated volume of tissues, and these images can generally be reproduced in multiple planes. CT is also generally superior at depicting the degree of mass effect and involved adjacent tissues. However, conspicuity of lesions in the thyroid and salivary glands can be quite variable and, not infrequently, may not be visible on CT. Similarly, artifact from dental amalgam and hardware can obscure large portions of the oral cavity mucosa, tongue, and oropharynx. While CT quality is somewhat dependent on the available equipment and reconstruction methods, all examinations are generally interpretable by a radiologist with appropriate training, and findings are generally reproducible across scanner platforms and institutions.

Given the accessibility, reproducibility, and relatively lower cost than MRI and PET, and general clear depiction of the primary tumor while thoroughly screening for node metastases (**Fig. 1**), contrast-enhanced CT is the primary imaging examination for the staging and restaging of most cancers in the head and neck. Situations in which CT may not be the optimal examination are outlined in the other sections of this article.

It is important for all providers to understand radiology reporting variance in tumor measurements. While the American Joint Committee on Cancer staging criteria rely on tumor and lymph node measurements in the greatest dimension,[1] many radiologists report measurements in the longest axial dimension, which can differ substantially from the greatest dimension in craniocaudal or oblique planes. There is a historical reason for this reporting discrepancy. CT images were originally acquired in the axial plan and could not be reconstructed into multiple planes. More recently, images were not reconstructed into multiple planes routinely because of data storage limitations. Only recently have images been routinely reconstructed in multiple planes. Radiologist practices and imaging criteria have thus been typically based on axial measurements. Oncologists and oncology surgeons should recognize such potential size discrepancies in radiology reports and encourage their

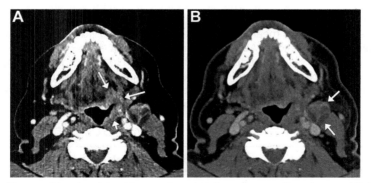

Fig. 1. A 60-year-old male with p16+ oropharyngeal squamous cell carcinoma. (*A*) Contrast-enhanced axial CT image in mucosal windows shows left glossotonsillar sulcus primary tumor (*arrows*). (*B*) Contrast-enhanced axial CT image in soft-tissue windows shows partially cystic/necrotic left level 2A lymph node metastasis.

radiologists to begin reporting greatest overall dimensions, at least in the setting of known or suspected cancer.

On CT images, morphologic features of lymph node necrosis or cystic change are considered the most reliable finding of metastatic involvement.[2] Clusters of three or more nodes in the drainage pathway of a primary tumor and abnormal rounded shape are both also predictors of metastatic involvement.[2] Multiple size criteria have been proposed and investigated for discriminating metastatic and benign lymph nodes; however, all encounter a somewhat arbitrary decision between sensitivity and specificity. The following size criteria are the commonly used ones for reporting a lymph node as suspicious for malignant involvement:

Maximum axial diameter: greater than 15 mm in level 1 and level 2; greater than 8 mm for retropharyngeal; and greater than 10 mm for all other nodes.

Minimum axial diameter: greater than 11 mm in level 2; greater than 5 mm for retropharyngeal; and greater than 10 mm for all other nodes.[2]

Recent research has focused on whether we can accurately determine extranodal extension without the need for intervention. Multiple features have been published as indicative of extranodal extension, but the criteria have varied by study, and the studies have been small. A recent meta-analysis indicates that infiltration of adjacent fat planes has the highest pooled specificity (94%), while central necrosis has the highest pooled sensitivity (81%); however, interobserver agreement is substantial.[3]

Variation in radiologist reporting is known,[4,5] can be confusing, and can make treatment decisions more difficult. Development of radiologist reporting lexicons and templates has aimed to reduce unwarranted variation. The Neck Imaging Reporting and Data Systems (NI-RADS) reporting recommendations and standardized reporting template were introduced in 2018 to help reduce unwarranted variation in the reporting of head and neck cancer restaging examinations.[6] The use of NI-RADS reporting is likely to become more commonplace, particularly at cancer institutions.

Acute adverse reactions to the types of iodinated intravenous contrast medications currently used in diagnostic imaging (low-osmolality contrast media) have been reported at a frequency of between 0.2% and 0.7% including both allergy-like and physiologic reactions.[7] Serious reactions are reported at a historical rate of 0.04%[8] with rare fatal reactions reported.[7] Patients with prior contrast reactions deemed to be at high risk are thought to benefit from premedication before subsequent injection of iodinated contrast media and guidelines are published.[7] Contrast-induced nephropathy, in which intravenous iodinated contrast causes acute kidney injury, is currently believed to be a real but rare entity. Contrast-induced nephropathy is often confused with postcontrast acute kidney injury, which is multifactorial and likely unrelated to but associated with administration of intravenous contrast.[7] Protocols for managing the risk of contrast-induced nephropathy vary by institution.

For those interested, briefly and in general, CT images are essentially density maps of body tissues calculated from the extent to which high-energy photons (ionizing radiation, as used in radiographic imaging) penetrate the tissues. CT images are currently acquired by spinning an x-ray tube and multiple x-ray detectors around a patient as the patient moves craniocaudally through the x-ray beam. The acquired data are then reconstructed into images using one of a variety of methods. The reconstruction process optimizes images for viewing different types of tissues, can generate a variety of slice thicknesses, and can generate images in any plane, conventionally in the anatomic axial, coronal, and sagittal planes. The American Association of Physicists in Medicine (AAPM)/Radiological Society of North America (RSNA) resident physics series includes a nice overview of CT physics by Mahesh.[9]

Positron emission tomography

PET is more expensive and more resource-intensive than CT. Moreover, it relies on the production and safe storage of radioactive materials. Its availability is limited in some rural parts of the United States and many parts of the world. The spatial resolution of PET is generally poor compared with the other imaging modalities. PET imaging is typically performed concurrently with CT. This CT is performed with a low-dose technique and is not a diagnostic CT examination. The low-dose CT has two functions: It serves as a density map for the computations required to create the PET images, and it enables soft-tissue localization of regions of ^{18}F-fluorodeoxyglucose (FDG)-avidity. A diagnostic neck CT, with intravenous contrast, should thus be performed in addition to PET for initial staging of primary head and neck cancers. A restaging PET that is positive may necessitate a subsequent diagnostic neck CT to fully evaluate the size and margins of the recurrence.

The most common radioisotope used for head and neck cancer imaging is FDG, a glucose analog that serves as a marker for relative cellular metabolic activity. Multiple studies have shown a substantial increase in rate of detection of primary tumor when FDG-PET is performed in the setting of a biopsy-proven lymph node squamous cell carcinoma metastases when a primary tumor is not seen on the contrast-enhanced CT examination or physical examination.[10] For nasopharyngeal cancer restaging, a meta-analysis has shown FDG-PET to be the best modality for diagnosis of local residual or recurrent cancer[11] (Fig. 2). Overall, FDG-PET has a high negative predictive value for response assessment and surveillance imaging in primary head and neck squamous cell carcinoma, but the positive predictive value has been reported low at under 60%[12]; pooled sensitivity is reported at 0.92 and 0.87, respectively.[13]

FDG-PET may also be useful for the workup of newly diagnosed head and neck squamous cell carcinoma in the clinically N0 neck. Several studies have shown that FDG-PET may increase detection of small lymph node metastases,[10] and a new study has shown a good negative predictive value that can potentially impact treatment

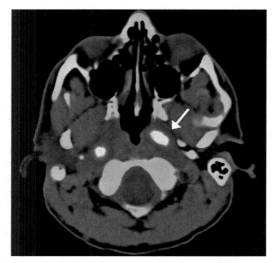

Fig. 2. A 38-year-old male with nasopharyngeal squamous cell carcinoma. Fused axial FDG-PET/CT image shows focal uptake in the region of the left nasopharynx primary tumor (*arrow*) and focal uptake in the region of a right retropharyngeal lymph node metastasis.

planning.[14] The use of FDG-PET for this purpose remains variable and debated in practice.

For iodine-refractory recurrent thyroid cancer, FDG-PET can be used for restaging.[15] FDG-PET can also be used for restaging medullary thyroid cancer, although ^{68}GA-DOTATOC-PET imaging and ^{18}F-FDOPA-PET imaging (radiopharmaceuticals that target somatostatin receptors and dopaminergic nerve terminals, respectively) are more sensitive and better used for this indication where these radioisotopes are available.[16] Note that traditional radioactive iodine imaging (both ^{129}I and ^{131}I) and other non-PET nuclear medicine imaging are fundamentally different from PET imaging and require different detector technologies and equipment.

To confirm a suspicion of glomus tumor/paraganglioma and to screen for paraganglioma in patients with succinate dehydrogenase complex subunits B (SDHB) mutations, ^{68}GA-DOTATATE-PET is the most sensitive examination.[17,18]

For those interested, briefly and in general, PET images are generated by detecting and localizing high-energy photons traveling in opposite directions that were created from the annihilation of a positron that was emitted from the nucleus of a radioactively decaying nucleotide. PET images are thus maps of relative functional uptake of the radiotracer. The AAPM/RSNA resident physics series includes a nice overview of PET physics by Votaw.[19]

Ultrasound

Ultrasound is a portable, relatively low-cost, widely available imaging modality that provides excellent resolution of soft tissues. It also provides real-time evaluation, making it ideal for image-guided biopsies. Image quality and identification of abnormalities are largely dependent on the sonographer and available equipment. Saved images are limited to those selected by the sonographer. Soft tissues deep to air and bone cannot be evaluated with ultrasound. Deeper tissue is more difficult to evaluate than more superficial tissue.

Ultrasound is the primary imaging examination for the evaluation of thyroid nodules and diagnosis of thyroid cancer.[20] Multiple thyroid nodule scoring and reporting criteria are in use.[21] Including patient criteria can increase precision of thyroid nodule risk assessment.[22] Ultrasound is also typically used for screening cervical lymph nodes in newly diagnosed thyroid cancer with a reasonable sensitivity and specificity for lateral compartment metastases but poor sensitivity for central compartment metastases.[23]

Palpable and other superficial salivary gland tumors can typically be well characterized with ultrasound,[24] while MRI is more appropriate for deeper tumors or when there is concern for tumor infiltration of surrounding structures or concern for perineural spread.

Ultrasound is generally the preferred imaging method to guide percutaneous biopsies of head and neck lesions because the needle location can be monitored in real time with appropriate lesion targeting and avoidance of blood vessels. Deep face, including deep lobe of the parotid, and skull base lesions are typically better accessed with CT guidance. Both fine-needle aspiration and core biopsies can be obtained with either ultrasound guidance or CT guidance (**Fig. 3**). A good review of these techniques has been published by Loevner.[25]

For those interested, briefly and in general, ultrasound images are generated by pulsing sound waves into the body and then calculating the time it takes for those pulses to reflect back to the body surface. The sound waves are generated, and reflections recorded, by a small transducer held on the surface of the body by a sonographer. Different tissues have different reflective properties. Margins between

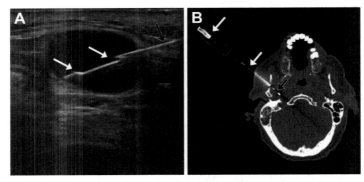

Fig. 3. (*A*) A 59-year-old male with metastatic prostate adenocarcinoma. Intraprocedural ultrasound image shows the core biopsy needle (*black arrow*) with the 1-cm biopsy tray (*white arrows*) within the circumscribed left supraclavicular lymph node. (*B*) An 85-year-old male with a mass in the deep lobe of the right parotid gland. Intraprocedural axial CT fluoroscopy image in bone windows shows the biopsy device and needle (*white arrows*) with the biopsy tray (*black arrow*) within the right deep parotid gland.

different tissue types are particularly reflective. A more in-depth overview of ultrasound physics is provided by Hangiandreou in the AAPM/RSNA resident physics tutorial series.[26]

Magnetic resonance imaging

MRI is more expensive and more resource-intensive than ultrasound or CT. While widely available in major United States medical centers and cities, it is not available in some rural locations in the United States and is not available in many parts of the world. For imaging of head and neck cancer, intravenous gadolinium-based contrast material can improve the visibility of tumor margins and abnormal lymph node morphology. In general, MRI can provide superior soft-tissue contrast and bone marrow evaluation compared with CT. MRI can be excellent for identifying and characterizing oral cavity, nasopharynx, salivary, and infiltrative tumors. However, MRI examination quality is highly dependent on the institution. Most stock MRI sequences available from vendors are not optimized for neck imaging, and thus many institutions use thick images with gaps between slices. Such imaging is suboptimal for evaluating the small structures in the head and neck.

MRI is the examination of choice for salivary gland tumors when there is concern for a fixed or infiltrative mass, nerve involvement, or perineural tumor spread (**Fig. 4**). Tumors of the major salivary glands can be difficult to see on CT. On ultrasound, infiltrating tumor and deep tumors can be difficult to appreciate, adjacent nerves cannot be located, and perineural spread cannot be evaluated. CT is often suitable for minor salivary glands, although MRI can be helpful in delineating the extent of soft-tissue or marrow involvement.[27] Perineural tumor spread is best evaluated with MRI.[28] The location of the facial nerve relative to parotid tumors can be accurately determined with MRI in many cases.[29]

MRI has largely replaced CT as the routine examination for staging of nasopharyngeal carcinoma.[30] The soft-tissue extent of tumor is generally more conspicuous on MRI. Furthermore, while CT can show permeative bone erosion in the skull base, loss of fat signal within the marrow on MRI has been more sensitive since the mid-1990s,[31] with substantially improved MRI imaging techniques since that time.

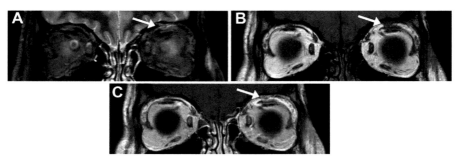

Fig. 4. A 59-year-old male with recurrent cutaneous squamous cell carcinoma. Coronal (*A*) short tau inversion recovery (STIR), (*B*) T1-weighted, and (*C*) T1-weighted postcontrast MRI images show thickening, inflammation around, and enhancement of left V1 (*arrows*) within the orbit, indicating perineural tumor spread.

For sinonasal tumors, a small study[32] and anecdotal cases suggest that MRI is more accurate in depicting involvement/breach of the periorbita with true orbital involvement.

For oral cavity cancers, artifact from dental amalgam and hardware can obscure large portions of the mucosa and tongue. There is frequently less artifact on MRI; coronal T2-weighted images with fat suppression often can clearly demonstrate the extent of tumor. MRI is highly sensitive for the detection of bone marrow invasion.[33] The use of MRI for preoperative depth-of-invasion or tumor thickness assessment may be useful,[34,35] but results have been unreliable, and CT may perform better[36,37] for a variety of reasons beyond the scope of this article. Ultimately, MRI is a useful adjunct to CT for oral cavity cancer when more information than what is discernible on the CT examination is needed.

In larynx and hypopharynx cancers, MRI has a higher sensitivity than CT for detecting cartilage invasion.[38] Dual-energy CT (which requires special CT equipment) can also be used to detect cartilage invasion[39] and may even be superior to MRI.[40] So MRI may be a useful additional examination when knowledge of cartilage invasion will change the recommended therapy.

Mild physiologic reactions to gadolinium-based contrast agents are common. Allergy-like reactions are uncommon with a reported frequency of 0.004% to 0.7%.[7] Severe, life-threatening, and fatal reactions to gadolinium-based contrast agents are exceedingly rare but do occur.[7] For patients with prior allergic reactions, there are no published studies to confirm whether premedication or agent change is efficacious in reducing the likelihood of a repeated reaction,[7] and institutional protocols thus vary. Nephrogenic systemic fibrosis has been associated with some gadolinium-based contrast agents, primarily in patients with renal failure on dialysis.[7] Institutional protocols for gadolinium-based contrast agent administration are often based on glomerular filtration rate but are also variable and determined in part on the available contrast agents.

For those interested, briefly and in general, MRI images are generated by characterizing the response of protons (primarily hydrogen atoms in water and fat molecules) to changes in the electromagnetic environment. This response varies based on the magnetic environment of local tissues and results in exceptional soft-tissue contrast. Essentially, for most MRI images, the body is placed in a large and strong magnetic field with which a proportion of protons align, radiofrequency waves are pulsed to disrupt the magnetic field and align the protons in the direction of the radiofrequency pulse, and then the machine records the time it takes for the protons to tip away from the direction of the radiofrequency pulse and the time it takes for the protons to realign with the large magnetic field. The AAPM/RSNA resident physics series includes a nice overview of MRI physics by Pooley.[41]

DISCUSSION

CT, PET, ultrasound, and MRI examinations all have roles in the staging and surveillance of cancers in the head and neck. Contrast-enhanced CT is generally the primary examination because of availability, cost, reproducibility, and good overall quality regardless of where performed. PET, ultrasound, and MRI have more specific and nuanced applications.

This review largely focuses on head and neck squamous cell carcinoma, thyroid cancer, and salivary gland cancers, but the same principles apply to sarcomas[42] as well as to invasive cutaneous cancers, metastases from primary solid tumors in other parts of the body, and lymphoproliferative disorders. Advanced imaging techniques can be helpful in specific situations, such as identifying parathyroid adenomas[43] or location of parotid tumor relative to facial nerve,[29] but require special protocols be set up by a knowledgeable radiologist and thus may not be readily available locally. Similarly, MRI quality is quite variable from site to site and is largely dependent on whether the local radiologists modify the scanner protocols to optimize the resolution for head and neck imaging.

Given the variation of imaging availability, imaging quality, and radiologist expertise, developing a good relationship with a local radiologist with experience in head and neck imaging is encouraged. Good interdisciplinary interactions with radiologist consultation can streamline the examination process and reduce the examination burden on patients by limiting the number and maximizing the quality of the examinations and image-guided interventions performed.

SUMMARY

CT, PET, ultrasound, and MRI examinations all have roles in the staging and surveillance of cancers in the head and neck. Contrast-enhanced CT is generally the primary examination because of availability, cost, reproducibility, and good overall quality regardless of where performed. PET, ultrasound, and MRI have more specific and nuanced applications. Good interdisciplinary interactions with radiologist consultation can streamline the examination process and reduce the examination burden on patients by limiting the number and maximizing the quality of the examinations and image-guided interventions performed.

CLINICS CARE POINTS

- Contrast-enhanced CT is generally the primary examination for staging and surveillance of head and neck cancers because of availability, cost, reproducibility, and good overall quality regardless of where performed.
- Ultrasound is the primary examination for thyroid and superficial salivary gland lesions.
- Ultrasound quality and lesion identification is highly dependent on the sonographer, and only limited images are saved for future review.
- PET has a variable role based on availability and provider preference but can help improve detection of some primary cancers and small metastases with a good negative predictive value for surveillance imaging.

- MRI is the examination of choice for deep salivary gland lesions and when there is concern for a fixed or infiltrative mass, bone involvement, or perineural tumor spread.

- MRI quality is quite variable from site to site and is largely dependent on whether the local radiologists modify the scanner protocols to optimize the resolution for head and neck imaging.

- Good interdisciplinary interactions with radiologist consultation can streamline the examination process and reduce the examination burden on patients by limiting the number and maximizing the quality of the examinations and image-guided interventions performed.

DISCLOSURE

The author has no disclosures.

REFERENCES

1. Lydiatt WM, Patel SG, O'Sullivan B, et al. Head and neck cancers—major changes in the American Joint Committee on cancer eighth edition cancer staging manual. Cancer J Clinician 2017;67(2):122–37.
2. Kelly HR, Curtin HD. Chapter 2 Squamous Cell Carcinoma of the Head and Neck—Imaging Evaluation of Regional Lymph Nodes and Implications for Management. Semin Ultrasound CT MRI 2017;38(5):466–78.
3. Park SI, Guenette JP, Suh CH, et al. The diagnostic performance of CT and MRI for detecting extranodal extension in patients with head and neck squamous cell carcinoma: a systematic review and diagnostic meta-analysis. Eur Radiol 2020. https://doi.org/10.1007/s00330-020-07281-y.
4. Shinagare AB, Lacson R, Boland GW, et al. Radiologist Preferences, Agreement, and Variability in Phrases Used to Convey Diagnostic Certainty in Radiology Reports. J Am Coll Radiol 2019;16(4 Pt A):458–64.
5. Cochon LR, Kapoor N, Carrodeguas E, et al. Variation in Follow-up Imaging Recommendations in Radiology Reports: Patient, Modality, and Radiologist Predictors. Radiology 2019;291(3):700–7.
6. Aiken AH, Rath TJ, Anzai Y, et al. ACR Neck Imaging Reporting and Data Systems (NI-RADS): A White Paper of the ACR NI-RADS Committee. J Am Coll Radiol 2018;15(8):1097–108.
7. ACR Committee on Drugs and Contrast Media. ACR manual on contrast media 2020. Available at: https://www.acr.org/Clinical-Resources/Contrast-Manual. Accessed June 6, 2021.
8. Katayama H, Yamaguchi K, Kozuka T, et al. Adverse reactions to ionic and nonionic contrast media. A report from the Japanese Committee on the Safety of Contrast Media. Radiology 1990;175(3):621–8.
9. Mahesh M. The AAPM/RSNA Physics Tutorial for Residents. RadioGraphics 2002; 22(4):949–62.
10. Goel R, Moore W, Sumer B, et al. Clinical Practice in PET/CT for the Management of Head and Neck Squamous Cell Cancer. AJR Am J Roentgenol 2017;209(2):289–303.
11. Liu T, Xu W, Yan W-L, et al. MRI for diagnosis of local residual or recurrent nasopharyngeal carcinoma, which one is the best? A systematic review. Radiother Oncol 2007;85(3):327–35.
12. Gupta T, Master Z, Kannan S, et al. Diagnostic performance of post-treatment FDG PET or FDG PET/CT imaging in head and neck cancer: a systematic review and meta-analysis. Eur J Nucl Med Mol Imaging 2011;38(11):2083.

13. Sheikhbahaei S, Taghipour M, Ahmad R, et al. Diagnostic Accuracy of Follow-Up FDG PET or PET/CT in Patients With Head and Neck Cancer After Definitive Treatment: A Systematic Review and Meta-Analysis. Am J Roentgenol 2015;205(3): 629–39.

14. Lowe VJ, Duan F, Subramaniam RM, et al. Multicenter Trial of [18F]fluorodeoxyglucose Positron Emission Tomography/Computed Tomography Staging of Head and Neck Cancer and Negative Predictive Value and Surgical Impact in the N0 Neck: Results From ACRIN 6685. J Clin Oncol 2019;37(20):1704–12.

15. Haslerud T, Brauckhoff K, Reisæter L, et al. F18-FDG-PET for recurrent differentiated thyroid cancer: a systematic meta-analysis. Acta Radiol 2016;57(10): 1193–200.

16. Brauckhoff K, Biermann M. Multimodal imaging of thyroid cancer. Curr Opin Endocrinol Diabetes Obes 2020;27(5):335–44.

17. Janssen I, Blanchet EM, Adams K, et al. Superiority of [68Ga]-DOTATATE PET/CT to Other Functional Imaging Modalities in the Localization of SDHB-Associated Metastatic Pheochromocytoma and Paraganglioma. Clin Cancer Res 2015; 21(17):3888–95.

18. Janssen I, Chen CC, Taieb D, et al. 68Ga-DOTATATE PET/CT in the Localization of Head and Neck Paragangliomas Compared with Other Functional Imaging Modalities and CT/MRI. J Nucl Med 2016;57(2):186–91.

19. Votaw JR. The AAPM/RSNA physics tutorial for residents. Physics of PET. *Radio-Graphics*. 1995;15(5):1179–90.

20. Haugen BR, Alexander EK, Bible KC, et al. 2015 American Thyroid Association Management Guidelines for Adult Patients with Thyroid Nodules and Differentiated Thyroid Cancer: The American Thyroid Association Guidelines Task Force on Thyroid Nodules and Differentiated Thyroid Cancer. Thyroid 2016;26(1):1–133.

21. Middleton WD, Teefey SA, Reading CC, et al. Comparison of Performance Characteristics of American College of Radiology TI-RADS, Korean Society of Thyroid Radiology TIRADS, and American Thyroid Association Guidelines. AJR Am J Roentgenol 2018;210(5):1148–54.

22. Angell TE, Maurer R, Wang Z, et al. A Cohort Analysis of Clinical and Ultrasound Variables Predicting Cancer Risk in 20,001 Consecutive Thyroid Nodules. J Clin Endocrinol Metab 2019;104(11):5665–72.

23. Zhao H, Li H. Meta-analysis of ultrasound for cervical lymph nodes in papillary thyroid cancer: Diagnosis of central and lateral compartment nodal metastases. Eur J Radiol 2019;112:14–21.

24. Lobo R, Hawk J, Srinivasan A. A Review of Salivary Gland Malignancies: Common Histologic Types, Anatomic Considerations, and Imaging Strategies. Neuroimaging Clin N Am 2018;28(2):171–82.

25. Loevner LA. Image-guided procedures of the head and neck: the radiologist's arsenal. Otolaryngol Clin North Am 2008;41(1). 231–250, viii.

26. Hangiandreou NJ. AAPM/RSNA Physics Tutorial for Residents: Topics in US. RadioGraphics 2003;23(4):1019–33.

27. Hiyama T, Kuno H, Sekiya K, et al. Imaging of Malignant Minor Salivary Gland Tumors of the Head and Neck. Radiographics 2021;41(1):175–91.

28. Moonis G, Cunnane MB, Emerick K, et al. Patterns of Perineural Tumor Spread in Head and Neck Cancer. Magn Reson Imaging Clin 2012;20(3):435–46.

29. Guenette JP, Ben-Shlomo N, Jayender J, et al. MR Imaging of the Extracranial Facial Nerve with the CISS Sequence. AJNR Am J Neuroradiol 2019;40(11): 1954–9.

30. Razek AAKA, King A. MRI and CT of Nasopharyngeal Carcinoma. Am J Roentgenol 2012;198(1):11–8.
31. Chong VFH, Fan YF. Skull base erosion in nasopharyngeal carcinoma: Detection by CT and MRI. Clin Radiol 1996;51(9):625–31.
32. Kim HJ, Lee TH, Lee H-S, et al. Periorbita: Computed Tomography and Magnetic Resonance Imaging Findings. Am J Rhinol 2006;20(4):371–4.
33. Abd El-Hafez YG, Chen C-C, Ng S-H, et al. Comparison of PET/CT and MRI for the detection of bone marrow invasion in patients with squamous cell carcinoma of the oral cavity. Oral Oncol 2011;47(4):288–95.
34. Suzuki N, Kuribayashi A, Sakamoto K, et al. Diagnostic abilities of 3T MRI for assessing mandibular invasion of squamous cell carcinoma in the oral cavity: comparison with 64-row multidetector CT. Dentomaxillofac Radiol 2019;48(4): 20180311.
35. Noorlag R, Klein NTJW, Delwel VEJ, et al. Assessment of tumour depth in early tongue cancer: Accuracy of MRI and intraoral ultrasound. Oral Oncol 2020; 110:104895.
36. Chin SY, Kadir K, Ibrahim N, et al. Correlation and accuracy of contrast-enhanced computed tomography in assessing depth of invasion of oral tongue carcinoma. Int J Oral Maxillofac Surg 2020. https://doi.org/10.1016/j.ijom.2020.09.025.
37. Baba A, Ojiri H, Ogane S, et al. Usefulness of contrast-enhanced CT in the evaluation of depth of invasion in oral tongue squamous cell carcinoma: comparison with MRI. Oral Radiol 2021;37(1):86–94.
38. Cho SJ, Lee JH, Suh CH, et al. Comparison of diagnostic performance between CT and MRI for detection of cartilage invasion for primary tumor staging in patients with laryngo-hypopharyngeal cancer: a systematic review and meta-analysis. Eur Radiol 2020;30(7):3803–12.
39. Forghani R, Levental M, Gupta R, et al. Different spectral hounsfield unit curve and high-energy virtual monochromatic image characteristics of squamous cell carcinoma compared with nonossified thyroid cartilage. AJNR Am J Neuroradiol 2015;36(6):1194–200.
40. Kuno H, Sakamaki K, Fujii S, et al. Comparison of MR Imaging and Dual-Energy CT for the Evaluation of Cartilage Invasion by Laryngeal and Hypopharyngeal Squamous Cell Carcinoma. Am J Neuroradiol 2018;39(3):524–31.
41. Pooley RA. Fundamental Physics of MR Imaging. RadioGraphics 2005;25(4): 1087–99.
42. Tran N-A, Guenette JP, Jagannathan J. Soft Tissue Special Issue: Imaging of Bone and Soft Tissue Sarcomas in the Head and Neck. Head Neck Pathol 2020;14(1):132–43.
43. Bunch PM, Randolph GW, Brooks JA, et al. Parathyroid 4D CT: What the Surgeon Wants to Know. Radiographics 2020;40(5):1383–94.

Robotic and Endoscopic Approaches to Head and Neck Surgery

Andrew J. Holcomb, MD[a], Jeremy D. Richmon, MD[b],*

KEYWORDS

- Robotic surgery • Head and neck cancer • da Vinci • Oropharyngeal cancer
- Laryngeal cancer • Human papillomavirus • Surgical robotics
- Transoral robotic surgery

KEY POINTS

- Robotic head and neck surgery emerged in the early 2000s as a minimally invasive alternative to radiotherapy-based treatments for oropharyngeal cancer.
- Transoral robotic surgery for human papillomavirus-mediated oropharyngeal cancer has comparable oncologic and functional outcomes relative to radiotherapy.
- Robotic surgery offers improved visualization, instrumentation, and ergonomics relative to endoscopic and microscopic approaches to the head and neck, although cost remains a concern.
- Future robotic systems will incorporate technologic innovation to further improve visualization, expand access, and even augment surgical decision-making through artificial intelligence.

INTRODUCTION

Incorporation of endoscopic and robotic technologies into head and neck surgery has been a gradual process over several decades by means of incremental contributions from a variety of sources. These techniques offer a number of advantages over traditional open approaches, including improved surgical safety, lower morbidity, and improved cosmesis. As technologic advancements continue to develop, further integration of these tools into surgical practice is inevitable. We discuss the history of endoscopic and robotic surgery, describe data supporting their safety and efficacy, outline their current role in the care of head and neck oncology patients, and describe novel uses of these technologies and future anticipated developments.

[a] Nebraska Methodist Hospital, 8303 Dodge Street Suite 305, Omaha, NE 68114, USA; [b] Mass Eye and Ear, Harvard Medical School, 243 Charles Street, Boston, MA 02114, USA
* Corresponding author.
E-mail address: Jeremy_richmon@meei.harvard.edu

Hematol Oncol Clin N Am 35 (2021) 875–894
https://doi.org/10.1016/j.hoc.2021.05.002
0889-8588/21/© 2021 Elsevier Inc. All rights reserved.

HISTORY

Historically, surgical management of oropharyngeal squamous cell carcinoma (OSCC) was associated with high morbidity and generally poor survival.[1] Although a transoral approach to selected tumors of the tonsil predated the use of modern robotic or endoscopic equipment,[2,3] its use was limited by challenges with access, lighting, and control of bleeding. Instead, radical approaches involving mandibulotomy, partial mandibulectomy, and lingual release were commonly used to access the oropharynx in the era spanning the mid to late 1900s.[1,4] These surgeries were disfiguring, and functional outcomes including speech intelligibility and dietary normalcy were poor, resulting in poor quality of life.[5] Furthermore, rates of severe or fatal complications were four to ten times greater in patients treated with surgery than for patients treated with radiation.[6] Surgery with adjuvant radiotherapy demonstrated improved local control relative to surgery alone, albeit without significant improvement in survival.[7–9] These findings, along with advances in radiation technology and the development of platinum chemotherapeutics, contributed to an eventual preference for concurrent chemoradiation in advanced OPSCC in the late 20th century.[10] Over the same time period, the incidence of OPSCC rose significantly worldwide, predominately in developed countries.[11] The role of human papillomavirus (HPV) infection in the pathophysiology of OPSCC was elucidated in the early 2000s, accounting for profound epidemiologic changes, with younger, healthier patients developing these tumors.[12–14] Higher survival among HPV-related OPSCC has contributed to a focus on functional outcomes of treatment and increased the desire for minimally invasive approaches to treat these tumors.

Laryngeal SCC was addressed with total laryngectomy beginning with Billroth in 1873,[15] although anesthetic limitations, antibiotic unavailability, and high surgical mortality contributed to favoring radiotherapy for laryngeal cancer early in the 20th century.[16] With advances in surgical technique and perioperative care, total laryngectomy with adjuvant radiation emerged as the standard of care for advanced laryngeal SCC until the mid-20th century, when open partial laryngeal surgery was popularized at some centers.[17] The landmark 1991 Veteran's Affairs Laryngeal Cancer Study Group trial established a new role for combined chemotherapy and radiation in the treatment of advanced laryngeal cancer with high rates of laryngeal preservation.[18] Further contribution of the Radiation Therapy Oncology Group 91-11 trial in 1993 then established concurrent chemoradiation as a standard of care surgical alternative for advanced laryngeal SCC.[19] The following decade yielded a trend toward nonsurgical therapy for laryngeal SCC.[20] Although the percentage of early versus late-stage laryngeal SCC remained relatively static over that time, early stage laryngeal cancer represents over half of all newly diagnosed cases annually, presenting a need for low-morbidity surgical approaches as an alternative to radiotherapy.

Although the use of microscopes dates to the 11th century, applications in otologic surgery began in the late 1800s.[21] Widespread acceptance of microscopic techniques in otologic surgery developed over the course of the mid-20th century, whereas uses in head and neck oncology remained limited. Jako and Strong described the use of a carbon dioxide (CO2) laser for endoscopic laryngeal tumor resection in the 1970s.[22] In 1993, Steiner published results of 240 patients treated for laryngeal cancer with transoral laser microsurgery (TLM), showing excellent results for patients with early stage glottic cancers.[23] He used a bivalved laryngoscope for tumor exposure, an operating microscope, and a micromanipulator attached to the microscope to deliver a CO2 laser. He described results from 48 base-of-tongue resections beginning in 1986, demonstrating 92% rate of return to a normal diet, no cases of tracheostomy, and significant functional improvements relative to open operative results.[24] This surgical approach required the surgeon to remove tumors in a piecemeal fashion, which deviated from traditional surgical tenets mandating en bloc tumor resection.[25] However, their results and those of others, including a multi-institutional study by Haughey and colleagues, have since validated the oncologic efficacy of this technique.[26–28] TLM has since been used for removal of select oropharyngeal and laryngeal tumors at a number of institutions.

The first endoscopes were used in 1806 in Vienna, consisting of candlelight reflected by a mirror through a tube into an eyepiece.[29] Subsequent innovations, including Edison's incandescent bulbs, led to the first application of endoscopes in sinus surgery in 1901,[30] when Hirschmann used a modified cystoscope to visualize the maxillary sinus.[31] The Hopkins rod lens system was patented in 1960 with significant improvements in aperture, light transmission, image quality, and the ability to take photographs.[32] Endoscopic approaches in the head and neck were not widely accepted until Messerklinger expanded application of endoscopes in sinus surgery.[33] A series of advances by Kennedy, Stammberger, Draf, and others led to the emergence of endoscopic sinus and skull surgery as a standard of care.[33] While microscopic techniques remain highly relevant for TLM and elsewhere in otolaryngology, endoscopy represented another step forward in minimally invasive surgery, offering dynamic and angled visualization permitting surgeons to look around corners, albeit with the sacrifice of the two-handed surgical technique in many cases.[34,35]

The use of surgical robotics dates to 1985, when the PUMA 560 robot was used for a robotic-assisted stereotactic brain biopsy.[36] This was followed by applications in a number of other body areas, including urology, general surgery, and cardiothoracic surgery.[37–39] The ZEUS Robotic Surgical System (Computer Motion Inc., Goleta, CA) and da Vinci Surgical System (Intuitive Surgical Inc., Sunnyvale, CA) were concurrently developed until Computer Motion Inc. was acquired by Intuitive Inc. in 2003 and the ZEUS platform was discontinued.[40] The da Vinci robot soon became the most widely used surgical robotics platform, its name paying homage to Leonardo da Vinci, the designer of the first robot in 1495.[41] Surgical robotics were first applied in the head and neck in an animal model in 2003 by Haus and colleagues[42] and by McLeod and Melder in 2005 with the removal of a vallecular cyst.[43]

Significant progress was then made by Hockstein, Weinstein, and O'Malley, who created a comprehensive strategy to explore the feasibility and safety of using the da Vinci robot to resect oropharyngeal tumors.[44] They devised a series of studies conducted at the University of Pennsylvania, first involving mannequin and cadaver models to establish that transoral robotic surgery (TORS) had an acceptable safety profile relative to conventional transoral surgery.[44] This was followed by canine experiments, with a focus on hemostasis and secretion management.[45–47] Finally, testing was performed on human subjects in a clinical trial, resecting both supraglottic and oropharyngeal tumors, achieving negative margins with preservation of critical neurovascular tumors and acceptable hemostasis.[48,49]

A structured training program to teach surgeons to perform TORS also originated with Weinstein and O'Malley, with an initial training workshop taking place in 2006. Subsequent development of TORS programs has occurred nationwide, and TORS has been incorporated into head and neck fellowship training (American Head and Neck Society).[50] The da Vinci Surgical System gained approval from the Food and Drug Administration (FDA) for treatment of benign and early T-stage malignant tumors of the oral cavity, pharynx, and larynx in 2009.[51] Utilization of TORS rapidly expanded, and its indications for a variety of otolaryngologic conditions have similarly grown.[52] A summary of technological advancements in robotic and endoscopic surgery is outlined in **Fig. 1**.

CURRENT ROBOTIC SYSTEMS

Surgical systems have continued refinement in the years since their first use in head and neck surgery. The da Vinci Si surgical system is one of the earlier iterations still broadly used among head and neck surgeons. This is a three-component system, the first being a patient cart, which uses three instrument arms, one that holds a digital endoscope for visualization of the surgical field, and the other two that hold a variety of surgical instruments (**Fig. 2**).[53] The second component is a surgeon console separate from the patient cart, where the surgeon controls movements of the surgical arms and the position and rotation of the endoscope (**Fig. 3**). A third component, the vision cart, allows the surgical assistant to share the console surgeon's endoscopic view (**Fig. 4**). Some systems include dual surgeon consoles, improving teaching capabilities and allowing seamless transition of instrument control from teacher to learner.[54]

The da Vinci Xi system was introduced in 2014 but has not been FDA approved in otolaryngology (**Fig. 5**). Nonetheless, it has been praised for its easier docking and narrower robotic arms relative to the Si system, with reports of comparable safety and improved surgical time.[55–57] The da Vinci SP system was most recently

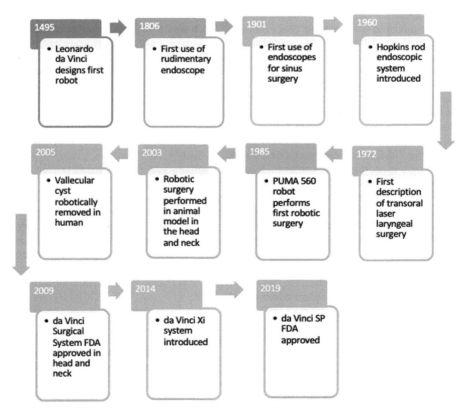

Fig. 1. A graphic timeline of major advances in robotic and endoscopic surgery.

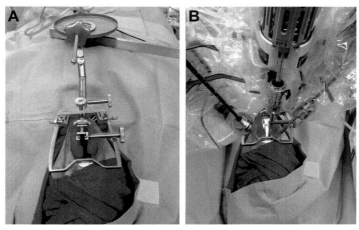

Fig. 2. (*A*) An oral retractor provides access for transoral robotic surgical instruments. (*B*) A 30-degree endoscope and two instruments attached to the patient cart are passed through the oral cavity to gain access to the oropharynx.

introduced in 2018 and subsequently FDA approved in 2019 for base-of-tongue resection and radical tonsillectomy (**Fig. 6**). This system uses a single-port 2.5-cm cannula with three working instruments and a fully wristed endoscope that can rotate 360°.[53] The addition of this useable third working arm allows for traction and countertraction to be simultaneously applied, improving surgical dissection.[58] The narrow parallel orientation of the instruments allows for greater access to the lower pharynx than previous models. The da Vinci SP has been shown to offer comparable safety to previous platforms and offers access to a broader range of sites within the head and neck, opening possibilities of expanded indications for TORS.[59,60]

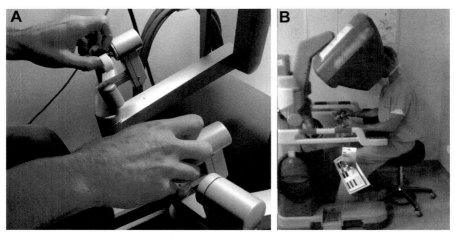

Fig. 3. (*A*) The surgeon's arms rest comfortably with manipulation of two wristed surgical instruments. (*B*) The surgeon console is adjustable to match the surgeon's ergonomic preferences.

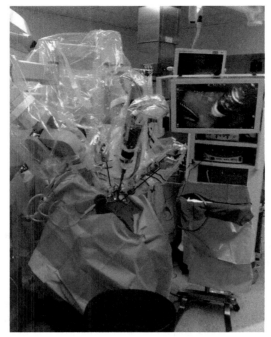

Fig. 4. The vision cart is positioned for optimal visualization by the surgical assistant and surgical technologist, who work at the patient's head of bed.

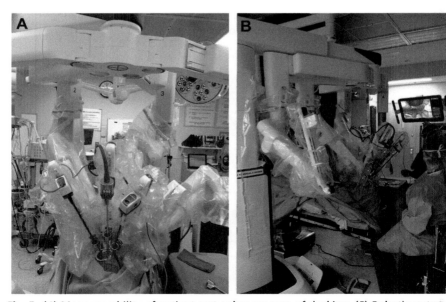

Fig. 5. (*A*) Maneuverability of patient cart enhances ease of docking. (*B*) Robotic system in use. Despite improved ergonomics, fourth working arm remains unusable because of limited transoral aperture.

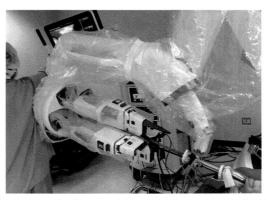

Fig. 6. Robot provides access for four working arms through a single 25-mm port.

ADVANTAGES AND LIMITATIONS OF ROBOTIC SURGERY

Robotic surgery offers a growing number of advantages over other endoscopic and microscopic techniques (**Table 1**).[41] The separate surgeon console and patient cart improves surgical ergonomics. High-definition dual-lens endoscopes provide a three-dimensional view, light intensity of up to 2450 lumens, and 10 to 15x magnification. This view is dynamic, and angled endoscopes allow for panoramic visualization, which compares favorably to microscopic approaches. Microscopic approaches also struggle with line-of-sight problems and instrument collisions due to the narrow working aperture through a laryngoscope. Robotic systems use wristed instruments that provide 7° of freedom and have rotational abilities that exceed those of the human hand, allowing for avoidance of line-of-sight problems and improving dexterity (**Fig. 7**). A broad range of working instruments are available for use in surgical robotics, including harmonic scalpels and electrocautery instruments, which have superior coagulative properties relative to the lasers used in TLM, thus reducing instrument switching and improving efficiency.[61] In comparison with endoscopic techniques, the dual lens scope is a key advantage, offering stereoscopic vision to the console surgeon. Robotic systems also allow a two-handed technique for the console surgeon, which allows for superior tissue handling relative to one-handed endoscopic approaches.

One source of loss of surgical dexterity in surgery is hand tremor, which can be significant during endoscopic surgery. Robotic surgical platforms can detect involuntary hand motions, discriminate these from voluntary hand motion, and provide tremor filtering to improve dexterity.[62,63] Perhaps even more relevant to improving surgical accuracy is motion scaling, whereby large hand movements are scaled down to small instrument movements. The combined effects of these features of robotic surgery have been shown to increase surgical accuracy.[64] Direct comparisons of robotic and laparoscopic surgical techniques have demonstrated reduced errors and improved task performance speed in robotic surgery.[65,66] In addition, robotic surgery complements nondominant hand performance to create virtual ambidexterity.[67]

A primary criticism of robotic surgery is expense, with system acquisition costs approaching 1.5 million dollars and annual service contracts in excess of 150,000 dollars.[68] Total procedural and inpatient costs to patients are roughly 22,000 dollars and exceed 55,000 dollars in total treatment cost when the potential of adjuvant therapy is considered.[69,70] Cost analyses have compared TORS to open surgery for treatment of

Table 1
Comparison of microscopic, endoscopic, and robotic surgical platforms

Feature	Platform		
	Microscope	Endoscope	Robotics
Visualization/Access	Fixed external point of view. Illumination limited by aperture of laryngoscope. Stereoscopic vision. Magnification alterable. Suffers from line-of-sight limitations	Dynamic endoscope position. Angled cameras offer panoramic view. Fixed magnification. Good illumination. Two-dimensional vision.	Dynamic endoscope position with fully wristed endoscopes in newer iterations. Angled cameras offer panoramic view. Stereoscopic (3D) vision. Dynamic magnification. Excellent illumination.
Instrumentation	Long instruments amplify tremor. Limited range of accessible instruments. Suffers from line-of-sight limitations. Lack of wristed instrumentation.	Single-handed surgery. Limited fulcrum ability amplifies tremor. Lack of wristed instrumentation.	Broad range of instruments. Tremor filtration and motion scaling improve dexterity. Wristed instruments minimize line-of-sight limitations. Lacks haptic feedback
Ergonomics	Manipulation of instruments requires abnormal hand positioning to avoid line-of-sight limitations, resulting in extremity fatigue	Abnormal body positioning, manipulation of rigid endoscopes and instruments results in surgeon fatigue	Surgeon console adjustable to optimize body position. Wristed, clutchable instruments with 7° of freedom improve hand positioning
Cost	Low to moderate	Low to moderate	High

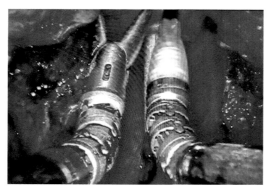

Fig. 7. Wristing allows excellent visualization of instrument tips without line-of-sight limitations.

OPSCC or identification of unknown primary surgery and have supported TORS as cost-effective.[71] Studies directly comparing TORS to nonsurgical therapy for OPSCC have produced conflicting results but generally support TORS as a cost-effective alternative to radiotherapy or chemoradiotherapy.[69,70,72] This limitation remains significant however because acquisition and maintenance costs may preclude cost-effective use of robotic surgical platforms at centers with a lower volume.[69]

TORS is also criticized for the bulky, straight working arms that may be difficult to maneuver within the pharynx. Newer iterations of robotic systems, including the da Vinci SP, have addressed these issues, offering expanded access using flexible endoscopes. The lack of haptic feedback, which includes touch and proprioception, is a third major limitation of robotic surgery, which can cause surgeons to apply greater compression or shear forces, leading to increased tissue injury or increased surgical error.[73] Direct comparisons have shown loss of haptic feedback of the da Vinci system compared with hand-held instruments.[74] A number of haptic feedback systems have been investigated, with some integrating multiple classes of human mechanoreceptors to simulate natural tactile and proprioceptive sensation.[75,76] These systems have been shown to reduce average and maximum grip force and to improve detection of vessels embedded within soft tissue. Further refinements may be incorporated into robotic surgical systems in future years.

CURRENT ROLE OF ROBOTIC SURGERY IN MANAGEMENT OF HEAD AND NECK CANCER

At present, TORS is primarily used to treat OPSCC. Primary surgery for T1-T2 OPSCC rose significantly from 2004 to 2014, with primary surgery selected for 33.3% of cases in 2014 according to data from the National Cancer Database.[77,78] Multiple studies have retrospectively compared TORS with or without adjuvant therapy to radiotherapy with or without chemotherapy for early stage OPSCC.[79–81] These studies demonstrated comparable survival outcomes between the two modalities. In light of the excellent survival outcomes among patients with HPV-related OPSCC regardless of treatment modality, focus has shifted toward treatment morbidity and quality of life.

Radiation and chemoradiation are associated with a number of short- and long-term toxicities, including mucositis, fatigue, xerostomia, dysphagia, osteoradionecrosis, cranial neuropathy, and trismus.[82,83] TORS is associated with significant morbidities as well, including pain, swallowing dysfunction, and bleeding risk. Retrospective data have suggested favorable functional outcomes in TORS relative to radiotherapy.[79] However, until recently, no prospective trials have compared oncologic or functional outcomes between TORS and primary radiation. The ORATOR (Early-stage Squamous Cell Carcinoma of the Oropharynx: Radiotherapy vs Trans-oral Robotic Surgery) trial was the first randomized trial to directly compare these treatment modalities, enrolling 68 patients with T1 or T2, N0–N2 HPV-related OPSCC.[84] Patients were randomized to receive either radiotherapy with addition of concurrent chemotherapy in N1-2 patients or TORS with neck dissection followed by adjuvant therapy based on pathologic findings. With a median follow-up duration of 25 months, no differences in overall survival or progression-free survival were observed between groups. However, patients in the radiotherapy arm had superior scores on the MD Anderson Dysphagia Inventory at 1 year. While these differences were statistically significant, they did not meet predefined thresholds of clinical significance. Other adverse events present in the radiation group included dysphagia, hearing loss, and mucositis. This is a small study with various limitations. These results contrast with findings of Hutcheson and colleagues, who reported on prospectively collected swallowing outcomes of patients with low- or intermediate-risk HPV-related OPSCC, albeit outside of a clinical trial.[85] In this study, which consisted of 75 TORS patients and 182 radiotherapy patients, they identified no significant difference in swallowing outcomes at 3 to 6 months between the two primary treatment modalities. Further comparative studies are needed on long-term toxicities of these treatment modalities.

Tremendous efforts are being made toward conscientious de-escalation of therapy for HPV-related OPSCC to balance minimization of treatment-related morbidity with preservation of favorable survival outcomes. The Eastern Cooperative Oncology Group 3311 multicenter trial examined treatment de-escalation among 519 patients undergoing TORS for clinical stage T1-T2, N1-2b, HPV-related OPSCC.[86] Patients with intermediate-risk tumors (clear/close margins, 2–4+ nodes, or extranodal extension ≤1 mm) were randomized to receive either 60 Gy or 50 Gy intensity-modulated radiation therapy. With an average of 103 patients per arm and a median follow-up of 31.8 months, 2-year progression-free survival was 95.0% in the group receiving 50 Gy and 95.9% in the group receiving 60 Gy. Furthermore, grade 3 or greater toxicities occurred in 15% in the lower dose arm and 25% in the higher dose arm. Other deintensification strategies, including further dose reduction or primary-site avoidance with adjuvant therapy, have been investigated in phase 2 clinical trials with promising results.[87,88] With the continued advancement of radiotherapy techniques, emergence of targeted molecular therapies, and refinement of robotic systems, the role of robotic surgery in treatment of oropharyngeal cancer will continue to evolve in the coming years.

Treatment of early stage laryngeal cancer remains heavily weighted toward TLM given the limited access to the larynx offered by earlier iterations of robotic systems. Nonetheless, TORS offers similar rates of positive margins and survival outcomes compared with TLM.[89] However, robotic supraglottic and even total laryngectomy have been described.[90–93] Newer iterations of robotic systems such as the da Vinci SP will undoubtedly expand indications for robotic surgery in addressing laryngeal pathology.

Robotic surgery is also relevant in identification of cancer of unknown primary (CUP), which comprises 2% to 5% of head neck cancers.[94] Although a thorough history and physical examination combined with lymph node fine-needle aspirate biopsy (FNAB) and appropriate imaging will identify a primary site in roughly 90% of cases of CUP, the remaining cases will require some form of upper endoscopy for primary site visualization.[95] If a primary site cannot be identified at the time of endoscopy, ipsilateral tonsillectomy is recommended, especially in cases where the HPV-related disease is suspected based on positivity of the biomarker p16 within an FNAB of the lymph node.[96] If a tumor is not identified within the tonsil, robotic lingual tonsillectomy is recommended by current American Society of Clinical Oncology guidelines and has been shown to identify a primary tumor in approximately 56% of these cases, with single-institution series reporting detection rates approximating 90%.[96–99] This has significant potential to provide appropriately selected patients with single-modality therapy or to limit radiotherapy fields in patients requiring multi-modality therapy.

EXPANDED USES OF ROBOTIC/ENDOSCOPIC TECHNIQUES

Robotic surgery has also been used for treatment of obstructive sleep apnea (OSA) for base-of-tongue reduction in which continuous positive airway pressure is not tolerable. Multiple studies have demonstrated safety and efficacy of TORS in patients with moderate to severe OSA, showing reductions in apnea hypopnea index, lowest oxygen saturation, and daytime sleepiness.[100–103] TORS avoids line-of-sight issues in conventional transoral access to the base of tongue and hypopharynx, allowing for applications in multilevel obstruction with good results even in patients who have failed previous surgery.[104] A variety of procedures have been safely performed using TORS, including base-of-tongue reduction, uvulopalatopharyngoplasty, and epiglottoplasty.[105] The future role of TORS for OSA in the era of hypoglossal nerve stimulation remains to be seen.[106]

Robotic and endoscopic surgery has been adapted to several other purposes within the head and neck. Perhaps the most extensively studied application is remote-access thyroid and parathyroid surgery, in which endoscopic approaches, including axillary, lateral neck, and breast incisions, have been described since the 1990s.[107–110] The primary advantage of these approaches is to avoid a visible cutaneous scar which may have a negative quality of life impact on select patients. In contrast to transoral approaches, these remote-access approaches are not less-invasive. These typically require CO_2 insufflation, suffer from restricted instrument movement and two-dimensional visualization, and have been associated with longer operative time, prolonged hospital length of stay, and increased postoperative pain.[111,112] The transoral endoscopic thyroidectomy, vestibular approach is the most commonly used approach today worldwide. This uses three small incisions in the lower lip to access the central neck. This can also be performed robotically (transoral robotic thyroidectomy) although this has not garnered as much enthusiasm. These approaches to the central neck are more direct than axillary or breast incisions, requiring less overall dissection, and the oral mucosal incisions heal without any visible scars. Although many continue to advocate for open approaches, cervical scars have been shown to adversely affect quality of life, and there is clearly a role for these approaches in properly selected patients.[113]

Robotic surgery has been applied to a number of additional purposes within otolaryngology, including access to the parapharyngeal space, skull base, retropharyngeal space, salivary glands, anterior cervical spine, and the lateral neck (**Fig. 8**).[114–121] TORS-assisted reconstruction of defects in the pharynx and other sites has also been described, using local, regional, and free flaps, with TORS offering minimally invasive access and precise suturing for flap inset.[122–125] As robotic systems continue to be refined and further studies assess the safety, efficacy, and cost-effectiveness of

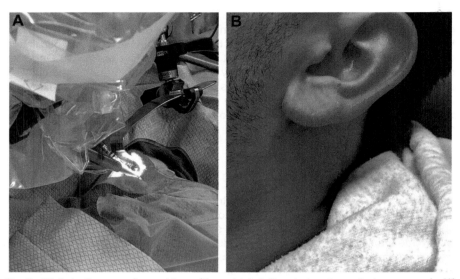

Fig. 8. (A) Robotic access for excision of branchial cleft cyst via retroauricular approach. (B) Postoperative image of surgical incision with excellent esthetic outcome.

these applications of TORS relative to traditional techniques, the role of robotic surgery in otolaryngology will undoubtedly continue to expand.

FUTURE DEVELOPMENTS IN ROBOTIC SURGERY

Future advances in robotic surgery will aid the surgeon in a number of ways, through progress in instrumentation to expand access or improve dexterity, through augmenting visualization to go beyond what the human eye can assess, and through data science innovations designed to augment surgical judgment. Flexible, miniaturized endoscopes and integration of haptic feedback into surgical systems will address major limitations of TORS. Integration of real-time imaging data into the visual field of the surgeon can create an augmented reality, allowing for surgical navigation and instrument tracking.[126] This has been shown to improve identification of phantom vessels and improve margin control in modeled scenarios.[127,128]

Narrow-band imaging uses light of specific blue and green wavelengths to improve surface visualization and has been shown to improve margin clearance in TORS.[129] Enhanced visualization of tumor margins or vascular structures using indocyanine green dye, which fluoresces under near-infrared light, has been used in robotic surgery within other body sites using the da Vinci FIREFLY system, but this requires a timed injection, and results in TORS have been unremarkable.[130,131] Time-resolved fluorescence spectroscopy exploits the distinct autofluorescence signature that results from tissue structure and biochemical profile distortion from neoplastic tissues. This has been shown to distinguish between malignant and nonmalignant tissues in oral cancers without an injectable label and has recently been integrated into TORS in experimental models.[132–134] Effective incorporation into robotic systems offers potential to improve margin control and also may assist surgeons in limiting excision of normal tissues, thus limiting treatment toxicity.

Surgical data science is an emerging field that aims to improve the quality of health care by harnessing the power of data to improve decision-making.[135] This has the potential to disrupt surgery in a number of ways, integrating data from a variety of sources to provide decision support at multiple time points before, during, and after surgery. Artificial intelligence has already shown promise in head and neck oncology and offers the potential to improve analysis of data beyond traditional statistical methods.[136–138] By integrating real-time and historical patient data, existing evidence from published literature and practice guidelines, and feedback from robotic systems, intraoperative techniques can be guided by a holistic application of all available data. Evolution of data science will be met with challenges related to data quantity and heterogeneity; however, as we progress toward a future of data sharing and interconnectedness, integration of data science into robotic surgery will almost certainly improve surgical outcomes.[139]

SUMMARY

Robotic and endoscopic surgery have become an essential part of head and neck surgery through a progression of technologic advancements and landmark studies that have demonstrated their usefulness and safety in a variety of applications. It is incumbent upon surgeons and oncologists alike to understand these technologies, including their history, strengths, and limitations, and to play a role in critical appraisal of new developments. Further technological advancements offer potential to improve patient safety, optimize treatment efficacy, and expand surgical indications to new frontiers.

CLINICS CARE POINT

- Patients with tumors of the oropharynx, larynx and hypopharynx deserve a mutli-disciplinary evaluation of treatment options including consideration of candidacy for minimally-invasive, transoral surgery.

DISCLOSURE

The authors have nothing to disclose.

REFERENCES

1. Foote RL, Olsen KD, Davis DL, et al. Base of tongue carcinoma: patterns of failure and predictors of recurrence after surgery alone. Head Neck 1993;15(4): 300–7.
2. Holsinger FC, McWhorter AJ, Ménard M, et al. Transoral lateral oropharyngectomy for squamous cell carcinoma of the tonsillar region: I. Technique, complications, and functional results. Arch Otolaryngol Head Neck Surg 2005;131(7): 583–91.
3. Laccourreye O, Hans S, Ménard M, et al. Transoral lateral oropharyngectomy for squamous cell carcinoma of the tonsillar region: II. An analysis of the incidence, related variables, and consequences of local recurrence. Arch Otolaryngol Head Neck Surg 2005;131(7):592–9.
4. Stanley RB. Mandibular lingual releasing approach to oral and oropharyngeal carcinomas. Laryngoscope 1984;94(5):596–600.
5. Harrison LB, Zelefsky MJ, Armstrong JG, et al. Performance status after treatment for squamous cell cancer of the base of tongue—a comparison of primary radiation therapy versus primary surgery. Int J Radiat Oncol Biol Phys 1994; 30(4):953–7.

6. Parsons JT, Mendenhall WM, Stringer SP, et al. Squamous cell carcinoma of the oropharynx: surgery, radiation therapy, or both. Cancer 2002;94(11):2967–80.
7. Weber RS, Gidley P, Morrison WH, et al. Treatment selection for carcinoma of the base of the tongue. Am J Surg 1990;160(4):415–9.
8. Gourin CG, Johnson JT. Surgical treatment of squamous cell carcinoma of the base of tongue. Head Neck 2001;23(8):653–60.
9. Nisi KW, Foote RL, Bonner JA, et al. Adjuvant radiotherapy for squamous cell carcinoma of the tongue base: improved local-regional disease control compared with surgery alone. Int J Radiat Oncol Biol Phys 1998;41(2):371–7.
10. Chen AY, Schrag N, Hao Y, et al. Changes in treatment of advanced oropharyngeal cancer, 1985–2001. Laryngoscope 2007;117(1):16–21.
11. Chaturvedi AK, Anderson WF, Lortet-Tieulent J, et al. Worldwide trends in incidence rates for oral cavity and oropharyngeal cancers. J Clin Oncol 2013; 31(36):4550–9.
12. Ang KK, Harris J, Wheeler R, et al. Human papillomavirus and survival of patients with oropharyngeal cancer. N Engl J Med 2010;363(1):24–35.
13. Westra WH. The changing face of head and neck cancer in the 21st century: the impact of HPV on the epidemiology and pathology of oral cancer. Head Neck Pathol 2009;3(1):78–81.
14. D'Souza G, Kreimer AR, Viscidi R, et al. Case–control study of human papillomavirus and oropharyngeal cancer. N Engl J Med 2007;356(19):1944–56.
15. Čoček A. The history and current status of surgery in the treatment of laryngeal cancer. Acta Med (Hradec Kralove) 2008;51(3):157–63.
16. Morrison LF. Carcinoma of the larynx. I. Carcinoma of the laryngopharynx. Laryngoscope 1952;62(1):53–60.
17. Kirchner JA. A historical and histological view of partial laryngectomy. Bull N Y Acad Med 1986;62(8):808–17.
18. Wolf G, Wolf GT, Fisher SG, et al. Induction chemotherapy plus radiation compared with surgery plus radiation in patients with advanced laryngeal cancer. N Engl J Med 1991;324(24):1685–90.
19. Forastiere AA, Goepfert H, Maor M, et al. Concurrent chemotherapy and radiotherapy for organ preservation in advanced laryngeal cancer. N Engl J Med 2003;349(22):2091–8.
20. Hoffman HT, Porter K, Karnell LH, et al. Laryngeal cancer in the United States: changes in demographics, patterns of care, and survival. Laryngoscope 2006; 116(S111):1–13.
21. Mudry A. The history of the microscope for use in ear surgery. Am J Otol 2000; 21(6):877–86.
22. Strong MS, Jako GJ. Laser surgery in the larynx. Early clinical experience with continuous CO 2 laser. Ann Otol Rhinol Laryngol 1972;81(6):791–8.
23. Steiner W. Results of curative laser microsurgery of laryngeal carcinomas. Am J Otolaryngol 1993;14(2):116–21.
24. Steiner W, Fierek O, Ambrosch P, et al. Transoral laser microsurgery for squamous cell carcinoma of the base of the tongue. Arch Otolaryngol Head Neck Surg 2003;129(1):36–43.
25. Harris AT, Tanyi A, Hart RD, et al. Transoral laser surgery for laryngeal carcinoma: has Steiner achieved a genuine paradigm shift in oncological surgery? Ann R Coll Surg Engl 2017;100(1):1–4.
26. Grant DG, Salassa JR, Hinni ML, et al. Carcinoma of the tongue base treated by transoral laser microsurgery, part one: untreated tumors, a prospective analysis of oncologic and functional outcomes. Laryngoscope 2006;116(12):2150–5.

27. Henstrom DK, Moore EJ, Olsen KD, et al. Transoral resection for squamous cell carcinoma of the base of the tongue. Arch Otolaryngol Head Neck Surg 2009; 135(12):1231–8.
28. Haughey BH, Hinni ML, Salassa JR, et al. Transoral laser microsurgery as primary treatment for advanced-stage oropharyngeal cancer: a United States multicenter study. Head Neck 2011;33(12):1683–94.
29. Prevedello DM, Doglietto F, Jane JA, et al. History of endoscopic skull base surgery: its evolution and current reality. J Neurosurg 2007;107(1):206–13.
30. Linder TE, Simmen D, Stool SE. Revolutionary inventions in the 20th century. The history of endoscopy. Arch Otolaryngol Head Neck Surg 1997;123(11):1161–3.
31. Hirschmann A. Uber Endoskopie der nase und deren Nebenhohlen. Arch Laryngol Rhinol 1903;14:195–202.
32. Cockett WS, Cockett AT. The Hopkins rod-lens system and the Storz cold light illumination system. Urology 1998;51(5A Suppl):1–2.
33. Draf W. Endoscopy of the paranasal sinuses: technique· typical findings therapeutic possibilities. Springer Science & Business Media; 2012.
34. Catapano D, Sloffer CA, Frank G, et al. Comparison between the microscope and endoscope in the direct endonasal extended transsphenoidal approach: anatomical study. J Neurosurg 2006;104(3):419–25.
35. Jagannathan J, Laws ER, Jane JA Jr. Advantages of the endoscope and transitioning from the microscope to the endoscope for endonasal approaches. In: Kassam AB, Gardner PA, editors. Endoscopic approaches to the skull base, Vol 26. Prog Neurol Surg. Basel, Karger; 2012. p. 7–20.
36. Kwoh YS, Hou J, Jonckheere EA, et al. A robot with improved absolute positioning accuracy for CT guided stereotactic brain surgery. IEEE Trans Biomed Eng 1988;35(2):153–60.
37. Davies BL, Hibberd RD, Coptcoat MJ, et al. A surgeon robot prostatectomy—a laboratory evaluation. J Med Eng Technol 1989;13(6):273–7.
38. Marescaux J, Smith MK, Fölscher D, et al. Telerobotic laparoscopic cholecystectomy: initial clinical experience with 25 patients. Ann Surg 2001;234(1):1–7.
39. Bodner J, Wykypiel H, Wetscher G, et al. First experiences with the da Vinci™ operating robot in thoracic surgery. Eur J Cardiothorac Surg 2004;25(5):844–51.
40. Badaan SR, Stoianovici D. Robotic systems: past, present, and future. In: Robotics in genitourinary surgery. Springer; 2011. p. 655–65.
41. Garas G, Arora A. Robotic head and neck surgery: history, technical evolution and the future. ORL J Otorhinolaryngol Relat Spec 2018;80(3–4):117–24.
42. Haus BM, Kambham N, Le D, et al. Surgical robotic applications in otolaryngology. Laryngoscope 2003;113(7):1139–44.
43. McLeod IK, Melder PC. Da Vinci robot-assisted excision of a vallecular cyst: a case report. Ear Nose Throat J 2005;84(3):170–2.
44. Hockstein NG, O'Malley BW Jr, Weinstein GS. Assessment of intraoperative safety in transoral robotic surgery. Laryngoscope 2006;116(2):165–8.
45. O'Malley BW Jr, Hockstein NG, Hockstein NG. Transoral robotic surgery (TORS): glottic microsurgery in a canine model. J Voice 2006;20(2):263–8.
46. Weinstein GS, O'malley BW Jr, Hockstein NG. Transoral robotic surgery: supraglottic laryngectomy in a canine model. Laryngoscope 2005;115(7):1315–9.
47. O'Malley BW Jr, Weinstein GS, Snyder W, et al. Transoral Robotic Surgery (TORS) for Base of Tongue Neoplasms. Laryngoscope 2006;116(8):1465–72.
48. Weinstein GS, O'Malley BW, Snyder W, et al. Transoral robotic surgery: supraglottic partial laryngectomy. Ann Otol Rhinol Laryngol 2007;116(1):19–23.

49. Weinstein GS, O'Malley BW, Snyder W, et al. Transoral robotic surgery: radical tonsillectomy. Arch Otolaryngol Head Neck Surg 2007;133(12):1220–6.

50. Gross ND, Holsinger FC, Magnuson JS, et al. Robotics in otolaryngology and head and neck surgery: Recommendations for training and credentialing: A report of the 2015 AHNS education committee, AAO-HNS robotic task force and AAO-HNS sleep disorders committee. Head Neck 2016;38 Suppl 1(S1): E151–8.

51. Poon H, Li C, Gao W, et al. Evolution of robotic systems for transoral head and neck surgery. Oral Oncol 2018;87:82–8.

52. Chen MM, Roman SA, Kraus DH, et al. Transoral robotic surgery: a population-level analysis. Otolaryngol Head Neck Surg 2014;150(6) 968–75.

53. Da Vinci Surgical Systems. Intuitive Surgical, I., 09/2020. Web. Available at: https://www.intuitive.com/en-us/products-and-services/da-vinci/systems. Accessed September 1, 2020.

54. Fernandes E, Elli E, Giulianotti P. The role of the dual console in robotic surgical training. Surgery 2014;155(1):1–4.

55. Fiacchini G, Vianini M, Dallan I, et al. Is the Da Vinci Xi system a real improvement for oncologic transoral robotic surgery? A systematic review of the literature. J Robot Surg 2020;15:1–12.

56. Gabrysz-Forget F, Mur T, Dolan R, et al. Perioperative safety, feasibility, and oncologic utility of transoral robotic surgery with da Vinci Xi platform. J Robot Surg 2020;14(1):85–9.

57. Gorphe P, Simon C. A systematic review and meta-analysis of margins in transoral surgery for oropharyngeal carcinoma. Oral Oncol 2019;98:69–77.

58. Chen MM, Orosco RK, Lim GC, et al. Improved transoral dissection of the tongue base with a next-generation robotic surgical system. Laryngoscope 2018;128(1):78–83.

59. Chan JYK, Tsang RK, Holsinger FC, et al. Prospective clinical trial to evaluate safety and feasibility of using a single port flexible robotic system for transoral head and neck surgery. Oral Oncol 2019;94:101–5.

60. Van Abel KM, Yin LX, Price DL, et al. One-year outcomes for da Vinci single port robot for transoral robotic surgery. Head Neck 2020;42(8):2077–87.

61. Moore EJ, Olsen KD, Kasperbauer JL. Transoral robotic surgery for oropharyngeal squamous cell carcinoma: a prospective study of feasibility and functional outcomes. Laryngoscope 2009;119(11):2156–64.

62. Kumar A, Kumar S, Kaushik A, et al. Real time estimation and suppression of hand tremor for surgical robotic applications. Microsystem Technologies; 2020. p. 1–7.

63. Veluvolu KC, Ang WT. Estimation and filtering of physiological tremor for real-time compensation in surgical robotics applications. Int J Med Robot 2010; 6(3):334–42.

64. Prasad SM, Prasad SM, Maniar HS, et al. Surgical robotics: impact of motion scaling on task performance. J Am Coll Surg 2004;199(6):863–8.

65. Zihni A, Gerull WD, Cavallo JA, et al. Comparison of precision and speed in laparoscopic and robot-assisted surgical task performance. J Surg Res 2018; 223:29–33.

66. Kim HJ, Choi GS, Park JS, et al. Comparison of surgical skills in laparoscopic and robotic tasks between experienced surgeons and novices in laparoscopic surgery: an experimental study. Ann Coloproctol 2014;30(2):71–6.

67. Choussein S, Srouji SS, Farland LV, et al. Robotic assistance confers ambidexterity to laparoscopic surgeons. J Minim Invasive Gynecol 2018;25(1):76–83.

68. Feldstein J, Schwander B, Roberts M, et al. Cost of ownership assessment for a da Vinci robot based on US real-world data. Int J Med Robot 2019;15(5):e2023.

69. Rudmik L, An W, Livingstone D, et al. Making a case for high-volume robotic surgery centers: A cost-effectiveness analysis of transoral robotic surgery. J Surg Oncol 2015;112(2):155–63.

70. Spellman J, Coulter M, Kawatkar A, et al. Comparative cost of transoral robotic surgery and radiotherapy (IMRT) in early stage tonsil cancer. Am J Otolaryngol 2020;41:102409.

71. Othman S, McKinnon BJ. Financial outcomes of transoral robotic surgery: A narrative review. Am J Otolaryngol 2018;39(4):448–52.

72. Rodin D, Caulley L, Burger E, et al. Cost-effectiveness analysis of radiation therapy versus transoral robotic surgery for oropharyngeal squamous cell carcinoma. Int J Radiat Oncol Biol Phys 2017;97(4):709–17.

73. Amirabdollahian F, Livatino S, Vahedi B, et al. Prevalence of haptic feedback in robot-mediated surgery: a systematic review of literature. J Robot Surg 2018; 12(1):11–25.

74. Friedrich DT, Dürselen L, Mayer B, et al. Features of haptic and tactile feedback in TORS-a comparison of available surgical systems. J Robot Surg 2018;12(1): 103–8.

75. Abiri A, Juo YY, Tao A, et al. Artificial palpation in robotic surgery using haptic feedback. Surg Endosc 2019;33(4):1252–9.

76. Abiri A, Pensa J, Tao A, et al. Multi-modal haptic feedback for grip force reduction in robotic surgery. Sci Rep 2019;9(1):1–10.

77. Cracchiolo JR, Baxi SS, Morris LG, et al. Increase in primary surgical treatment of T1 and T2 oropharyngeal squamous cell carcinoma and rates of adverse pathologic features: National Cancer Data Base. Cancer 2016;122(10):1523–32.

78. Zhan KY, Puram SV, Li MM, et al. National treatment trends in human papillomavirus–positive oropharyngeal squamous cell carcinoma. Cancer 2020;126(6):1295–305.

79. Yeh DH, Tam S, Fung K, et al. Transoral robotic surgery vs. radiotherapy for management of oropharyngeal squamous cell carcinoma - A systematic review of the literature. Eur J Surg Oncol 2015;41(12):1603–14.

80. De Virgilio A, Costantino A, Mercante G, et al. Transoral robotic surgery and intensity-modulated radiotherapy in the treatment of the oropharyngeal carcinoma: A systematic review and meta-analysis. Eur Arch Otorhinolaryngol 2020;278(5):1321–35.

81. De Almeida JR, Byrd JK, Wu R, et al. A systematic review of transoral robotic surgery and radiotherapy for early oropharynx cancer: a systematic review. Laryngoscope 2014;124(9):2096–102.

82. Dong Y, Ridge JA, Li T, et al. Long-term toxicities in 10-year survivors of radiation treatment for head and neck cancer. Oral Oncol 2017;71:122–8.

83. Dong Y, Ridge JA, Ebersole B, et al. Incidence and outcomes of radiation-induced late cranial neuropathy in 10-year survivors of head and neck cancer. Oral Oncol 2019;95:59–64.

84. Nichols AC, Theurer J, Prisman E, et al. Radiotherapy versus transoral robotic surgery and neck dissection for oropharyngeal squamous cell carcinoma (ORATOR): an open-label, phase 2, randomised trial. Lancet Oncol 2019; 20(10):1349–59.

85. Hutcheson KA, Warneke CL, Yao CMKL, et al. Dysphagia after primary transoral robotic surgery with neck dissection vs nonsurgical therapy in patients with low-

to intermediate-risk oropharyngeal cancer. JAMA Otolaryngol Head Neck Surg 2019;145(11):1053–63.

86. Ferris RL, Flamand Y, Weinstein GS, et al. Transoral robotic surgical resection followed by randomization to low-or standard-dose IMRT in resectable p16+ locally advanced oropharynx cancer: a trial of the ECOG-ACRIN Cancer Research Group (E3311). American Society of Clinical Oncology 2020; 38(15_suppl):6500-6500.

87. Ma DJ, Price KA, Moore EJ, et al. Phase II evaluation of aggressive dose de-escalation for adjuvant chemoradiotherapy in human papillomavirus–associated oropharynx squamous cell carcinoma. J Clin Oncol 2019;37(22): 1909–18.

88. Swisher-McClure S, Lukens JN, Aggarwal C, et al. A Phase 2 Trial of Alternative Volumes of Oropharyngeal Irradiation for De-intensification (AVOID): Omission of the Resected Primary Tumor Bed After Transoral Robotic Surgery for Human Papilloma Virus–Related Squamous Cell Carcinoma of the Oropharynx. Int J Radiat Oncol Biol Phys 2020;106(4):725–32.

89. Hanna J, Brauer PR, Morse E, et al. Is robotic surgery an option for early T-stage laryngeal cancer? Early nationwide results. Laryngoscope 2020;130(5): 1195–201.

90. Smith RV, Schiff BA, Sarta C, et al. Transoral robotic total laryngectomy. Laryngoscope 2013;123(3):678–82.

91. Krishnan G, Krishnan S. Transoral robotic surgery total laryngectomy: evaluation of functional and survival outcomes in a retrospective case series at a single institution. ORL J Otorhinolaryngol Relat Spec 2017;79(4):191–201.

92. Ozer E, Alvarez B, Kakarala K, et al. Clinical outcomes of transoral robotic supraglottic laryngectomy. Head Neck 2013;35(8):1158–61.

93. Olsen SM, Moore EJ, Koch CA, et al. Transoral robotic surgery for supraglottic squamous cell carcinoma. Am J Otolaryngol 2012;33(4):379–84.

94. Eskander A, Ghanem T, Agrawal A. AHNS Series: Do you know your guidelines? Guideline recommendations for head and neck cancer of unknown primary site. Head Neck 2018;40(3):614–21.

95. Motz K, Qualliotine JR, Rettig E, et al. Changes in unknown primary squamous cell carcinoma of the head and neck at initial presentation in the era of human papillomavirus. JAMA Otolaryngol Head Neck Surg 2016;142(3):223–8.

96. Maghami E, Ismaila N, Alvarez A, et al. Diagnosis and Management of Squamous Cell Carcinoma of Unknown Primary in the Head and Neck: ASCO Guideline. J Clin Oncol 2020;38(22):2570–96.

97. Fu TS, Foreman A, Goldstein DP, et al. The role of transoral robotic surgery, transoral laser microsurgery, and lingual tonsillectomy in the identification of head and neck squamous cell carcinoma of unknown primary origin: a systematic review. J Otolaryngol Head Neck Surg 2016;45(1):28.

98. Mehta V, Johnson P, Tassler A, et al. A new paradigm for the diagnosis and management of unknown primary tumors of the head and neck: a role for transoral robotic surgery. Laryngoscope 2013;123(1):146–51.

99. Graboyes EM, Sinha P, Thorstad WL, et al. Management of human papillomavirus–related unknown primaries of the head and neck with a transoral surgical approach. Head Neck 2015;37(11):1603–11.

100. Arora A, Chaidas K, Garas G, et al. Outcome of TORS to tongue base and epiglottis in patients with OSA intolerant of conventional treatment. Sleep Breath 2016;20(2):739–47.

101. Chiffer RC, Schwab RJ, Keenan BT, et al. Volumetric MRI analysis pre- and post-Transoral robotic surgery for obstructive sleep apnea. Laryngoscope 2015; 125(8):1988–95.
102. Toh ST, Han HJ, Tay HN, et al. Transoral robotic surgery for obstructive sleep apnea in Asian patients: a Singapore sleep centre experience. JAMA Otolaryngol Head Neck Surg 2014;140(7):624–9.
103. Hoff PT, Glazer TA, Spector ME. Body mass index predicts success in patients undergoing transoral robotic surgery for obstructive sleep apnea. ORL J Otorhinolaryngol Relat Spec 2014;76(5):266–72.
104. Garas G, Kythreotou A, Georgalas C, et al. Is transoral robotic surgery a safe and effective multilevel treatment for obstructive sleep apnoea in obese patients following failure of conventional treatment(s)? Ann Med Surg (Lond) 2017;19:55–61.
105. Tamaki A, Rocco JW, Ozer E. The future of robotic surgery in otolaryngology - head and neck surgery. Oral Oncol 2020;101:104510.
106. Yu JL, Mahmoud A, Thaler ER. Transoral robotic surgery versus upper airway stimulation in select obstructive sleep apnea patients. Laryngoscope 2019; 129(1):256–8.
107. Ikeda Y, Takami H, Niimi M, et al. Endoscopic thyroidectomy by the axillary approach. Surg Endosc 2001;15(11):1362–4.
108. Park YL, Han WK, Bae WG. 100 cases of endoscopic thyroidectomy: breast approach. Surg Laparosc Endosc Percutan Tech 2003;13(1):20–5.
109. Shimizu K, Akira S, Jasmi AY, et al. Video-assisted neck surgery: endoscopic resection of thyroid tumors with a very minimal neck wound. J Am Coll Surg 1999;188(6):697–703.
110. Sebag F, Palazzo FF, Harding J, et al. Endoscopic lateral approach thyroid lobectomy: safe evolution from endoscopic parathyroidectomy. World J Surg 2006;30(5):802–5.
111. Tan CT, Cheah WK, Delbridge L. "Scarless" (in the neck) endoscopic thyroidectomy (SET): an evidence-based review of published techniques. World J Surg 2008;32(7):1349–57.
112. Chen C, Huang S, Huang A, et al. Total endoscopic thyroidectomy versus conventional open thyroidectomy in thyroid cancer: a systematic review and meta-analysis. Ther Clin Risk Manag 2018;14:2349–61.
113. Arora A, Swords C, Garas G, et al. The perception of scar cosmesis following thyroid and parathyroid surgery: A prospective cohort study. Int J Surg 2016; 25:38–43.
114. Chan JY, Tsang RK, Eisele DW, et al. Transoral robotic surgery of the parapharyngeal space: a case series and systematic review. Head Neck 2015;37(2): 293–8.
115. Chan JY, Richmon JD. Transoral robotic surgery (TORS) for benign pharyngeal lesions. Otolaryngol Clin North Am 2014;47(3):407–13.
116. Walvekar RR, Peters G, Hardy E, et al. Robotic-assisted transoral removal of a bilateral floor of mouth ranulas. World J Surg Oncol 2011;9(1):78.
117. Razavi C, Pascheles C, Samara G, et al. Robot-assisted sialolithotomy with sialendoscopy for the management of large submandibular gland stones. Laryngoscope 2016;126(2):345–51.
118. Liang LM, Lin XZ, Shao XJ, et al. Trans-oral robotic submandibular gland removal. Zhonghua Kou Qiang Yi Xue Za Zhi 2019;54(4):263–5.
119. Molteni G, Greco MG, Presutti L. Transoral robotic-assisted surgery for the approach to anterior cervical spine lesions. Eur Arch Otorhinolaryngol 2017; 274(11):4011–6.

120. Bearelly S, Prendes BL, Wang SJ, et al. Transoral robotic-assisted surgical excision of a retropharyngeal parathyroid adenoma: A case report. Head Neck 2015;37(11):E150–2.

121. Carrau RL, Prevedello DM, de Lara D, et al. Combined transoral robotic surgery and endoscopic endonasal approach for the resection of extensive malignancies of the skull base. Head Neck 2013;35(11):E351–8.

122. Bonawitz SC, Duvvuri U. Robot-assisted oropharyngeal reconstruction with free tissue transfer. J Reconstr Microsurg 2012;28(7):485–90.

123. Bonawitz SC, Duvvuri U. Robotic-assisted FAMM flap for soft palate reconstruction. Laryngoscope 2013;123(4):870–4.

124. Holcomb AJ, Richmon JD. Transoral robotic salvage oropharyngectomy with submental artery island flap reconstruction. Head Neck 2020;43(2):E13–9.

125. Hatten KM, Brody RM, Weinstein GS, et al. Defining the role of free flaps for transoral robotic surgery. Ann Plast Surg 2018;80(1):45–9.

126. Pratt P, Arora A. Transoral robotic surgery: image guidance and augmented reality. ORL J Otorhinolaryngol Relat Spec 2018;80(3–4):204–12.

127. Liu WP, Richmon JD, Sorger JM, et al. Augmented reality and cone beam CT guidance for transoral robotic surgery. J Robot Surg 2015;9(3):223–33.

128. Chan JYK, Holsinger FC, Liu S, et al. Augmented reality for image guidance in transoral robotic surgery. J Robot Surg 2020;14(4):579–83.

129. Vicini C, Montevecchi F, D'Agostino G, et al. A novel approach emphasising intra-operative superficial margin enhancement of head-neck tumours with narrow-band imaging in transoral robotic surgery. Acta Otorhinolaryngol Ital 2015;35(3):157–61.

130. Scott-Wittenborn N, Jackson RS. Intraoperative imaging during minimally invasive transoral robotic surgery using near-infrared light. Am J Otolaryngol 2018;39(2):220–2.

131. Daskalaki D, Aguilera F, Patton K, et al. Fluorescence in robotic surgery. J Surg Oncol 2015;112(3):250–6.

132. Meier JD, Xie H, Sun Y, et al. Time-resolved laser-induced fluorescence spectroscopy as a diagnostic instrument in head and neck carcinoma. Otolaryngol Head Neck Surg 2010;142(6):838–44.

133. Gorpas D, Phipps J, Bec J, et al. Autofluorescence lifetime augmented reality as a means for real-time robotic surgery guidance in human patients. Sci Rep 2019;9(1):1187–9.

134. Sun Y, Phipps JE, Meier J, et al. Endoscopic fluorescence lifetime imaging for in vivo intraoperative diagnosis of oral carcinoma. Microsc Microanal 2013; 19(4):791–8.

135. Maier-Hein L, Vedula SS, Speidel S, et al. Surgical data science for next-generation interventions. Nat Biomed Eng 2017;1(9):691–6.

136. Bur AM, Holcomb A, Goodwin S, et al. Machine learning to predict occult nodal metastasis in early oral squamous cell carcinoma. Oral Oncol 2019;92:20–5.

137. Bur AM, Shew M, New J. Artificial intelligence for the otolaryngologist: a state of the art review. Otolaryngol Head Neck Surg 2019;160(4):603–11.

138. Kann BH, Hicks DF, Payabvash S, et al. Multi-institutional validation of deep learning for pretreatment identification of extranodal extension in head and neck squamous cell carcinoma. J Clin Oncol 2020;38(12):1304–11.

139. Warren E. Strengthening research through data sharing. N Engl J Med 2016; 375(5):401–3.

Lip and Oral Cavity Squamous Cell Carcinoma

Adam Howard, MD, Nishant Agrawal, MD, Zhen Gooi, MBBS*

KEY WORKS

- Lip cancer • Oral cavity cancer • Squamous cell carcinoma • Head and neck cancer

KEY POINTS

- There should be a low threshold to biopsy nonhealing lip or oral ulcers, especially in those with risk factors.
- Physical examination and appropriate imaging are crucial for accurate clinical staging.
- Surgical resection of the primary lesion, with neck dissection when indicated, is the recommended treatment of lip and oral cavity cancer.
- Adjuvant radiation or chemoradiation should be performed when indicated by adverse histopathologic features.

INTRODUCTION

Epidemiology

Cancers of the lip and oral cavity are the most common nonmelanoma head and neck cancer in the world, with approximately 350,000 new cases each year worldwide.[1] For example, South Central Asia and some regions of Oceania demonstrate the highest incidence at 12.9 to 21.2 per 100,000 for men and 4.5 to 12 per 100,000 for women. This incidence contrasts with the incidence in North America, shown to be 6.3 per 100,000 for men and 2.4 per 100,000 for women.[1] Roughly 15,000 to 20,000 new cases of mucosal lip and oral cavity cancers are diagnosed each year in the United States.[2] The incidence of SCC in every anatomic subsite of the oral cavity has been decreasing over the last decade in the United States with the exception of the anterior tongue and alveolar ridge, which have both increased in incidence.[2] Approximately 90% of mucosal lip and oral cavity malignancies are squamous cell carcinoma (SCC).[2] The male/female ratio is about 2:1, and most cases present between 65 and 84 years of age.[3,4]

Anatomy and Risk Factors

The oral cavity begins with the mucosal lip and extends to the junction of the hard and soft palate. The subsites of the oral cavity, in order of descending frequency of cancer,

University of Chicago, 5841 South Maryland Avenue, MC 1035, Chicago, IL 60637, USA
* Corresponding author.
E-mail address: zgooi@surgery.bsd.uchicago.edu

Hematol Oncol Clin N Am 35 (2021) 895–911
https://doi.org/10.1016/j.hoc.2021.05.003
0889-8588/21/© 2021 Elsevier Inc. All rights reserved.
hemonc.theclinics.com

are the oral tongue tissue anterior to the circumvallate papillae, the floor of mouth, alveolar ridge, hard palate, buccal mucosa, and retromolar trigone.[2] It is important to distinguish mucosal lip cancer from cutaneous lip cancer, because the 2 entities have different pathophysiology and prognostic implications. Mucosal lip cancers originate from the internal vermillion or the wet lip, which has a thin mucosal epithelium and is rich in capillaries and minor salivary glands. In contrast, the cutaneous lip or external vermillion demonstrates a thick keratinizing epidermis, similar to the rest of the skin of the head and neck.[2] Both types of lip cancer share sun exposure as a risk factor; however, tobacco and alcohol use are also risk factors for mucosal lip and oral cavity cancers. Other risk factors for oral cavity SCC include immunosuppression, betel quid chewing, and certain rare genetic syndromes such as Fanconi anemia and Howel-Evans syndrome. Fanconi anemia is an autosomal recessive disorder resulting from mutations in several genes responsible for DNA repair. Many patients with Fanconi anemia develop hematologic malignancy early in life, but those who reach adulthood are at especially high risk for head and neck cancer.[5] Howel-Evans syndrome is an autosomal dominant disease characterized by thickening of the skin of the hands and feet. These patients are at extremely high risk for esophageal cancer and also at risk for oral cancer, particularly of the tongue.[6]

Outcomes

Cutaneous lip SCC has a very promising 95% five-year overall survival, partly due to low cervical node metastatic rates of 2% to 5%[7–9]; this contrasts with a 5-year survival rate of about 60% to 65% for all stages of oral cavity cancers.[9] However, survival outcomes differ dramatically for those with localized oral cavity carcinoma versus regional or distant metastases. The 5-year survival rate for localized disease is about 80%, in contrast to a 40% to 50% and less than 10% 5-year survival for those with regional and distant metastases, respectively.[9–12] Regional nodal metastases (both clinical and occult) are present in up to 40% of oral cavity SCCs, and distant metastases are present in around 2% to 3% of cases.[9–12]

Outcomes for mucosal lip SCC fall between cutaneous lip and oral cavity. Five-year overall survival rates are 85% to 95% for stage I and II lip SCC and 40% to 70% for stage III and IV disease.[13–15] However, regional metastases are more common than cutaneous lip SCC and range between 10% and 20% for all mucosal lip SCCs.[7,9,13,14,16] Mucosal lip SCC tends to present at earlier stages than oral cavity SCC given the prominent and noticeable anatomic region. This review focuses on the diagnosis, workup, and treatment options for mucosal lip and oral cavity SCC.

DISCUSSION
Presentation and Diagnosis

SCC of the lip accounts for about 10% to 20% of all oral cavity cancers.[2,17] Lip SCC most frequently begins as ulcerative lesions known as actinic cheilosis. Data from the Survival Epidemiology End Results database (SEER) from 1973 to 2012 revealed that about 90% of all lip SCCs were of the lower lip, 8% to 9% were of the upper lip, and 1% to 2% were of the oral commissure.[17] Lip SCCs often present early given their visible location. Workup for any lip or oral cavity cancer begins with a thorough history and physical examination. It is important to determine the epicenter and extent of the primary tumor, and the patient should be evaluated for regional cervical lymphadenopathy. Any nonhealing ulcerative lesion of the lip or oral cavity warrants a biopsy for histopathologic analysis. Diagnosis of SCC is ultimately achieved with tissue biopsy. Cancerous and precancerous lesions of the lip and oral cavity exist on a spectrum of varying degrees of dysplasia, to carcinoma in situ, and finally invasive carcinoma. Mild dysplasia can often be observed clinically, whereas severe dysplasia and carcinoma in situ are generally managed similar to early-stage invasive SCC and warrant definitive treatment.

Oral cavity SCC includes cancer of the tongue, floor of mouth, alveolar ridge, hard palate, and retromolar trigone (**Fig. 1**). Of these subsites, the tongue is the most common location for SCC.[1,18] In the Western world, the floor of mouth is the second most common subsite; however, in regions where betel quid usage is high the buccal mucosa is the second most common subsite.[19] Risk factors for oral cavity cancer include tobacco use (smoking and chewing), alcohol use, and betel quid chewing. All 3 of these risk factors act synergistically when used simultaneously.[19] The use of betel quid is prevalent in South East Asia and migrant Asian communities around the world. Similar to lip SCC, oral cavity SCC is usually preceded by a white or red mucosal change known as leukoplakia or erythroplakia, respectively.[20] These potentially malignant lesions should be biopsied given the risk of harboring invasive carcinoma and risk for transformation over time. Findings on physical examination concerning for cancer include ulceration, necrosis, friability and bleeding, submucosal firmness, and tenderness.

Workup and Staging

Imaging recommendations for lip and oral cavity SCC are constantly evolving. The 2 main imaging modalities used are computed tomography (CT) and MRI. Both modalities rely on intravenous contrast to distinguish malignancy from surrounding tissue. Tumors of the lip and oral cavity that are less than 2 cm in size (T1) are often not visualized on either CT or MRI. Tumors of the lip and oral cavity that are more than 2 cm in size (T2 and higher) have a greater likelihood of invading adjacent subsites and higher rates of cervical metastases.[7,13,14,16] Current National Comprehensive Cancer Network (NCCN) guidelines recommend cross-sectional imaging for all newly diagnosed head and neck cancers,[21] which can be accomplished by CT and/or MRI. CT scans have the advantage of being more available, being cheaper and faster, and providing high resolution of bony anatomy.[22] MRI images are superior at characterizing local soft tissue involvement, depth of invasion, perineural invasion, and bone

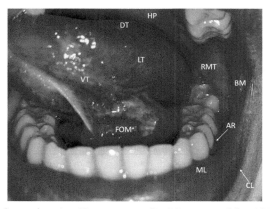

Fig. 1. Subsites of the oral cavity. CL, cutaneous lip; ML, mucosal lip; FOM, floor of mouth; VT, ventral tongue; LT, lateral tongue; DT, dorsal tongue; HP, hard palate; RMT, retromolar trigone; BM, buccal mucosa; AR, alveolar ridge.

marrow involvement.[23,24] Both modalities are equally effective at evaluating the neck for cervical metastases. PET/CT is an imaging modality used to evaluate locoregional disease as well as distant metastases. Multiple studies have demonstrated superior sensitivity with PET/CT over CT or MRI in identifying further regional and distant metastases in patients with a clinically positive lymph node.[25,26] The most recent NCCN guidelines recommend advanced-stage lip and oral cavity cancers (T3/4 and/or > N0) be evaluated with full-body PET/CT as well as CT of the chest for higher resolution of potential mediastinal, perihilar, and pulmonary metastases.[21]

Head and neck cancers are staged using the American Joint Committee on Cancer 8th edition TNM system, which is the most up-to-date and uniformly accepted staging method. This system incorporates size of tumor, involvement of adjacent structures, and regional neck metastases based on physical examination and imaging (Table 1). An important difference between the seventh and eighth editions of lip and oral cavity staging is the inclusion of depth of invasion (DOI) as a tumor staging criteria. Nodal staging is determined by the number, size and laterality, and absence or presence of extranodal involvement of lymph nodes (Tables 2 and 3). Patients without clinical or radiographic evidence of distant metastases are M0.

Treatment and Outcomes

Lip squamous cell carcinoma

Treatment strategies for lip and oral cavity SCC are similar. The NCCN guidelines recommend upfront surgical resection with adjuvant therapy as indicated by pathologic condition for both lip and oral cavity SCC.[21] Surgery for both types of cancer involves resecting the primary tumor along with a margin of healthy-appearing tissue. The recommended margin for lip SCC is 1 cm.[21] The NCCN defines adequate margins as having 1 cm of visible and palpable normal mucosa from the gross tumor, to allow for clear frozen margins and at least 5 mm of clear margins on permanent histopathologic analysis.[21] A close margin on permanent analysis indicates microscopic invasive tumor within 5 mm of the resected margin. A positive margin indicates invasive tumor or carcinoma in situ identified at the resection margin.[21]

When adverse features such as close margins (<5 mm), perineural invasion (PNI), lymphovascular invasion (LVI) or multiple lymph node metastasis are present on histopathologic analysis, current NCCN guidelines recommend use of adjuvant radiotherapy (RT).[21] Indications for adjuvant chemoradiotherapy (CRT) include extranodal extension (ENE) after neck dissection or positive margins on pathologic analysis of

Table 1 T staging for lip and oral cavity carcinoma based on AJCC 8th edition TNM staging system	
Tumor Staging	Extent of Disease
Tis	Carcinoma in situ
T1	Tumor ≤2 cm with DOI ≤5 mm
T2	Tumor ≤2 cm with DOI >5 mm or tumor >2 cm and ≤4 cm with DOI ≤10 mm
T3	Tumor >2 cm and ≤4 cm with DOI >10 mm or tumor >4 cm with DOI ≤10 mm
T4a	Tumor >4 cm with DOI >10 mm or tumor invades adjacent structures: cortical bone of maxilla or mandible, maxillary sinus, skin of the face
T4	Tumor invades masticator space, pterygoid plates, skull base, and/or encases internal carotid artery

Abbreviation: AJCC, American Joint Committee on Cancer; DOI, depth of invasion.

Table 2
Clinical N staging for lip and oral cavity carcinoma based on AJCC 8th edition TNM staging system

Clinical Lymph Node Staging	Extent of Disease
cN0	No regional lymph node metastasis
cN1	Single ipsilateral lymph node metastasis ≤3 cm in greatest dimension and ENE(−)
cN2a	Metastasis in single ipsilateral lymph node >3 cm and <6 cm and ENE(−)
cN2b	Metastases in multiple ipsilateral lymph nodes, none larger than 6 cm and all ENE(−)
cN2c	Metastases in bilateral or contralateral lymph nodes, none larger than 6 cm and all ENE(−)
cN3a	Metastasis in any lymph node larger than 6 cm and ENE(−)
cN3b	Metastasis in any lymph node with clinically overt ENE(+)

the primary tumor. Re-resection is the preferred approach to close or positive margins when feasible.

There have been no randomized controlled trials to date that compare surgery to nonsurgical treatment of lip SCC. Multiple database reviews have demonstrated improved overall survival with surgical treatment compared with nonsurgical approaches for all oral cavity cancers.[27–30] However, most of these studies lack subgroup analysis to specifically compare treatment outcomes for lip SCC. One recent analysis of the National Cancer Database (NCDB) found that lip cancers of all stages treated with surgery had superior 5-year overall survival rates compared with those treated with nonsurgical approaches (70.2% vs 44.5%, respectively).[31] However, many retrospective studies have shown that surgery and RT provide similar overall survival and local control rates for early-stage lip SCC.[32–34]

Table 3
Pathologic N staging for lip and oral cavity carcinoma based on AJCC 8th edition TNM staging system

Pathologic Lymph Node Staging	Extent of Disease
pN0	No regional lymph node metastasis
pN1	Single ipsilateral lymph node metastasis ≤3 cm in greatest dimension and ENE(−)
pN2a	Metastasis in single ipsilateral lymph node >3 cm and ≤6 cm and ENE(−) **or single ipsilateral lymph node ≤3 cm and ENE(+)**
pN2b	Metastasis in multiple ipsilateral lymph nodes, none larger than 6 cm and all ENE(−)
pN2c	Metastases in bilateral or contralateral lymph nodes, none larger than 6 cm and all ENE(−)
pN3a	Metastasis in any lymph node larger than 6 cm and ENE(−)
pN3b	**Metastasis in any lymph node >3 cm and ENE(+), or multiple ipsilateral lymph nodes of any size with ENE(+), or any number of contralateral lymph nodes ENE(+)**

Entries in bold indicate differences from clinical N staging.

Advantages of surgery include histopathologic analysis of the primary tumor and cervical lymph nodes for identification of adverse features. These results can direct the need for adjuvant treatment and would not be obtained with RT alone. The implications of surgical resection include esthetic and functional considerations, including microstomia, oral incompetence, and poor cosmetic outcomes. However, there are a multitude of reconstructive options and techniques that can help minimize the morbidity of surgical resection of the lip.[35] Reconstruction of lip defects not amenable to primary closure can be achieved with locoregional flaps or free tissue transfer for larger resections. Advantages of RT include preserving the natural function and appearance of the mouth and lips and the avoidance of perioperative risks of anesthesia and surgery. Disadvantage of RT include the need for multiple encounters to treatment completion and the risk of early and late RT sequelae such as xerostomia, dysphagia, and osteoradionecrosis (ORN). Overall, the current NCCN guidelines recommend surgical resection of early-stage lip SCC for those who are amenable and suitable for surgery, with RT reserved for those who decline surgery or are not suitable for general anesthesia.[21]

Treatment of the neck in early-stage lip SCC is generally not indicated in patients with clinical N0 stage tumor. Early-stage lip SCC has a low (5%–10%) incidence of occult metastases rates based on existing data in the literature.[7,9,13,14] Therefore, elective neck dissection for cT1N0 or cT2N0 is not recommended by NCCN guidelines.[21] A fine-needle aspiration biopsy can be considered in patients with early T stage tumor with an indeterminate cervical lymph node on imaging studies. However, any patient with clinically or radiologically evident cervical metastases requires treatment of the neck by therapeutic neck dissection or definitive radiation. Studies have shown that sentinel lymph node biopsy (SLNB) can be an effective method for evaluating patients with early-stage lip SCC who are at higher risk for cervical metastasis.[36–38] Patients with early-stage lip SCC who are at higher risk for cervical metastases include those with T2 primary lesions and with tumor thickness greater than 4 mm.[36] Various randomized controlled trials have shown that SLNB is not inferior to elective neck dissection, in terms of overall and recurrence-free survival, for early-stage lip and oral cavity SCC.[38–40] Current NCCN guidelines recommend considering SLNB for T1/T2 N0 lip and oral cavity SCC with a depth of invasion less than 4 mm.[21]

Early-stage lip SCC can generally be treated with single-modality therapy (surgery or RT alone), whereas advanced-stage disease requires multimodality therapy. Surgical resection is still the preferred approach based on NCCN guidelines.[21] Advanced primary tumors present with more local tissue destruction and cosmetic deformity. Many advanced-stage tumors also harbor adverse pathologic features such as PNI and LVI,[41,42] which are indications for adjuvant RT. Moreover, advanced-stage primary lesions also have higher rates of cervical metastases, either occult or clinically evident. Therefore, the current NCCN guidelines recommend elective ipsilateral neck dissection for cT3N0 and cT4N0 lip SCC. Bilateral neck dissection should be performed for lesions approaching or crossing midline.[21] Patients who are unfit for surgery or have unresectable disease (cT4b) have the treatment options of either definitive chemoradiation or clinical trial enrollment.[21]

The presence of one or more cervical metastasis is the single most important prognostic factor for lip SCC.[43,44] An estimated 5% to 10% of early T stage lip SCC (T1 and T2) will have lymph node metastases.[45] Most metastases are found in level I; however, levels II and III are also at risk for metastases and should be addressed when neck treatment is performed.[46] Higher T stage lesions (T3 and T4) and lesions of the oral commissure were found to be more likely to present with cervical metastases, up to 15% to 23%.[45,46]

Survival outcomes for early-stage lip cancers are generally favorable. Five-year overall survival rates for stage I and II lip SCC are estimated to be 85% to 95%, whereas 5-year overall survival for stage III and IV disease are about 40% to 70%.[13,14] This steep decline in overall survival for advanced-stage disease is believed to be associated with the presence of cervical metastasis. Five-year survival for all lip SCC is around 80% to 90%, aligning more closely with early-stage disease as these are more common than advanced stage.[13,14]

Oral cavity squamous cell carcinoma

Pretreatment multidisciplinary evaluation by speech and language pathologists (SLPs), nutritionists, and dentists is essential for patients with oral cavity SCC. Many patients with head and neck cancer present with significant weight loss and low nutritional intake. The NCCN recommends considering starting enteral nutritional support for select patients before and during treatment; this includes patients who have pain on swallowing, have lost 5% of their body weight over the previous month, or lost 10% of their body weight over 6 months.[47] Speech and language pathologists are instrumental at determining which patients may eat safely by clinical and radiographic evaluation of swallow function. Dental evaluation before treatment is essential to treat dental carries, dentoalveolar infection, and mitigate the risks of ORN with any anticipated radiation therapy.[48]

Current NCCN guidelines recommend surgical resection for early-stage oral cavity SCC.[21] Adequate surgical margins of 1 cm should be obtained during resection. Surgery provides the advantage of pathologic staging to direct adjuvant therapy when indicated. Adverse pathologic features that warrant adjuvant RT include LVI, PNI, close margins (<5 mm), pT3 or greater, pN2 or greater, and nodal disease in levels IV or V.[10,21,49,50] Re-resection is the preferred approach for close or positive surgical margins when feasible. Adjuvant CRT should be considered for unresectable positive margins or when ENE is present.[21] Definitive RT for early oral cavity SCC is an option for patients who are unsuitable for surgery, refuse surgery, or for recurrent disease not amenable to resection (**Table 4**).

Advanced oral cavity tumors often require free tissue transfer for reconstruction of the postresection defect. The goals of free tissue transfer for reconstruction are to provide bulk to the defect cavity, to restore function of the resected structures, and to maintain cosmesis as much as possible.[51] Options for soft tissue transfer only include radial forearm and anterolateral thigh free flaps. These options are useful when reconstructing soft tissue defects such as lip, oral tongue, and floor of mouth. Resection of bony structures of the oral cavity, such as the mandible or maxilla, may require fibula- or scapula-free flaps to restore function and cosmesis of the resected bone.

Management of mandibular bone is an important consideration in patients with alveolar ridge, retromolar trigone, and floor of mouth SCC. There exist 2 treatment consideration approaches for resecting tumors abutting or involving mandibular bone. Marginal mandibulectomy involves removing the superior portion of the mandibular bone while maintaining the overall continuity of the mandible. Segmental mandibulectomy involves complete removal of a segment of mandibular bone, which results in discontinuity of the remaining mandibular segments. Segmental mandibulectomy generally requires free tissue transfer for reconstruction, often bone-containing tissue such as a fibula-free flap. This process is opposed to marginal mandibulectomy, which does not require as extensive reconstruction. The exposed mandible from a marginal mandibulectomy may be amenable to skin graft closure, locoregional flaps, or free soft tissue transfer for reconstruction.

Table 4
Staging, treatment, and outcomes for early-stage lip and oral cavity cancer

Site	Overall Stage	T	N	Treatment of Tumor	Treatment of Neck	5-y Overall Survival
Lip	Stage I	T1	N0	**Surgery** ± adjuvant therapy based on adverse pathologic features	Observe. Consider SLNB	90%–100%
Lip	Stage II	T2	N0	**Surgery** ± adjuvant therapy based on adverse pathologic features	Observe. Consider SLNB	85%–95%
Oral cavity	Stage 1	T1	N0	**Surgery** ± adjuvant therapy based on adverse pathologic features	DOI <4 mm: observe. Consider SLNB DOI ≥4 mm: elective neck dissection	~80%
Oral cavity	Stage II	T2	N0	**Surgery** ± adjuvant therapy based on adverse pathologic features	Elective neck dissection	~70%

Bolded significance is to emphasize surgery as the primary modality of therapy.

A recent meta-analysis reviewed results from 15 articles comparing marginal to segmental mandibulectomy. This study found that tumors with medullary bone involvement treated with marginal mandibulectomy had lower 2-year and 5-year disease-free survival (DFS).[52] Involvement of medullary bone not only may be evident in preoperative imaging but also can be clinically evident if a patient has clinical involvement of the inferior alveolar nerve on examination manifested by paresthesia or numbness of the lower jaw region. The investigators conclude that marginal mandibulectomy is reasonable for tumors encroaching on, adherent to, or superficially invading the mandibular cortex.[52] Segmental mandibulectomy should be performed when there is deep invasion of the mandibular cortex, invasion of medullary bone, or when obtaining appropriate oncologic margins would necessitate leaving less than 1 cm of height of the remaining mandibular bone.[52] In select patient groups, such as those with prior radiation to the head and neck or edentulous patients, it may be reasonable to perform segmental mandibulectomy even for superficially invading tumors because these patients are at higher risk of ORN and pathologic fractures following marginal mandibulectomy.

The presence of cervical nodal metastases has been shown to be the most important prognostic factor for oral cavity SCC. The presence of a single cervical metastasis reduces overall survival by about half compared with equal tumor-stage patients without cervical metastases.[53] Current NCCN guidelines recommend elective neck dissection in early-stage oral cavity cancers with depth of invasion greater than 3 mm.[21] Multiple prospective studies have shown that tumors with DOI 4 mm or greater have increased risk of both clinically positive and occult metastases on elective neck dissections.[54–57] When selective neck dissection is performed for lip and oral cavity SCC, all lymph node-bearing tissue should be removed from neck levels I to III and possibly superior level V.[21] Level IV may be addressed during a neck dissection in select cases such as advanced tumor stage or a clinically node-positive neck.

The results of a large randomized controlled trial evaluating elective neck dissection versus therapeutic neck dissection in early-stage oral cavity cancer without clinical cervical metastases were recently reported. This study demonstrated significantly higher overall survival (80.0% vs 67.5%) and DFS (69.5% vs 45.9%) in patients who received elective neck dissection compared with therapeutic neck dissection.[58] In addition, a meta-analysis from 2011 demonstrated that elective neck dissection in early-stage oral cavity SCC significantly reduced disease-specific mortality.[59] Bilateral neck treatment should be performed for tumors approaching or crossing midline when neck treatment is indicated.

Current NCCN guidelines state that the depth of invasion and a positive SLNB are the 2 most reliable predictors of occult metastases. Therefore, SLNB can be considered for tumors with DOI 3 mm or less.[21] Multiple studies, including randomized controlled trials, have demonstrated sensitivity and specificity between 90% and 100% in SLNB and equivalent overall and recurrence-free survival compared with elective neck dissection for early-stage oral cavity SCC.[38–40,60,61] Patients with early-stage oral cavity SCC who are at high risk for occult cervical metastases should undergo elective neck dissection. Features that would place patients into this high-risk group include tumor size (T2 at higher risk) and DOI greater than 3 mm.[54,55,62,63]

Treatment of advanced-stage oral cavity SCC is generally accomplished via multimodality therapy. The preferred approach is surgery with adjuvant RT or CRT depending on the pathologic condition or nonsurgical options for select cases.[21] Several studies have demonstrated improved survival outcomes. Multiple studies have demonstrated improved survival outcomes with surgery and appropriate adjuvant therapy as opposed to definitive RT or CRT for advanced oral cavity SCC.[29,64] One prospective trial evaluating this topic randomized 119 patients to receive either concurrent chemoradiotherapy (CCRT) or surgery followed by postoperative radiotherapy (PORT). The study found a significantly higher 5-year disease-specific survival and lower distant recurrence rate in favor of surgery plus PORT.[64] Limitations of this study are that it ended early due to poor accrual and that the oral cavity SCC data were based on subset analysis, leading to small subject numbers. A large multiinstitutional retrospective review also demonstrated higher 5-year overall, disease-specific, disease-free, and metastasis-free survival in patients who received surgery with PORT or postoperative chemoradiotherapy compared with RT or CCRT alone.[29] In addition, these studies include selection bias in that the patients selected for surgery likely have better functional status and are fit to undergo general anesthesia and major surgery; this is compared with the patients who receive definitive RT or CRT who are more likely to have inoperable cancers, reduced functional status, and existing comorbidities contributing to the poorer survival rates.

There are potential advantages of concurrent CRT over surgery in select patients with advanced oral cavity SCC. These advantages are largely due to the significant morbidity entailed with total or near-total removal of critical structures in the oral cavity. For example, total glossectomies required for certain T3/T4 oral tongue cancers can lead to high rates of dysphagia, aspiration, and speech difficulties. Multiple institutions have investigated nonsurgical approaches to select T4 oral cavity cancers to preserve organ function while achieving oncologic control.[30,65] Data supporting the use of CCRT for advanced-stage oral cavity SCC is limited to retrospective reviews. These studies demonstrate no significant difference in 5-year overall survival and either disease-specific or DFS between surgery and CRT arms.[30,65] Long-term complication rates between the 2 groups were similar in both studies. One significant disadvantage of CCRT for advanced oral cavity SCC is the risk of ORN. The rates of ORN with CCRT for advanced oral cavity SCC are estimated to be 5% to 20%.[48,66–69]

Induction chemotherapy followed by either surgery or definitive CRT has been investigated through multiple clinical trials. Data from these trials suggest that induction chemotherapy followed by definitive treatment does not improve overall survival, locoregional control, or distant control.[70–72] However, patients with favorable response on pathologic analysis after induction followed by surgery did have improved OS, LRC, and DC compared with patients with unfavorable response to induction chemotherapy.[70,71] The decision to pursue nonsurgical treatment of advanced-stage oral cavity SCC should be made by the patient after extensive discussion of the risks and benefits of both approaches. The NCCN still recommends upfront surgical resection, with reservation of CCRT for select patients who decline or are unfit for surgery.[21]

Survival outcomes for oral cavity SCC have improved over the past 5 decades, thanks to advances in surgery and reconstruction, radiation therapy, and chemotherapy. Database and large retrospective reviews have demonstrated fairly consistent survival outcomes for patients with oral cavity SCC.[27,31,73,74] As expected, survival is the highest for early-stage disease and decreases dramatically for advanced-stage disease. Patients with stage I and II disease have an estimated 70% to 80% 5-year overall survival rates when treated with surgery and appropriate adjuvant therapy.[10–12,27,31,73–75] Five-year overall survival rates for stage III disease are around 60% to 65%, which then decreases to 35% to 45% for stage IV disease[10–12,28,31,74,75] (**Table 5**).

Surveillance for lip and oral cavity SCC is done primarily by routine physical examinations given the accessibility to these anatomic regions; however, imaging is used to compliment regular examinations. The NCCN guidelines recommend a physical examination every 1 to 3 months during the first year after treatment. This schedule can be extended to 1 examination every 2 to 6 months during year 2 and then every 4 to 8 months during years 3 to 5. After 5 years without recurrence, the patient can be examined yearly.[21] Posttreatment imaging is recommended by NCCN guidelines and should be obtained 3 months after completion of definitive treatment.[21] Ideally, imaging identical to the pretreatment modality should be obtained, with consideration for the usage of PET/CT in the case of locoregionally advanced disease. A meta-analysis of PET/CT after the treatment of head and neck cancer demonstrated that the imaging study should be obtained no earlier than 10 weeks after completion of treatment, to maximize sensitivity and specificity.[76] Furthermore, the investigators found no adverse effect on survival when PET/CT was obtained at 12 weeks compared with 8 to 10 weeks after completion of treatment.[76]

Studies reviewing the efficacy of posttreatment imaging have demonstrated reasonable sensitivity and negative predictive value at detecting recurrence but have failed to demonstrate an increase in survival.[77,78] Repeat imaging at 6 months after treatment is recommended, although there is little evidence to support long-term imaging (>6 months after completion of treatment) in patients who have negative 3- and 6-month posttreatment imaging.[79,80] However, the NCCN guidelines acknowledge that given anatomic or regional changes from treatment, detection of recurrence with physical examination alone may be difficult. Therefore, it is recommended that select patients have annual imaging using the pretreatment modality when physical examination is limited by anatomic changes or treatment effect until 5 years after completion of treatment.[21]

Patients with lip and oral cavity SCC who undergo multimodality treatment should be followed closely by a SLP, nutritionist, and dentist. These patients are at uniquely high risk for swallowing dysfunction particularly after major oral cavity reconstruction followed by RT or CRT. These issues can cause malnutrition, poor wound healing, and

Table 5
Staging, treatment, and outcomes for advanced-stage lip and oral cavity cancer

Overall Stage	T	N	Treatment of Tumor	Treatment of Neck	5-y Overall Survival
III	T1-2	N1	**Surgery + adjuvant RT** (CRT for positive margins or ENE+)	Ipsilateral or bilateral neck dissection based on tumor location	Lip: 50%–70%
	T3	N0-1			Oral cavity: 60%–65%
IVa	T1-3	N2	**Surgery + adjuvant RT** (CRT for positive margins or ENE+)	Ipsilateral or bilateral neck dissection based on tumor location	Lip: 40%–60%
	T4a	N0-2	Consider definitive CRT		Oral cavity: 35%–45%
IVb	Any T T4b	N3	**Surgery + adjuvant RT or CRT**	Consider bilateral neck dissection/ RT	Lip: 40%–60%
		Any N	Consider definitive CRT		Oral cavity: 35%–45%
IVc	Any T	Any N + M1	**Clinical trial preferred**	**Clinical trial preferred**	<10%

Bolded significance is to emphasize that advanced stage cancer require multimodality treatment.

increase enteral feeding tube dependence. The NCCN guidelines recommend evaluation of patients by SLP and nutritionist following completion of treatment to evaluate swallowing function, nutrition status, and the need for enteral tube feeding supplementation.[21] Regular dental follow-up after treatment completion is also critical for proactive treatment of dental caries and dental rehabilitation.

SUMMARY

Lip and oral cavity SCC share similarities in risk factors, presentation, and recommended treatment options. Lip and oral SCC usually arise from progressive dysplasia and can often be identified often as nonhealing ulcerative lesions. High clinical suspicion and early biopsy for tissue diagnosis is important for detecting lip and oral SCC at early stages. Lip and oral cavity SCC are staged base on tumor characteristics, presence of neck lymph node metastases, and distant metastases. Surgery is generally the recommended treatment of lip and oral cavity SCC. Adjuvant RT or CRT is based on histopathologic analysis of the tumor and neck lymph nodes when neck dissection is performed. Nonsurgical treatment can be considered for advanced-stage oral cavity SCC in patients who have unresectable disease or in whom the expected functional outcomes are anticipated to be poor even with reconstruction. Survival outcomes for lip and oral cavity SCC are good for early-stage disease and decrease quite dramatically for advanced-stage disease.

CLINICS CARE POINTS

- Nonhealing lip and oral cavity lesions should be biopsied, especially if the patient has risk factors for cancer.
- Appropriate workup with imaging for clinical staging is imperative to provide prognostic information for the patient.
- Surgical excision of lip and oral cavity SCC is the preferred treatment option, with reconstruction and adjuvant therapy as indicated.
- Early-stage lip tumors may be amenable to radiation therapy in patients who decline surgery or are unfit for surgery.
- Advanced-stage oral cavity tumors, especially those of the oral tongue, may be amenable for treatment with concurrent CRT with the goal of organ preservation without compromising survival outcomes.

DISCLOSURE

Nothing to disclose.

REFERENCES

1. Bray F, Ferlay J, Soerjomataram I, et al. Global cancer statistics 2018: GLOBOCAN estimates of incidence and mortality worldwide for 36 cancers in 185 countries. CA Cancer J Clin 2018;68(6):394–424.
2. Ellington TD, Henley SJ, Senkomago V, et al. Trends in Incidence of Cancers of the Oral Cavity and Pharynx - United States 2007-2016. MMWR Morb Mortal Wkly Rep 2020;69(15):433–8.
3. Aupérin A. Epidemiology of head and neck cancers: an update. Curr Opin Oncol 2020;32(3):178–86.

4. Miller KD, Nogueira L, Mariotto AB, et al. Cancer treatment and survivorship statistics, 2019. CA Cancer J Clin 2019;69(5):363–85.
5. Furquim CP, Pivovar A, Amenábar JM, et al. Oral cancer in Fanconi anemia: Review of 121 cases. Crit Rev Oncol Hematol 2018;125:35–40.
6. Blaydon DC, Etheridge SL, Risk JM, et al. RHBDF2 mutations are associated with tylosis, a familial esophageal cancer syndrome. Am J Hum Genet 2012;90(2): 340–6.
7. Rowe DE, Carroll RJ, Day CL. Prognostic factors for local recurrence, metastasis, and survival rates in squamous cell carcinoma of the skin, ear, and lip. Implications for treatment modality selection. J Am Acad Dermatol 1992;26(6):976–90.
8. Mourouzis C, Boynton A, Grant J, et al. Cutaneous head and neck SCCs and risk of nodal metastasis - UK experience. J Craniomaxillofac Surg 2009;37(8):443–7.
9. Cooper JS, Porter K, Mallin K, et al. National Cancer Database report on cancer of the head and neck: 10-year update. Head Neck 2009;31(6):748–58.
10. Zanoni DK, Montero PH, Migliacci JC, et al. Survival outcomes after treatment of cancer of the oral cavity (1985-2015). Oral Oncol 2019;90:115–21.
11. Rogers SN, Brown JS, Woolgar JA, et al. Survival following primary surgery for oral cancer. Oral Oncol 2009;45(3):201–11.
12. Listl S, Jansen L, Stenzinger A, et al. Survival of patients with oral cavity cancer in Germany. PLoS One 2013;8(1):e53415.
13. Ozturk K, Gode S, Erdogan U, et al. Squamous cell carcinoma of the lip: survival analysis with long-term follow-up. Eur Arch Otorhinolaryngol 2015;272(11): 3545–50.
14. Bilkay U, Kerem H, Ozek C, et al. Management of lower lip cancer: a retrospective analysis of 118 patients and review of the literature. Ann Plast Surg 2003; 50(1):43–50.
15. Biasoli É, Valente VB, Mantovan B, et al. Lip Cancer: A Clinicopathological Study and Treatment Outcomes in a 25-Year Experience. J Oral Maxillofac Surg 2016; 74(7):1360–7.
16. Califano L, Zupi A, Massari PS, et al. Lymph-node metastasis in squamous cell carcinoma of the lip. A retrospective analysis of 105 cases. Int J Oral Maxillofac Surg 1994;23(6 Pt 1):351–5.
17. Han AY, Kuan EC, Mallen-St Clair J, et al. Epidemiology of Squamous Cell Carcinoma of the Lip in the United States: A Population-Based Cohort Analysis. JAMA Otolaryngol Head Neck Surg 2016;142(12):1216–23.
18. Society AC. Cancer facts & figures 2015. Atlanta, GA: American Cancer Society; 2015.
19. Krishna Rao SV, Mejia G, Roberts-Thomson K, et al. Epidemiology of oral cancer in Asia in the past decade–an update (2000-2012). Asian Pac J Cancer Prev 2013;14(10):5567–77.
20. Chi AC, Day TA, Neville BW. Oral cavity and oropharyngeal squamous cell carcinoma–an update. CA Cancer J Clin 2015;65(5):401–21.
21. Pfister DG, Spencer S, Adelstein D, et al. Head and Neck Cancers, Version 2.2020, NCCN Clinical Practice Guidelines in Oncology. J Natl Compr Canc Netw 2020;18(7):873–98.
22. Law CP, Chandra RV, Hoang JK, et al. Imaging the oral cavity: key concepts for the radiologist. Br J Radiol 2011;84(1006):944–57.
23. Chung TS, Yousem DM, Seigerman HM, et al. MR of mandibular invasion in patients with oral and oropharyngeal malignant neoplasms. AJNR Am J Neuroradiol 1994;15(10):1949–55.

24. Bouhir S, Mortuaire G, Dubrulle-Berthelot F, et al. Radiological assessment of mandibular invasion in squamous cell carcinoma of the oral cavity and oropharynx. Eur Ann Otorhinolaryngol Head Neck Dis 2019;136(5):361–6.

25. Sun R, Tang X, Yang Y, et al. 18)FDG-PET/CT for the detection of regional nodal metastasis in patients with head and neck cancer: a meta-analysis. Oral Oncol 2015;51(4):314–20.

26. Rohde M, Nielsen AL, Johansen J, et al. Head-to-Head Comparison of Chest X-Ray/Head and Neck MRI, Chest CT/Head and Neck MRI, and. J Nucl Med 2017;58(12):1919–24.

27. Ellis MA, Graboyes EM, Wahlquist AE, et al. Primary Surgery vs Radiotherapy for Early Stage Oral Cavity Cancer. Otolaryngol Head Neck Surg 2018;158(4): 649–59.

28. Spiotto MT, Jefferson G, Wenig B, et al. Differences in Survival With Surgery and Postoperative Radiotherapy Compared With Definitive Chemoradiotherapy for Oral Cavity Cancer: A National Cancer Database Analysis. JAMA Otolaryngol Head Neck Surg 2017;143(7):691–9.

29. Zhang H, Dziegielewski PT, Biron VL, et al. Survival outcomes of patients with advanced oral cavity squamous cell carcinoma treated with multimodal therapy: a multi-institutional analysis. J Otolaryngol Head Neck Surg 2013;42:30.

30. Tangthongkum M, Kirtsreesakul V, Supanimitjaroenporn P, et al. Treatment outcome of advance staged oral cavity cancer: concurrent chemoradiotherapy compared with primary surgery. Eur Arch Otorhinolaryngol 2017;274(6):2567–72.

31. Fujiwara RJT, Burtness B, Husain ZA, et al. Treatment guidelines and patterns of care in oral cavity squamous cell carcinoma: Primary surgical resection vs. nonsurgical treatment. Oral Oncol 2017;71:129–37.

32. de Visscher JG, Botke G, Schakenraad JA, et al. A comparison of results after radiotherapy and surgery for stage I squamous cell carcinoma of the lower lip. Head Neck 1999;21(6):526–30.

33. de Visscher JG, van den Elsaker K, Grond AJ, et al. Surgical treatment of squamous cell carcinoma of the lower lip: evaluation of long-term results and prognostic factors–a retrospective analysis of 184 patients. J Oral Maxillofac Surg 1998;56(7):814–20 [discussion: 820–1].

34. de Visscher JG, Grond AJ, Botke G, et al. Results of radiotherapy for squamous cell carcinoma of the vermilion border of the lower lip. A retrospective analysis of 108 patients. Radiother Oncol 1996;39(1):9–14.

35. Dougherty W, Givi B, Jameson MJ, et al. AHNS Series - Do you know your guidelines? Lip cancer. Head Neck 2017;39(8):1505–9.

36. Sollamo EM, Ilmonen SK, Virolainen MS, et al. Sentinel lymph node biopsy in cN0 squamous cell carcinoma of the lip: A retrospective study. Head Neck 2016; 38(Suppl 1):E1375–80.

37. Chone CT, Magalhes RS, Etchehebere E, et al. Predictive value of sentinel node biopsy in head and neck cancer. Acta Otolaryngol 2008;128(8):920–4.

38. Garrel R, Poissonnet G, Moyà Plana A, et al. Equivalence Randomized Trial to Compare Treatment on the Basis of Sentinel Node Biopsy Versus Neck Node Dissection in Operable T1-T2N0 Oral and Oropharyngeal Cancer. J Clin Oncol 2020;38(34):4010–8.

39. Schilling C, Stoeckli SJ, Haerle SK, et al. Sentinel European Node Trial (SENT): 3-year results of sentinel node biopsy in oral cancer. Eur J Cancer 2015;51(18): 2777–84.

40. Moya-Plana A, Aupérin A, Guerlain J, et al. Sentinel node biopsy in early oral squamous cell carcinomas: Long-term follow-up and nodal failure analysis. Oral Oncol 2018;82:187–94.
41. Adel M, Kao HK, Hsu CL, et al. Evaluation of Lymphatic and Vascular Invasion in Relation to Clinicopathological Factors and Treatment Outcome in Oral Cavity Squamous Cell Carcinoma. Medicine (Baltimore) 2015;94(43):e1510.
42. Jardim JF, Francisco AL, Gondak R, et al. Prognostic impact of perineural invasion and lymphovascular invasion in advanced stage oral squamous cell carcinoma. Int J Oral Maxillofac Surg 2015;44(1):23–8.
43. Agostini T, Spinelli G, Arcuri F, et al. Metastatic Squamous Cell Carcinoma of the Lower Lip: Analysis of the 5-Year Survival Rate. Arch Craniofac Surg 2017;18(2):105–11.
44. Gooris PJ, Vermey A, de Visscher JG, et al. Supraomohyoid neck dissection in the management of cervical lymph node metastases of squamous cell carcinoma of the lower lip. Head Neck 2002;24(7):678–83.
45. Bhandari K, Wang DC, Li SC, et al. Primary cN0 lip squamous cell carcinoma and elective neck dissection: Systematic review and meta-analysis. Head Neck 2015;37(9):1392–400.
46. Vartanian JG, Carvalho AL, de Araújo Filho MJ, et al. Predictive factors and distribution of lymph node metastasis in lip cancer patients and their implications on the treatment of the neck. Oral Oncol 2004;40(2):223–7.
47. Ehrsson YT, Langius-Eklöf A, Laurell G. Nutritional surveillance and weight loss in head and neck cancer patients. Support Care Cancer 2012;20(4):757–65.
48. Lee IJ, Koom WS, Lee CG, et al. Risk factors and dose-effect relationship for mandibular osteoradionecrosis in oral and oropharyngeal cancer patients. Int J Radiat Oncol Biol Phys 2009;75(4):1084–91.
49. Huang SH, O'Sullivan B. Oral cancer: Current role of radiotherapy and chemotherapy. Med Oral Pathol Oral Cir Bucal 2013;18(2):e233–40.
50. Huang TY, Hsu LP, Wen YH, et al. Predictors of locoregional recurrence in early stage oral cavity cancer with free surgical margins. Oral Oncol 2010;46(1):49–55.
51. Chim H, Salgado CJ, Seselgyte R, et al. Principles of head and neck reconstruction: an algorithm to guide flap selection. Semin Plast Surg 2010;24(2):148–54.
52. Gou L, Yang W, Qiao X, et al. Marginal or segmental mandibulectomy: treatment modality selection for oral cancer: a systematic review and meta-analysis. Int J Oral Maxillofac Surg 2018;47(1):1–10.
53. Robbins KT, Ferlito A, Shah JP, et al. The evolving role of selective neck dissection for head and neck squamous cell carcinoma. Eur Arch Otorhinolaryngol 2013;270(4):1195–202.
54. Asakage T, Yokose T, Mukai K, et al. Tumor thickness predicts cervical metastasis in patients with stage I/II carcinoma of the tongue. Cancer 1998;82(8):1443–8.
55. Fukano H, Matsuura H, Hasegawa Y, et al. Depth of invasion as a predictive factor for cervical lymph node metastasis in tongue carcinoma. Head Neck 1997;19(3):205–10.
56. Fakih AR, Rao RS, Borges AM, et al. Elective versus therapeutic neck dissection in early carcinoma of the oral tongue. Am J Surg 1989;158(4):309–13.
57. Kligerman J, Lima RA, Soares JR, et al. Supraomohyoid neck dissection in the treatment of T1/T2 squamous cell carcinoma of oral cavity. Am J Surg 1994;168(5):391–4.
58. D'Cruz AK, Vaish R, Kapre N, et al. Elective versus Therapeutic Neck Dissection in Node-Negative Oral Cancer. N Engl J Med 2015;373(6):521–9.

59. Fasunla AJ, Greene BH, Timmesfeld N, et al. A meta-analysis of the randomized controlled trials on elective neck dissection versus therapeutic neck dissection in oral cavity cancers with clinically node-negative neck. Oral Oncol 2011;47(5): 320–4.

60. Alkureishi LW, Ross GL, Shoaib T, et al. Sentinel node bicpsy in head and neck squamous cell cancer: 5-year follow-up of a European multicenter trial. Ann Surg Oncol 2010;17(9):2459–64.

61. Govers TM, Hannink G, Merkx MA, et al. Sentinel node bicpsy for squamous cell carcinoma of the oral cavity and oropharynx: a diagnostic meta-analysis. Oral Oncol 2013;49(8):726–32.

62. Iype EM, Sebastian P, Mathew A, et al. The role of selective neck dissection (I-III) in the treatment of node negative (N0) neck in oral cancer. Oral Oncol 2008; 44(12):1134–8.

63. Thiele OC, Seeberger R, Flechtenmacher C, et al. The role of elective supraomohyoidal neck dissection in the treatment of early, node-negative oral squamous cell carcinoma (OSCC): a retrospective analysis of 122 cases. J Craniomaxillofac Surg 2012;40(1):67–70.

64. Iyer NG, Tan DS, Tan VK, et al. Randomized trial comparing surgery and adjuvant radiotherapy versus concurrent chemoradiotherapy in patients with advanced, nonmetastatic squamous cell carcinoma of the head and neck: 10-year update and subset analysis. Cancer 2015;121(10):1599–607.

65. Stenson KM, Kunnavakkam R, Cohen EE, et al. Chemoradiation for patients with advanced oral cavity cancer. Laryngoscope 2010;120(1):93–9.

66. Peterson DE, Doerr W, Hovan A, et al. Osteoradionecrosis in cancer patients: the evidence base for treatment-dependent frequency, current management strategies, and future studies. Support Care Cancer 2010;18(8):1089–98.

67. Beadle BM, Liao KP, Chambers MS, et al. Evaluating the impact of patient, tumor, and treatment characteristics on the development of jaw complications in patients treated for oral cancers: a SEER-Medicare analysis. Head Neck 2013; 35(11):1599–605.

68. Aarup-Kristensen S, Hansen CR, Forner L, et al. Osteoradionecrosis of the mandible after radiotherapy for head and neck cancer: risk factors and dose-volume correlations. Acta Oncol 2019;58(10):1373–7.

69. Owosho AA, Tsai CJ, Lee RS, et al. The prevalence and risk factors associated with osteoradionecrosis of the jaw in oral and oropharyngeal cancer patients treated with intensity-modulated radiation therapy (IMRT): The Memorial Sloan Kettering Cancer Center experience. Oral Oncol 2017;64:44–51.

70. Bossi P, Lo Vullo S, Guzzo M, et al. Preoperative chemotherapy in advanced resectable OCSCC: long-term results of a randomized phase III trial. Ann Oncol 2014;25(2):462–6.

71. Zhong LP, Zhang CP, Ren GX, et al. Long-term results of a randomized phase III trial of TPF induction chemotherapy followed by surgery and radiation in locally advanced oral squamous cell carcinoma. Oncotarget 2015;6(21):18707–14.

72. Chinn SB, Spector ME, Bellile EL, et al. Efficacy of induction selection chemotherapy vs primary surgery for patients with advanced oral cavity carcinoma. JAMA Otolaryngol Head Neck Surg 2014;140(2):134–42.

73. Sowder JC, Cannon RB, Buchmann LO, et al. Treatment-related determinants of survival in early-stage (T1-2N0M0) oral cavity cancer: A population-based study. Head Neck 2017;39(5):876–80.

74. Guntinas-Lichius O, Wendt T, Buentzel J, et al. Head and neck cancer in Germany: a site-specific analysis of survival of the Thuringian cancer registration database. J Cancer Res Clin Oncol 2010;136(1):55–63.
75. Carvalho AL, Ikeda MK, Magrin J, et al. Trends of oral and oropharyngeal cancer survival over five decades in 3267 patients treated in a single institution. Oral Oncol 2004;40(1):71–6.
76. Isles MG, McConkey C, Mehanna HM. A systematic review and meta-analysis of the role of positron emission tomography in the follow up of head and neck squamous cell carcinoma following radiotherapy or chemoradiotherapy. Clin Otolaryngol 2008;33(3):210–22.
77. Roman BR, Goldenberg D, Givi B, (AHNS) ECoAHaNS. AHNS Series–Do you know your guidelines? Guideline recommended follow-up and surveillance of head and neck cancer survivors. Head Neck 2016;38(2):168–74.
78. Spector ME, Chinn SB, Rosko AJ, et al. Diagnostic modalities for distant metastasis in head and neck squamous cell carcinoma: are we changing life expectancy? Laryngoscope 2012;122(7):1507–11.
79. Heineman TE, Kuan EC, St John MA. When should surveillance imaging be performed after treatment for head and neck cancer? Laryngoscope 2017;127(3):533–4.
80. Ho AS, Tsao GJ, Chen FW, et al. Impact of positron emission tomography/computed tomography surveillance at 12 and 24 months for detecting head and neck cancer recurrence. Cancer 2013;119(7):1349–56.

Cancer of the Oropharynx and the Association with Human Papillomavirus

Eleni M. Rettig, MD[a,b,c,]*, Rosh K.V. Sethi, MD, MPH[a,b,c]

KEYWORDS

- Oropharynx cancer • Head and neck cancer • Human papillomavirus
- Deintensification

KEY POINTS

- HPV-positive and HPV-negative oropharyngeal cancer (OPC) are distinct disease entities, with unique staging, epidemiology, and prognosis.
- In general, early stage OPC is treated with surgery or radiation, whereas later-stage OPC is treated with a combination of radiation, chemotherapy, and surgery.
- HPV-positive OPC has a significantly improved prognosis compared with HPV-negative OPC. However, HPV tumor status should not affect treatment outside of a clinical trial setting.
- Several promising biomarkers for HPV-positive OPC are under investigation for use in screening, risk stratification, and surveillance.
- HPV vaccination likely prevents oral HPV infection, the precursor to HPV-OPC, and should be encouraged for males and females.

INTRODUCTION

Squamous cell carcinoma (SCCa) of the oropharynx (OPC) is now considered as two distinct disease entities: human papillomavirus (HPV)-negative disease caused by tobacco and alcohol use, and HPV-positive disease caused by the sexually transmitted infection HPV.[1] Although HPV-negative OPC has decreased in incidence with lower prevalence of tobacco smoking, the incidence of HPV-positive OPC continues to rise in the United States and other developed countries.[2,3] These entities have unique but overlapping risk factors, epidemiologic trends, staging systems, and survival outcomes, with HPV-positive tumor status conferring a significant survival benefit compared with HPV-negative disease. Treatment of OPC entails a combination of

[a] Division of Otolaryngology–Head and Neck Surgery, Department of Surgery, Brigham and Women's Hospital, 45 Francis Street, ASB-2, Boston, MA 02115, USA; [b] Center for Head and Neck Oncology, Dana-Farber Cancer Institute, Boston, MA, USA; [c] Department of Otolaryngology Head and Neck Surgery, Harvard Medical School, Boston, MA, USA
* Corresponding author. Division of Otolaryngology–Head and Neck Surgery, Department of Surgery, Brigham and Women's Hospital, 45 Francis Street, ASB-2, Boston, MA 02115.
E-mail address: emrettig@bwh.harvard.edu

Hematol Oncol Clin N Am 35 (2021) 913–931
https://doi.org/10.1016/j.hoc.2021.05.004
0889-8588/21/© 2021 Elsevier Inc. All rights reserved.

hemonc.theclinics.com

surgery, radiation, and chemotherapy, and can result in significant morbidity. Although treatment guidelines remain identical regardless of HPV tumor status at present, ongoing trials will determine whether treatment of HPV-related disease may be safely deintensified to maintain favorable survival outcomes with decreased morbidity. Emerging HPV-related biomarkers are under study as tools that may inform screening, diagnosis, treatment, and surveillance for HPV-positive OPC.

EPIDEMIOLOGY
Incidence

The epidemiology of OPC in the United States is largely characterized by the emergence of the HPV-positive OPC epidemic that began in the early 2000s. OPC, like other head and neck SCCa, was historically strongly associated with tobacco and alcohol use, such that the incidence of OPC was stable in the late twentieth century as tobacco use rates began to decline (annual percentage change [APC] in age-adjusted incidence/100,000 person-years for 1975–1999 = 0.10; $P>.05$).[4] However, around 2000, while the incidence of other head and neck SCCa decreased,[5] the OPC incidence began to rise dramatically (APC = 2.6; $P<.05$ for 2000–2017),[4] particularly among men and White individuals (**Fig. 1**A, B). This rise in OPC incidence has been unequivocally linked to the increasing proportion of OPCs caused by HPV,[2] especially HPV type 16, which accounts for more than 90% of HPV-positive OPCs.[6] Although early studies reported the proportion of HPV positivity among OPCs to be

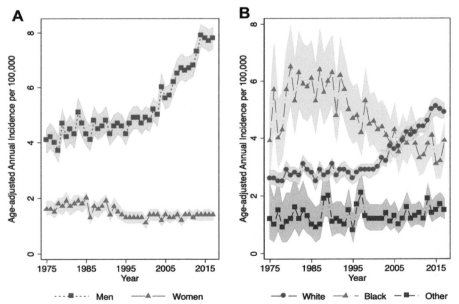

Fig. 1. Incidence of OPC by (A) sex and (B) race, 1975 to 2017 in the United States. Incidence rates are per 100,000 and age-adjusted to the 2000 US Standard Population. Shaded regions represent 95% confidence intervals. (From Database: Surveillance, Epidemiology, and End Results (SEER) Program (www.seer.cancer.gov) SEER*Stat Database: Incidence - SEER Research Data, 9 Registries, Nov 2019 Sub (1975-2017) - Linked To County Attributes - Time Dependent (1990-2017) Income/Rurality, 1969-2018 Counties, National Cancer Institute, DCCPS, Surveillance Research Program, released April 2020, based on the November 2019 submission.)

50% to 60%,[7–10] contemporary studies report closer to 80% or greater HPV positivity.[11–13] Importantly, OPC has now surpassed cervical cancer as the most common HPV-related cancer in the United States. Between 2013 and 2017, the age-adjusted annual US incidence of all OPCs was 5.1 per 100,000 persons, representing 19,775 yearly cases overall, compared with 12,143 yearly cases of cervical cancer.[14] Current projections predict a continued increase for at least the next decade, with greater than 30,000 annual incident cases by the year 2029.[15] Similar incidence trends have been observed in other developed countries.[3,16]

Risk Factors

Both HPV-positive and HPV-negative OPC are most common among men, middle-aged or older individuals, and those with a history of smoking. However, there are distinct differences in demographic trends between the two groups that relate to the natural history of HPV-positive versus HPV-negative disease.

The primary risk factor for HPV-negative OPC is tobacco smoking, with nearly three times increased risk among former smokers and almost 13 times increased risk among current smokers, compared with never-smokers.[17] Alcohol drinking further increases the risk, in a synergistic fashion with smoking.[1,18] Approximately 75% of individuals with HPV-negative OPC have a history of tobacco smoking.[9]

In contrast, the primary risk factor for HPV-positive OPC is infection with oncogenic HPV.[1] Because HPV is a sexually transmitted infection, HPV-positive OPC is most strongly linked to sexual behaviors, and in particular to oral sexual behaviors.[1,19,20] Individuals with more than 10 lifetime oral sex partners have a greater than four-fold increased risk of HPV-positive OPC.[20] Indeed, the dramatic rise in HPV-positive OPC incidence has been attributed to the sexual revolution of the 1950s and 1960s, with the resultant younger average age of sexual debut and increase in prevalence of oral sexual behaviors.[21–25] Many of the demographic trends unique to HPV-positive OPC (eg, higher incidence among Whites, men, and certain age groups) are attributed to differences in oral sexual behaviors among these populations.[25]

Although never-smokers are much more likely to have HPV-positive disease, smoking does continue to play an important role in risk of HPV-positive OPC, with approximately 40% increased risk among former smokers and 200% increased risk among current smokers.[17] Approximately 50% to 60% of HPV-positive OPC patients report ever smoking.[1,9,17] Unlike the synergistic effect observed for smoking and alcohol, smoking and HPV seem to have an independent, additive effect in increasing risk of OPC.[26] Marijuana use has also been linked to risk of HPV-positive OPC, although the role of marijuana in the context of other risk factors is not well understood.[1,20,27]

Demographic Characteristics

OPC afflicts primarily men in the United States (see **Fig. 1**A), with a four-fold male predominance among HPV-positive OPCs compared with a three-fold male predominance for HPV-negative disease.[5] With regard to race, OPC incidence was previously highest among Black individuals in the United States, but is now highest among Whites (see **Fig. 1**B).[5] This is attributable to the growth of the largely White HPV-positive OPC patient population: from 2010 to 2015, approximately 90% of 28,653 HPV-positive OPCs reported in the US National Cancer Database were diagnosed in White patients.[12]

The mean age of OPC patients is around 60 years, with most patients diagnosed between 50 and 75 years.[13] HPV-positive OPC patients were initially observed to be significantly younger than HPV-negative patients.[1,9] However, recent studies have described increases in the mean age of the HPV-positive OPC patients as the proportion of OPCs caused by HPV increases among the elderly,[13,28] predicting an impending shift in the burden of disease to a largely elderly population.[15] This shift is attributable to an age cohort effect (eg, the aging of the populations that experienced the widespread shifts in sexual norms of the mid-twentieth century).[15]

Many reports have described an association of socioeconomic status with HPV tumor status among OPC patients, with higher measures of educational attainment and income among HPV-positive patients.[1,29] In addition, HPV-positive OPC patients tend to have fewer comorbidities than those with HPV-negative disease.[1,13]

ANATOMY AND HISTOLOGY

The oropharynx is located between the nasopharynx and hypopharynx and encompasses multiple subsites including the palatine tonsils, posterior tonsillar pillars, tongue base, lingual tonsils, vallecula, soft palate, and posterior pharyngeal wall (**Fig. 2**). It is contiguous anteriorly with the oral cavity, with its anterior border demarcated by the anterior tonsillar pillars and circumvallate papillae. The inferior border of the oropharynx is the hyoid bone and pharyngoepiglottic folds, and the superior limit is the posterior border of the soft palate. The base of tongue lacks a deep fascial plane and is attached to the root of the oral tongue anteriorly and to the epiglottis posteriorly. The palatine tonsils are covered by fascia on the deep aspect separating them from underlying pharyngeal musculature.

There is a dense vascular network that supplies the oropharynx from multiple branches of the external carotid artery, including the ascending pharyngeal, facial, lingual, and greater palatine arteries. Lymphatic channels in the oropharynx drain to lymph nodes located in neck levels two through four.

Unique to the oropharynx is a large volume of lymphoid tissue known as Waldeyer's ring. This is a circumferential band of mucosal-associated lymphoid tissue that includes most prominently the lingual and palatine tonsils, and lymphoid tissue in the

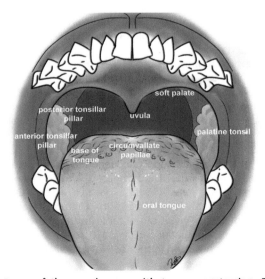

Fig. 2. Clinical anatomy of the oropharynx with tongue protrusion. The subsites of the oropharynx are depicted in this graphic including the palatine tonsils laterally, base of tongue posterior to the circumvallate papillae (*circles on tongue*), posterior tonsillar pillars, soft palate/uvula, and posterior pharyngeal wall. Original artwork, no copyright necessary.

palatopharyngeal arch behind the soft palate and posterior pharyngeal wall. Both the palatine and lingual tonsils are characterized by lymphoepithelium, with extensive crypts and shallow tubules lined by reticulated epithelium and laden with lymphoid nodules.[30] There are between 10 and 30 branched crypts per palatine tonsil that are estimated to increase their surface area up to 300 cm^2.[30] The lingual tonsil crypts are significantly less dense and are shallower than their palatine counterparts.[30] In contrast, the posterior wall and soft palate mucosal surfaces are comprised of nonkeratinized stratified squamous epithelium. Of note, HPV-positive OPC arises almost exclusively in the lymphatic tissue of the palatine and lingual tonsils, whereas HPV-negative disease also affects the mucosa of the soft palate and pharyngeal wall.

DIAGNOSIS AND WORK-UP
Presentation

Consistent with other head and neck cancers, patients with OPC may present with a constellation of symptoms including odynophagia, referred pain to the ears (otalgia), globus sensation, dysphagia, bleeding from the mouth or nose, palpable neck mass, exophytic mass in the oropharynx, tonsillar asymmetry on clinical examination, or voice changes. Patients with HPV-positive OPC often present with a painless lateral neck mass, whereas those with HPV-negative disease more commonly complain of throat pain.[31]

Work-up

Patients with suspected OPC should be evaluated in a multidisciplinary setting with team members from otolaryngology–head and neck surgery, medical oncology, radiation oncology, speech and language therapy, and a registered dietician. A complete history and physical should be obtained. Unique to the oropharynx, the examiner should query about history of palatine or lingual tonsillectomy.

A complete head and neck examination should be performed. The superior and posterior aspect of the oropharynx, including the soft palate, uvula, and palatine tonsils, are examined through the oral cavity and with depression of the oral tongue (see **Fig. 2**). The base of tongue and lingual tonsils are difficult to visualize without the aid of a laryngeal mirror or fiberoptic laryngoscope. Given the cryptic anatomy of the lymphoid tissue in the base of tongue and palatine tonsils, and risk of submucosal masses not readily visualized, manual palpation of these structures should be attempted. The neck should be palpated, and fixation and size of enlarged lymph nodes noted.

Imaging of the head and neck remains a vital tool in the work-up of OPC. Contrast-enhanced computed tomography (CT) and MRI may elucidate the extent of nodal involvement, proximity of enlarged nodes to critical structures in the neck, and the extent of the primary lesion including involvement of adjacent subsites or structures. PET/CT provides anatomic and metabolic information to assess, or in some cases identify, the primary tumor site, and remains a highly sensitive tool when assessing regional and distant metastatic disease burden.[32]

In patients with a known or suspected OPC, current National Comprehensive Cancer Network (NCCN) guidelines mandate pathologic confirmation. This may be performed with in-office biopsy, if amenable, or operative direct laryngoscopy with biopsy. Fine-needle aspiration biopsy of regional neck disease should also be performed. All specimens should be tested for high-risk HPV, as per guidelines from the College of American Pathologists and NCCN.[33,34] The gold standard for detection is HPV E6/E7 mRNA and HPV DNA detection by polymerase chain reaction and in situ hybridization.[35–37] Commonly, immunohistochemical testing for p16 is performed, which is an accurate and widely available surrogate marker for high-risk HPV infection and prognosis when there is at least 70% nuclear and cytoplasmic expression with moderate to strong intensity.[33,38]

Work-up of Unknown Primary

Head and neck SCCa of unknown primary (CUP) is defined as one or more lymph nodes in the head and neck region (with the exception of isolated supraclavicular lymph nodes) with biopsy-proven SCCa in the absence of a clinically or radiographically identifiable primary tumor. Although these cases represent only 1% to 3% of all new head and neck cancers, greater than 90% are HPV-positive.[39,40] Of note, HPV-positive CUP is currently staged and managed as HPV-positive OPC.

The work-up of CUP should include a thorough history and physical examination, with assessment of oropharyngeal and potential nonoropharyngeal primary sites including the scalp and non-hair-bearing skin. PET/CT is particularly helpful when trying to identify the primary tumor before examination under anesthesia with directed biopsies, and has been shown to detect 25% to 55% of primary tumors among patients with no identifiable primary after prior clinical and radiographic work-up.[41–43]

In patients where a primary site is not identified on in-office examination and imaging, it is appropriate to proceed with examination under anesthesia and directed biopsies. Triple endoscopy is the historical standard, with examination of the oral cavity, oropharynx, larynx and hypopharynx, nasopharyngoscopy, and upper esophagoscopy, in addition to deep palpation of the oropharyngeal subsites. Directed biopsies of suspicious sites identified on imaging or with physical examination should be performed and sent for frozen-section analysis. Prior studies have assessed the utility of ipsilateral deep tonsil biopsies versus tonsillectomy, with the latter favored for primary tumor detection.[44]

Strategies for identification of CUP have evolved significantly and are greatly improved with algorithmic approaches. The addition of lingual tonsillectomy with transoral robotic surgery (TORS) or transoral laser microsurgery has been shown to significantly improve primary tumor detection, with rates as high as 78%.[45–47] The implications of primary site identification are numerous, including the potential for definitive surgical resection and ability to minimize treatment toxicity by avoiding radiation to the hypopharynx or larynx.

Staging

The American Joint Committee on Cancer eighth edition staging schema is used to stage patients with OPC (**Fig. 3**). Notably, this edition provides a new staging algorithm for HPV-positive OPC that is separate from the staging for HPV-negative OPC, categorized by the surrogate and more readily available biomarker p16. This major change acknowledged the improved prognosis and distinct prognostic parameters for patients with HPV-positive tumors.[48] Staging for p16-positive disease no longer includes T4b disease, defines clinical nodal stage by size and laterality, and defines pathologic nodal stage strictly by number of lymph nodes. Unlike nodal staging for p16-negative disease, pathologic and clinical nodal staging for p16-positive disease omit consideration of extranodal extension (ENE).

MANAGEMENT

Although HPV status has impacted OPC staging and prognostication, current treatment guidelines do not endorse significant differences in management algorithms for HPV-positive and HPV-negative disease. Treatment deintensification has been

p16+ Clinical Staging				
T Category	N0	N1	N2	N3
T0	N/A	I	II	III
T1	I	I	II	III
T2	I	I	II	III
T3	II	II	II	III
T4	III	III	III	III

p16+ Pathologic Staging			
T Category	N0	N1	N2
T0	N/A	I	II
T1	I	I	II
T2	I	I	II
T3	II	II	III
T4	II	II	III

p16- Clinical/Pathologic Staging				
T Category	N0	N1	N2	N3
T1	I	III	IVa	IVb
T2	II	III	IVa	IVb
T3	III	III	IVa	IVb
T4a	IVa	IVa	IVa	IVb
T4b	IVb	IVb	IVb	IVb

Fig. 3. Clinical and pathologic staging for p16-positive and p16-negative oropharyngeal squamous cell carcinoma. (*Data from* AJCC Cancer Staging Manual, Eighth Edition [2017].)

studied or is currently under investigation in multiple clinical trials, which are discussed later.

Early Stage Oropharyngeal Cancer

Surgery or radiation therapy are the primary treatment options for early stage OPC. Treatment is often unimodal but there are indications for multimodality therapy in select cases, with cisplatin-based chemotherapy occasionally playing a role. Early stage is defined as T1-2, N0-1 for HPV-negative disease, and T1-2, N0 or single node less than or equal to 3 cm for HPV-positive disease. Surgery and radiation should include treatment of the primary tumor and ipsilateral neck. Contralateral neck dissection is performed if the tumor is at or approaches midline. Similarly, contralateral neck radiation is administered in cases with more than minimal involvement of the soft palate or tongue base by the primary tumor.[49]

Surgical approaches to the oropharynx have improved significantly since the introduction of transoral laser microsurgery and TORS, which allow for excellent exposure and transoral access to the soft palate, base of tongue, and palatine tonsils with minimal morbidity.[50,51] Robotic surgery and its use in head and neck surgery is discussed elsewhere in this issue. Postoperative adjuvant radiation or chemoradiation is considered for patients with evidence of adverse features on final pathology including positive margins, close margins, ENE, pT3 or pT4 primary tumor, one positive node greater than 3 cm (p16-positive disease), pN2 or N3 nodal disease, perineural invasion, vascular invasion, lymphatic invasion, or nodal disease in levels IV or V.[34,52] Surgical reresection should be considered for patients with positive margins.

There is ongoing discussion about indications for adjuvant therapy in patients with HPV-positive OPC. Although ENE is considered an indication for adjuvant systemic therapy and radiation therapy based on data from RTOG 9501 and EORTC 22931 trials,[53] these trials were limited by absence of HPV or p16 status, and inclusion of multiple subsites.[54] Therefore, omission of systemic therapy and postoperative adjuvant radiation alone may be considered for HPV-positive patients staged cT1-2, cN0-1 (single node ≤3 cm) with ENE on final pathology (category IIB recommendation by NCCN).[34]

With regard to definitive radiation, chemotherapy may be given concurrently for early T-stage tumors in p16-negative patients with T1-2, N1 disease and p16-positive patients with T2, N1 (single node ≤3 cm) disease. However this is considered a level IIB recommendation by the NCCN because of limited number of patients with N1 disease in the phase III randomized GORTEC trial comparing 5-year survival and late toxicity for patients with stage III or IV oropharynx SCCa randomized to radiation alone versus concomitant chemoradiation.[34,55]

The choice between surgical and radiation-based definitive treatment is made based on disease characteristics, patient preferences, and available expertise. Comparison of surgery versus radiation for early stage OPC is the subject of ongoing clinical studies. The only randomized control trial to date is the phase II ORATOR trial, which randomized patients with T1-T2, N0-2 OPC SCCa to definitive radiotherapy (with chemotherapy if N1-N2) or TORS with neck dissection (with adjuvant chemoradiation therapy as determined by pathology).[56] The primary outcome was swallowing-related quality-of-life outcomes at 1 year. Patients treated with radiation exhibited superior swallowing outcomes at 1 year compared with patients who underwent TORS; however, this was not a clinically meaningful difference.[56] Additional studies with longer-term follow-up are necessary to understand differences in outcomes between surgical and radiation-based treatment of early stage OPC, particularly in the context of the evolving landscape of deintensified treatment of HPV-positive OPC.

Late Stage (III/IV)

Concurrent chemotherapy and radiation therapy are the mainstay of treatment of advanced p16-positive and -negative oropharyngeal SCCa.[52,55] Surgical resection followed by adjuvant therapy, as indicated, may be considered for appropriately selected patients with resectable disease. Concurrent chemoradiation therapy is preferred over surgery for p16-positive patients with T4 or N3 disease because of high likelihood of requiring triple modality therapy (surgery, radiation, and chemotherapy), which causes significant morbidity.[34] Induction chemotherapy is considered a category III recommendation for treatment of advanced OPC.

DEINTENSIFICATION OF THERAPY FOR HUMAN PAPILLOMAVIRUS–POSITIVE OROPHARYNGEAL CANCER

HPV-positive tumor status confers significantly improved survival after diagnosis of OPC when compared with HPV-negative disease, with most studies reporting around 50% to 70% decreased risk of death for HPV-positive disease.[10] The observed 2-year overall survival (OS) for all HPV-positive OPCs included in SEER diagnosed from 2010 to 2016 (n = 9791) was 87.8% (95% confidence interval, 87.1%–88.6%), compared with 66.8% for HPV-negative OPCs (95% confidence interval, 65.1%–68.5%; n = 3530).[57] Low-risk HPV-positive OPC, with limited burden of nodal disease and minimal smoking history, is associated with greater than 90% survival at 3 years.[9] HPV-positive OPC also carries lower risk of recurrence and second primary tumors than HPV-negative disease.[9]

Currently, treatment guidelines remain essentially identical for OPC regardless of HPV tumor status.[58] However, the excellent survival outcomes for most HPV-positive OPC patients, combined with the acute and chronic morbidity of head and neck cancer treatments, have prompted a host of clinical trials designed to examine whether deintensified treatment regimens can reduce toxicities while maintaining excellent survival rates. Various strategies that deintensify one or several aspects of treatment (surgery, radiation, and systemic therapy) have been, or are being, examined. Several recently completed studies are discussed here and summarized in **Table 1**, but multiple additional trials are ongoing and have been comprehensively reviewed elsewhere.[59,60]

Several trials have used a strategy of initial transoral surgery, most commonly with minimally invasive robotic platforms, and neck dissection followed by decreased dose or field of radiation, with the degree of radiation de-escalation stratified according to pathologic features. MC1273 was a trial at Mayo Clinic that evaluated a dramatically decreased adjuvant radiation dose of 30 or 36 Gy (vs standard of 66–72 Gy),[34] and replaced cisplatin with docetaxel. Two-year outcomes were excellent, with progression-free survival (PFS) of 91.1% and OS of 98.7%, which was comparable with a historical cohort from the same institution.[62,63] ECOG 3311 was a multicenter trial that randomized intermediate-risk patients to either 50 or 60 Gy. Both groups likewise had excellent outcomes, with 2-year PFS of 95% and 95.9%, respectively.[64]

Two trials evaluated a decreased definitive radiation dose of 60 Gy. NCT02281955 spearheaded by the University of North Carolina included cisplatin for high-risk disease, and demonstrated 2-year PFS of 86% and OS of 95%.[65] NRG-HN002 randomized patients to either 60 Gy radiation alone or with cisplatin. The radiation alone group had 2-year PFS of 87.6%, but this did not meet the pre-established acceptability criteria and thus was not considered suitable for inclusion in future clinical trials; the radiation with cisplatin group had 2-year PFS of 90.5%.[66]

Two other large randomized trials, RTOG 1016 and De-ESCALaTE-HPV, evaluated the substitution of cetuximab for cisplatin as a strategy to reduce toxicity with the better-tolerated cetuximab. Unfortunately, both trials demonstrated significantly worse survival outcomes for the cetuximab group, without significance differences in toxicity.[67,71] Finally, the use of induction chemotherapy response as a tool to risk-stratify patients into more or less intensive treatment groups showed promise in the OPTIMA trial from the University of Chicago,[70] and in ECOG 1308.[69]

Despite the excellent prognosis of HPV-positive OPC, around 15% to 25% of patients experience recurrence, and the failure of cetuximab to successfully replace cisplatin in RTOG 1016[67] and De-ESCALaTE-HPV[71] is a sobering caution that not all deintensification strategies result in adequate treatment. Critical to the success of deintensification efforts is precise risk stratification; that is, the categorization of patients into higher- and lower-risk groups based on various characteristics, such as burden of tumor and nodal disease, presence and degree of ENE, tobacco use history, and possibly response to induction chemotherapy. Other potential strategies may rely on trends in dynamic biomarkers, such as circulating tumor HPV DNA (ctHPV DNA), or high-resolution on-treatment imaging.

Although treatment guidelines for HPV-positive OPC may evolve in the future based on the results of the many deintensification trials already completed or still underway, it is important to emphasize that deintensification of treatment should currently only take place in the carefully controlled clinical trial setting.[58]

Table 1
Selected completed deintensification trials for HPV-positive oropharyngeal squamous cell carcinoma

Trial	Description	Phase	Eligibility	N	Outcomes
Transoral surgery with deintensified adjuvant therapy					
AVOID Trial[61] (University of Pennsylvania)	Postoperative RT avoiding primary tumor site Concurrent cisplatin for ENE	Single-arm, phase II	p16+ pT1-2N1-3[a] Favorable primary site pathology	60	2-y local RFS 97.9% 2-y OS 100% Low toxicity
MC 1273[62,63] (Mayo Clinic)	Aggressive decrease in postoperative RT: 30 Gy or 36 Gy depending on risk Docetaxel instead of cisplatin with RT	Single-arm, phase II	p16+ ≤10 pk-yrs Negative margins	80	2-y PFS 91.1% 2-y OS 98.7% Low toxicity
ECOG 3311[64] (multicenter)	Risk stratification according to pathology after surgery Intermediate-risk group randomized to 50 Gy or 60 Gy	Randomized, phase II	p16+ cT1-2, stage III/IV[a] No matted neck nodes	353 total; 206 randomized	2-y PFS: 50 Gy: 95% 60 Gy: 95.9%
Deintensified (chemo)RT					
NCT02281955 (University of North Carolina, multicenter)[65]	60 Gy RT Concurrent weekly cisplatin for >T2 >N1[a]	Single-arm, phase II	p16+ T0-3N0-2[a] Minimal or remote smoking	114	2-y PFS 86% 2-y OS 95% Favorable QOL outcomes
NRG-HN002 (Multicenter)[66]	60 Gy RT Randomized to either RT alone or RT + weekly cisplatin	Randomized, phase II	p16+ T1-2N1-N2b or T3N0-N2b[a] ≤10 pk-yrs	306	RT alone arm with inferior PFS, did not meet 2-y PFS acceptability criteria: RT alone: 87.6% RT + cisplatin: 90.5% Lower acute toxicity in RT alone group
Deintensified chemotherapy					

Trial	Design	Eligibility	Treatment	N	Results
RTOG 1016[67] (multicenter)	Randomized, phase III Noninferiority	p16+ T1-2N2a-N3 or T3-4N0-3[a]	Standard RT Randomized to either concurrent cetuximab or cisplatin	805	5-y PFS and OS worse for cetuximab than cisplatin: PFS: 67.3% vs 78.4% OS: 77.9% vs 84.6% Toxicities similar
De-ESCALaTE-HPV[68] (multicenter)	Randomized, phase III	p16+ T3-4N0 or T1-4N1-3[a] <10 pk-yrs	Standard RT Randomized to either concurrent cetuximab or cisplatin	334	2-y OS and recurrence worse for cetuximab than cisplatin: OS: 89.4% vs 97.5% Recurrence: 16.1% vs 6% Toxicities similar
Induction chemotherapy with response-based deintensification of (chemo)radiation					
ECOG 1308[69] (multicenter)	Phase II	HPV16+ and/or p16+ Stage III-IV[a] Resectable	Induction chemo[b], risk stratified by response Complete response: low-dose RT (54 Gy) + cetuximab Less than complete response: standard-dose RT (69.3 Gy) + cetuximab	80	2-y survival for low-dose (54 Gy) RT group: PFS 80% OS 95% Improved swallowing and nutrition among low-dose group
OPTIMA[70] (University of Chicago)	Phase II	HPV+ T1-4N2-3 or T3-4N0-3[a]	Induction chemo[c], risk stratified by response, T, N, and smoking Treatment groups: RT50: 50 Gy RT CRT45: 45 Gy RT + chemo[c] CRT75: 75 Gy + chemo[c]	62	2-y survival: PFS 94.5% OS 98% Lower toxicity with greater deintensification

Abbreviations: PFS, progression-free survival; pk-yrs, pack-years of smoking; QOL, quality of life; RFS, recurrence-free survival; RT, radiation therapy.
[a] American Joint Committee on Cancer seventh edition staging; all trials excluded patients with distant metastatic disease (M1).
[b] Induction chemotherapy with cisplatin, paclitaxel, and cetuximab.
[c] Induction chemotherapy with carboplatin and nab-paclitaxel; concurrent chemotherapy with paclitaxel, 5-fluorouracil, and hydroxyurea.

BIOMARKERS, SCREENING, AND PREVENTION CONSIDERATIONS FOR HUMAN PAPILLOMAVIRUS–POSITIVE OROPHARYNGEAL CANCER

The viral etiology of HPV-positive OPC affords novel opportunities for prevention, screening, risk stratification, and surveillance that are not applicable to nonvirally mediated head and neck cancers.

Prevention

HPV vaccines were initially developed for prevention of HPV-related anogenital cancers. There are three approved vaccines: (1) the bivalent (HPV16/18), (2) quadrivalent (HPV16/18/6/11), and (3) nonavalent (HPV16/18/6/11/31/33/45/52/58); only the nonavalent vaccine is currently distributed in the United States.[72] The vaccine has been recommended for females age 11 or 12 years since 2006, but was not recommended for routine use in males until 2011.[73] Although it is not yet certain whether HPV vaccination is efficacious against HPV-positive OPCs, initial evidence does demonstrate a protective effect against oncogenic oral HPV infection, the precursor to HPV-positive OPC.[73–75] However, vaccine uptake in the United States is lagging, especially among males. In 2019, 71.5% of adolescents aged 13 to 17 in the United States had received at least one of the three-dose vaccine series, and only 54.2% received all three doses.[76] These rates are increasing, but there is room for improvement: uptake of the Tdap vaccine among adolescents, for comparison, was 90.2% in 2019.[76] With the recent approval of HPV vaccination for males and slow uptake, vaccination is not expected to have a significant effect on HPV-positive OPC incidence rates for several decades at least.[77]

Screening and HPV16 E6 Serology

The incidence of cervical cancer, overwhelmingly caused by HPV, has decreased significantly in the United States because of highly successful screening measures.[78] There is currently no analogous screening for HPV-positive OPC, but there are several biomarkers under study that may one day allow for screening of high-risk groups. The most promising HPV-positive OPC screening biomarker to date is seropositivity to the HPV16 E6 antigen, which is observed in approximately 90% of patients with known HPV-OPC and has more than 95% specificity for determining HPV-positive tumor status.[79–81] HPV16 E6 seropositivity has also been detected in 26.2% to 42.3% of blood samples collected before diagnosis of HPV-positive OPC, even up to 28 years before diagnosis, compared with just 0.4% to 0.6% of blood samples from control subjects without cancer.[82–84] One small study has reported the de novo detection of an asymptomatic HPV-positive OPC using E6 serology as a screening tool.[85] Oral infection with oncogenic HPV types is another possible screening biomarker under study, with good specificity but only moderate sensitivity.[80,86,87]

However, the incidence of HPV-OPC remains sufficiently low that the positive predictive value of HPV16 E6 seropositivity would likely not exceed 1% per year even among the highest-incidence group of white men, resulting in a high number of false-positive screens.[77] Furthermore, there is uncertainty over how to manage a positive screen in the absence of clinically detectable disease, because HPV-positive OPC has no known precancerous lesion that would be amenable to early treatment. For these and other reasons, screening is not yet practicable for HPV-positive OPC, but it remains an area of active investigation.[77]

Biomarkers for Risk Stratification and Surveillance

Several dynamic biomarkers of HPV-positive OPC are emerging as important tools for post-treatment surveillance, and even potentially for risk stratification to guide treatment. These biomarkers include ctHPV DNA and oncogenic oral HPV DNA detection.

ctHPV DNA has been detected in blood samples from most (88%–100%) patients with HPV-positive OPC, and has been correlated with burden of disease, response to treatment, and recurrence.[88–92] In the post-treatment surveillance setting, the assay has excellent predictive properties: a recent report indicated a 100% negative predictive value (single test) and 94% positive predictive value (two consecutive tests) of ctHPV DNA for detecting recurrent HPV-positive OPC.[93]

Oncogenic HPV DNA detection in oral rinses has also been associated with response to treatment and is predictive of recurrence after treatment. However, it is less sensitive than ctHPV DNA for HPV-positive disease (54%–81%) and for recurrence (43%), is subject to variability by anatomic location of disease, and is complicated by the presence of bystander oral HPV infections.[94,95]

Both ctHPV DNA copy number and oral HPV DNA viral load are dynamic measures that have been observed to change during treatment.[88,95] The kinetics of these biomarkers may in the future serve as a tool to guide therapy in real-time, such that favorable biomarker profiles would prompt deintensified treatment and unfavorable profiles would indicate higher-risk disease.

SUMMARY

Oropharynx SCCa comprises two distinct disease entities, HPV-negative and HPV-positive OPC, with unique risk factors, demographic characteristics, epidemiologic trends, and staging systems. Although HPV-negative OPC is decreasing in incidence, HPV-positive OPC incidence has increased dramatically since the early 2000s. HPV-positive OPC has significantly improved survival compared with HPV-negative disease, which has prompted multiple trials of deintensified treatment designed to minimize toxicities. However, deintensification of treatment should currently only take place in a clinical trial setting. Several promising biomarkers for HPV-positive OPC are under investigation for use in screening, risk stratification, and surveillance.

CLINICS CARE POINTS

- HPV-positive and HPV-negative OPC are distinct disease entities, with unique staging, epidemiology, and prognosis.
- HPV-positive OPC typically has excellent prognosis, with 2-year overall survival of 87.8% compared with 66.8% for HPV-negative OPC.
- In general, early stage OPC is treated with surgery or radiation, whereas later-stage OPC is treated with a combination of radiation, chemotherapy, and surgery.
- HPV tumor status should not affect treatment outside of a clinical trial setting.
- Several promising biomarkers for HPV-positive OPC are under investigation for use in screening, risk stratification, and surveillance.
- HPV vaccination likely prevents oral HPV infection, the precursor to HPV-OPC, and should be encouraged for males and females.

DISCLOSURE

The authors have nothing to disclose.

REFERENCES

1. Gillison ML, D'Souza G, Westra W, et al. Distinct risk factor profiles for human papillomavirus type 16–positive and human papillomavirus type 16–negative head and neck cancers. J Natl Cancer Inst 2008;100(6):407–20.
2. Chaturvedi AK, Engels EA, Pfeiffer RM, et al. Human papillomavirus and rising oropharyngeal cancer incidence in the United States. J Clin Oncol 2011; 29(32):4294–301.
3. Chaturvedi AK, Anderson WF, Lortet-Tieulent J, et al. Worldwide trends in incidence rates for oral cavity and oropharyngeal cancers. J Clin Oncol 2013; 31(36):4550–9.
4. Surveillance, Epidemiology, and End Results (SEER) Program. SEER*Stat Database: incidence - SEER Research data, 9 Registries, Nov 2019 Sub (1975-2017) - linked to county attributes - time dependent (1990-2017) income/rurality, 1969-2018 Counties, National Cancer Institute, DCCPS, surveillance research program, released April 2020, based on the November 2019 submission 2020. Available at: Www.Seer.Cancer.Gov.
5. Fakhry C, Krapcho M, Eisele DW, et al. Head and neck squamous cell cancers in the United States are rare and the risk now is higher among white individuals compared with black individuals. Cancer 2018;124(10):2125–33.
6. Fakhry C, Fung N, Tewari SR, et al. Unique role of HPV16 in predicting oropharyngeal cancer risk more than other oncogenic oral HPV infections. Oral Oncol 2020; 111:104981.
7. Gillison MLML, Koch WWM, Capone RB, et al. Evidence for a causal association between human papillomavirus and a subset of head and neck cancers. J Natl Cancer Inst 2000;92(9):709–20.
8. Fakhry C, Westra WH, Li S, et al. Improved survival of patients with human papillomavirus-positive head and neck squamous cell carcinoma in a prospective clinical trial. J Natl Cancer Inst 2008;100(4):261–9.
9. Ang KK, Harris J, Wheeler R, et al. Human papillomavirus and survival of patients with oropharyngeal cancer. N Engl J Med 2010;363(1):24–35.
10. Benson E, Li R, Eisele D, et al. The clinical impact of HPV tumor status upon head and neck squamous cell carcinomas. Oral Oncol 2014;50(6):565–74.
11. Fakhry C, Blackford AL, Neuner G, et al. Association of oral human papillomavirus DNA persistence with cancer progression after primary treatment for oral cavity and oropharyngeal squamous cell carcinoma. JAMA Oncol 2019;5(7): 985–92.
12. Faraji F, Rettig EM, Tsai H, et al. The prevalence of human papillomavirus in oropharyngeal cancer is increasing regardless of sex or race, and the influence of sex and race on survival is modified by human papillomavirus tumor status. Cancer 2019;125(5):761–9.
13. Rettig EM, Zaidi M, Faraji F, et al. Oropharyngeal cancer is no longer a disease of younger patients and the prognostic advantage of human papillomavirus is attenuated among older patients: analysis of the National Cancer Database. Oral Oncol 2018;83:147–53.
14. Cancers associated with human papillomavirus, United States—2013–2017. Available at: https://www.cdc.gov/cancer/uscs/pdf/USCS-DataBrief-No18-September2020-h.pdf. Accessed January 18, 2021.
15. Tota JE, Best AF, Zumsteg ZS, et al. Evolution of the oropharynx cancer epidemic in the United States: moderation of increasing incidence in younger individuals and shift in the burden to older individuals. J Clin Oncol 2019;37(18):1538–46.

16. Forman D, de Martel C, Lacey CJ, et al. Global burden of human papillomavirus and related diseases. Vaccine 2012;30:F12–23.
17. Chaturvedi AK, D'Souza G, Gillison ML, et al. Burden of HPV-positive oropharynx cancers among ever and never smokers in the U.S. population. Oral Oncol 2016; 60:61–7.
18. Blot WJ, McLaughlin JK, Winn DM, et al. Smoking and drinking in relation to oral and pharyngeal cancer. Cancer Res 1988;48(3282–3287):7.
19. D'Souza G, Kreimer AR, Viscidi R, et al. Case–control study of human papillomavirus and oropharyngeal cancer. N Engl J Med 2007;356(19):1944–56.
20. Drake VE, Fakhry C, Windon MJ, et al. Timing, number, and type of sexual partners associated with risk of oropharyngeal cancer. Cancer 2021;127(7):1029–38.
21. Bajos N, Bozon M, Beltzer N, et al. Changes in sexual behaviours: from secular trends to public health policies. AIDS 2010;24(8):1185–91.
22. Turner CFP, Danella RDP, Rogers SM. Sexual behavior in the United States, 1930-1990: trends and methodological problems. Sex Transm Dis 1995;22(3):173–90.
23. Finer LB. Trends in premarital sex in the United States, 1954–2003. Public Health Rep 2007;122(1):73–8.
24. Schmidt G, Sigusch V. Changes in sexual behavior among young males and females between 1960–1970. Arch Sex Behav 1972;2(1):27–45.
25. D'Souza G, Cullen K, Bowie J, et al. Differences in oral sexual behaviors by gender, age, and race explain observed differences in prevalence of oral human papillomavirus infection. PLoS One 2014;9(1):e86023.
26. Anantharaman D, Muller DC, Lagiou P, et al. Combined effects of smoking and HPV16 in oropharyngeal cancer. Int J Epidemiol 2016;45(3):752–61.
27. Liu C, Sadat SH, Ebisumoto K, et al. Cannabinoids promote progression of HPV-positive head and neck squamous cell carcinoma via p38 MAPK activation. Clin Cancer Res 2020;26(11):2693–703.
28. Windon MJ, D'Souza G, Rettig EM, et al. Increasing prevalence of human papillomavirus-positive oropharyngeal cancers among older adults: HPV-OPSCC increasing among older adults. Cancer 2018;124(14):2993–9.
29. Liederbach E, Kyrillos A, Wang C-H, et al. The national landscape of human papillomavirus-associated oropharynx squamous cell carcinoma. Int J Cancer 2017;140(3):504–12.
30. Fossum CC, Chintakuntlawar AV, Price DL, et al. Characterization of the oropharynx: anatomy, histology, immunology, squamous cell carcinoma and surgical resection. Histopathology 2017;70(7):1021–9.
31. McIlwain WR, Sood AJ, Nguyen SA, et al. Initial symptoms in patients with HPV-positive and HPV-negative oropharyngeal cancer. JAMA Otolaryngol Neck Surg 2014;140(5):441.
32. Benchaou M, Lehmann W, Slosman DO, et al. The role of FDG-PET in the preoperative assessment of N-staging in head and neck cancer. Acta Otolaryngol (Stockh) 1996;116(2):332–5.
33. Lewis JS, Beadle B, Bishop JA, et al. Human papillomavirus testing in head and neck carcinomas: guideline from the College of American Pathologists. Arch Pathol Lab Med 2018;142(5):559–97.
34. NCCN clinical practice guidelines in oncology (NCCN guidelines): head and neck cancer. Version 1.2021. Available at: https://www.nccn.org/professionals/physician_gls/pdf/head-and-neck.pdf. Accessed March 21, 2021.
35. Jordan RC, Lingen MW, Perez-Ordonez B, et al. Validation of methods for oropharyngeal cancer HPV status determination in US cooperative group trials. Am J Surg Pathol 2012;36(7):945–54.

36. Weinberger PM, Yu Z, Haffty BG, et al. Molecular classification identifies a subset of human papillomavirus-associated oropharyngeal cancers with favorable prognosis. J Clin Oncol 2006;24(5):736–47.
37. Cantley RL, Gabrielli E, Montebelli F, et al. Ancillary studies in determining human papillomavirus status of squamous cell carcinoma of the oropharynx: a review. Pathol Res Int 2011;2011:1–7.
38. Singhi AD, Westra WH. Comparison of human papillomavirus in situ hybridization and p16 immunohistochemistry in the detection of human papillomavirus-associated head and neck cancer based on a prospective clinical experience. Cancer 2010;116(9):2166–73.
39. Keller LM, Galloway TJ, Holdbrook T, et al. p16 status, pathologic and clinical characteristics, biomolecular signature, and long-term outcomes in head and neck squamous cell carcinomas of unknown primary: HPV-associated SCC of unknown primary. Head Neck 2014;36(12):1677–84.
40. Motz K, Qualliotine JR, Rettig E, et al. Changes in unknown primary squamous cell carcinoma of the head and neck at initial presentation in the era of human papillomavirus. JAMA Otolaryngol Neck Surg 2016;142(3):223.
41. Johansen J, Buus S, Loft A, et al. Prospective study of 18FDG-PET in the detection and management of patients with lymph node metastases to the neck from an unknown primary tumor. Results from the DAHANCA-13 study. Head Neck 2008;30(4):471–8.
42. Rudmik L, Lau HY, Matthews TW, et al. Clinical utility of PET/CT in the evaluation of head and neck squamous cell carcinoma with an unknown primary: a prospective clinical trial. Head Neck 2011;33(7):935–40.
43. Miller FR, Karnad AB, Eng T, et al. Management of the unknown primary carcinoma: long-term follow-up on a negative PET scan and negative panendoscopy. Head Neck 2008;30(1):28–34.
44. Lapeyre M, Malissard L, Peiffert D, et al. Cervical lymph node metastasis from an unknown primary: is a tonsillectomy necessary? Int J Radiat Oncol Biol Phys 1997;39(2):291–6.
45. Ryan JF, Motz KM, Rooper LM, et al. The impact of a stepwise approach to primary tumor detection in squamous cell carcinoma of the neck with unknown primary: unknown primary detection. Laryngoscope 2019;129(7):1610–6.
46. Nagel TH, Hinni ML, Hayden RE, et al. Transoral laser microsurgery for the unknown primary: role for lingual tonsillectomy: transoral laser microsurgery for unknown primary. Head Neck 2014;36(7):942–6.
47. Farooq S, Khandavilli S, Dretzke J, et al. Transoral tongue base mucosectomy for the identification of the primary site in the work-up of cancers of unknown origin: systematic review and meta-analysis. Oral Oncol 2019;91:97–106.
48. Lydiatt W, Patel S, O'Sullivan B, et al. Head and neck cancers-major changes in the American Joint Committee on cancer eighth edition cancer staging manual. CA Cancer J Clin 2017;67(2):122–37.
49. Tsai CJ, Galloway TJ, Margalit DN, et al. Ipsilateral radiation for squamous cell carcinoma of the tonsil: American Radium Society appropriate use criteria executive summary. Head Neck 2021;43(1):392–406.
50. Cracchiolo JR, Baxi SS, Morris LG, et al. Increase in primary surgical treatment of T1 and T2 oropharyngeal squamous cell carcinoma and rates of adverse pathologic features: National Cancer Data Base: increase in primary surgery for T1-T2 OPSCC. Cancer 2016;122(10):1523–32.
51. Parsons JT, Mendenhall WM, Stringer SP, et al. Squamous cell carcinoma of the oropharynx: surgery, radiation therapy, or both. Cancer 2002;94(11):2967–80.

52. Sher DJ, Adelstein DJ, Bajaj GK, et al. Radiation therapy for oropharyngeal squamous cell carcinoma: executive summary of an ASTRO evidence-based clinical practice guideline. Pract Radiat Oncol 2017;7(4):246–53.

53. Cooper JS, Pajak TF, Forastiere AA, et al. Postoperative concurrent radiotherapy and chemotherapy for high-risk squamous-cell carcinoma of the head and neck. N Engl J Med 2004;350(19):1937–44.

54. Sinha P, Piccirillo JF, Kallogjeri D, et al. The role of postoperative chemoradiation for oropharynx carcinoma: a critical appraisal of the published literature and National Comprehensive Cancer Network guidelines: adjuvant therapy in oropharynx cancer. Cancer 2015;121(11):1747–54.

55. Denis F, Garaud P, Bardet E, et al. Final results of the 94–01 French head and neck oncology and radiotherapy group randomized trial comparing radiotherapy alone with concomitant radiochemotherapy in advanced-stage oropharynx carcinoma. J Clin Oncol 2004;22(1):69–76.

56. Nichols AC, Theurer J, Prisman E, et al. Radiotherapy versus transoral robotic surgery and neck dissection for oropharyngeal squamous cell carcinoma (ORATOR): an open-label, phase 2, randomised trial. Lancet Oncol 2019; 20(10):1349–59.

57. Surveillance, Epidemiology, and End Results (SEER) Program. SEER*Stat Database: incidence - SEER 18 regs Custom data head and neck (select schemas with HPV recode and additional treatment fields), Nov 2018 Sub (2010-2016) - linked to county attributes - total U.S., 1969-2017 counties, National Cancer Institute, DCCPS, Surveillance Research Program, released April 2019, based on the November 2018 submission 2020. Available at: Www.Seer.Cancer.Gov.

58. Adelstein DJ, Ismaila N, Ku JA, et al. Role of treatment deintensification in the management of p16+ oropharyngeal cancer: ASCO provisional clinical opinion. J Clin Oncol 2019;37(18):1578–89.

59. Bigelow EO, Seiwert TY, Fakhry C. Deintensification of treatment for human papillomavirus-related oropharyngeal cancer: current state and future directions. Oral Oncol 2020;105:104652.

60. Strohl MP, Wai KC, Ha PK. De-intensification strategies in HPV-related oropharyngeal squamous cell carcinoma: a narrative review. Ann Transl Med 2020;8(23): 1601.

61. Swisher-McClure S, Lukens JN, Aggarwal C, et al. A phase 2 trial of alternative volumes of oropharyngeal irradiation for de-intensification (AVOID): omission of the resected primary tumor bed after transoral robotic surgery for human papilloma virus–related squamous cell carcinoma of the oropharynx. Int J Radiat Oncol 2020;106(4):725–32.

62. Ma DJ, Price KA, Moore EJ, et al. Phase II evaluation of aggressive dose de-escalation for adjuvant chemoradiotherapy in human papillomavirus–associated oropharynx squamous cell carcinoma. J Clin Oncol 2019;37(22):1909–18.

63. Moore EJ, Abel KMV, Routman DM, et al. Human papillomavirus oropharynx carcinoma: aggressive de-escalation of adjuvant therapy. Head Neck 2021;43(1): 229–37.

64. Ferris RL, Flamand Y, Weinstein GS, et al. Transoral robotic surgical resection followed by randomization to low- or standard-dose IMRT in resectable p16+ locally advanced oropharynx cancer: a trial of the ECOG-ACRIN Cancer Research Group (E3311). J Clin Oncol 2020;38(15_suppl):6500.

65. Chera BS, Amdur RJ, Green R, et al. Phase II trial of de-intensified chemoradiotherapy for human papillomavirus–associated oropharyngeal squamous cell carcinoma. J Clin Oncol 2019;37(29):2661–9.

66. Yom SS, Torres-Saavedra P, Caudell JJ, et al. Reduced-dose radiation therapy for HPV-associated oropharyngeal carcinoma (NRG oncology HN002). J Clin Oncol 2021;39(9):956–65.

67. Gillison ML, Trotti AM, Harris J, et al. Radiotherapy plus cetuximab or cisplatin in human papillomavirus-positive oropharyngeal cancer (NRG Oncology RTOG 1016): a randomised, multicentre, non-inferiority trial. Lancet 2019;393(10166): 40–50.

68. Mehanna H, Robinson M, Hartley A, et al. Radiotherapy plus cisplatin or cetuximab in low-risk human papillomavirus-positive oropharyngeal cancer (De-ESCA-LaTE HPV): an open-label randomised controlled phase 3 trial. Lancet 2019; 393(10166):51–60.

69. Marur S, Li S, Cmelak AJ, et al. E1308: phase II trial of induction chemotherapy followed by reduced-dose radiation and weekly cetuximab in patients with HPV-associated resectable squamous cell carcinoma of the oropharynx— ECOG-ACRIN Cancer Research Group. J Clin Oncol 2017;35(5):490–7.

70. Seiwert TY, Foster CC, Blair EA, et al. OPTIMA: a phase II dose and volume de-escalation trial for human papillomavirus-positive oropharyngeal cancer. Ann Oncol 2019;30(2):297–302.

71. Mehanna H, Robinson M, Hartley A, et al. Radiotherapy plus cisplatin or cetuximab in low-risk human papillomavirus-positive oropharyngeal cancer (De-ESCA-LaTE HPV): an open-label randomised controlled phase 3 trial. Lancet 2019; 393(10166):51–60.

72. Meites E, Szilagyi PG, Chesson HW, et al. Human papillomavirus vaccination for adults: updated recommendations of the advisory Committee on Immunization Practices. MMWR Morb Mortal Wkly Rep 2019;68(32):5.

73. Chaturvedi AK, Graubard BI, Broutian T, et al. Effect of prophylactic human papillomavirus (HPV) vaccination on oral HPV infections among young adults in the United States. J Clin Oncol 2018;36(3):262–7.

74. Herrero R, Quint W, Hildesheim A, et al. Reduced prevalence of oral human papillomavirus (HPV) 4 years after bivalent HPV vaccination in a randomized clinical trial in Costa Rica. PLoS One 2013;8(7):e68329.

75. Hirth JM, Chang M, Resto VA, et al. Prevalence of oral human papillomavirus by vaccination status among young adults (18–30 years old). Vaccine 2017;35(27): 3446–51.

76. Elam-Evans LD, Yankey D, Singleton J, et al. National, regional, state and selected local area vaccination coverage among adolescents aged 13-17 years—United States, 2019. MMWR Recomm Rep 2020;69(33):1109–16.

77. Kreimer AR, Shiels M, Fakhry C, et al. Screening for human papillomavirus-driven oropharyngeal cancer: considerations for feasibility and strategies for research. Cancer 2018;124(9):1859–66.

78. Islami F, Fedewa SA, Jemal A. Trends in cervical cancer incidence rates by age, race/ethnicity, histological subtype, and stage at diagnosis in the United States. Prev Med 2019;123:316–23.

79. Holzinger D, Wichmann G, Baboci L, et al. Sensitivity and specificity of antibodies against HPV16 E6 and other early proteins for the detection of HPV16-driven oropharyngeal squamous cell carcinoma. Int J Cancer 2017;140(12):2748–57.

80. D'Souza G, Clemens G, Troy T, et al. Evaluating the utility and prevalence of HPV biomarkers in oral rinses and serology for HPV-related oropharyngeal cancer. Cancer Prev Res (Phila) 2019;12(10):689–700.

81. Lang Kuhs KA, Kreimer AR, Trivedi S, et al. Human papillomavirus 16 E6 antibodies are sensitive for human papillomavirus–driven oropharyngeal cancer and are associated with recurrence. Cancer 2017;123(22):4382–90.
82. Kreimer AR, Johansson M, Yanik EL, et al. Kinetics of the human papillomavirus type 16 E6 antibody response prior to oropharyngeal cancer. J Natl Cancer Inst 2017;109(8):1–9.
83. Kreimer AR, Johansson M, Waterboer T, et al. Evaluation of human papillomavirus antibodies and risk of subsequent head and neck cancer. J Clin Oncol 2013; 31(21):2708–15.
84. Kreimer AR, Ferreiro-Iglesias A, Nygard M, et al. Timing of HPV16-E6 antibody seroconversion before OPSCC: findings from the HPVC3 consortium. Ann Oncol 2019;30(8):1335–43.
85. Waterboer T, Brenner N, Gallagher R, et al. Early detection of human papillomavirus–driven oropharyngeal cancer using serology from the study of prevention of anal cancer. JAMA Oncol 2020;6(11):1806.
86. Gipson BJ, Robbins HA, Fakhry C, et al. Sensitivity and specificity of oral HPV detection for HPV-positive head and neck cancer. Oral Oncol 2018;77:52–6.
87. D'Souza G, Clemens G, Strickler HD, et al. Long-term persistence of oral HPV over 7 years of follow-up. JNCI Cancer Spectr 2020;4(5):pkaa047.
88. Chera BS, Kumar S, Beaty BT, et al. Rapid clearance profile of plasma circulating tumor HPV Type 16 DNA during chemoradiotherapy correlates with disease control in HPV-associated oropharyngeal cancer. Clin Cancer Res 2019;25(15): 4682–90.
89. Hanna GJ, Supplee JG, Kuang Y, et al. Plasma HPV cell-free DNA monitoring in advanced HPV-associated oropharyngeal cancer. Ann Oncol 2018;29(9):1980–6.
90. Lee JY, Garcia-Murillas I, Cutts RJ, et al. Predicting response to radical (chemo) radiotherapy with circulating HPV DNA in locally advanced head and neck squamous carcinoma. Br J Cancer 2017;117(6):876–83.
91. Jeannot E, Becette V, Campitelli M, et al. Circulating human papillomavirus DNA detected using droplet digital PCR in the serum of patients diagnosed with early stage human papillomavirus-associated invasive carcinoma. J Pathol Clin Res 2016;2(4):201–9.
92. Jensen KK, Grønhøj C, Jensen DH, et al. Circulating human papillomavirus DNA as a surveillance tool in head and neck squamous cell carcinoma: a systematic review and meta-analysis. Clin Otolaryngol 2018;43(5):1242–9.
93. Chera BS, Kumar S, Shen C, et al. Plasma circulating tumor HPV DNA for the surveillance of cancer recurrence in HPV-associated oropharyngeal cancer. J Clin Oncol 2020;38(11):1050–8.
94. Rettig EM, Wentz A, Posner MR, et al. Prognostic implication of persistent human papillomavirus type 16 DNA detection in oral rinses for human papillomavirus-related oropharyngeal carcinoma. JAMA Oncol 2015;1(7):907–15.
95. Fakhry C, Blackford AL, Neuner G, et al. Association of oral human papillomavirus DNA persistence with cancer progression after primary treatment for oral cavity and oropharyngeal squamous cell carcinoma. JAMA Oncol 2019;5(7):985.

Cancer of the Larynx and Hypopharynx

Kristen A. Echanique, MD[a], Lauran K. Evans, MD, MPH[a], Albert Y. Han, MD, PhD[a], Dinesh K. Chhetri, MD[b], Maie A. St. John, MD, PhD[b],*

KEYWORDS

- Larynx • Hypopharynx • Laryngeal carcinoma • Squamous cell carcinoma

KEY POINTS

- Laryngeal and hypopharyngeal carcinomas are associated with high morbidity and mortality; despite decreases in incidence, survival rates have only minimally improved in past decades.
- Landmark trials have established laryngeal preservation treatment strategies that avoid total laryngectomy and instead use chemotherapy and radiation for advanced laryngeal cancers.
- Immune response via tumor-infiltrating T lymphocytes is critical to the carcinogenesis and recurrence of laryngeal cancer. As such, immunomodulators such as pembrolizumab have shown promise as an adjunct treatment in laryngeal/hypopharyngeal malignancy.
- A multidisciplinary team of providers is essential in diagnosis, management, and survivorship of laryngeal and hypopharyngeal cancer, which can lead to devastating quality-of-life impairments including the inability to speak and swallow.

STATE OF LARYNGEAL AND HYPOPHARYNGEAL SQUAMOUS CELL CARCINOMA TREATMENT: A HISTORIC OVERVIEW OF A FIELD IN TRANSITION

Care of the patient with advanced laryngeal and hypopharyngeal carcinoma has evolved drastically over the years from a primarily surgical approach in the 1980s and early 1990s to a laryngeal preserving approach today. Large prospective, randomized controlled trials such as the Radiation Therapy Oncology Group 91-11 (RTOG 91-11) trial[1] and the US Veterans Affairs trial[2] have been transformational and have changed the way locally advanced laryngeal cancers are treated. These trials ushered in a paradigm shift in therapeutic approaches to advanced laryngeal cancers, advocating for laryngeal preservation protocols in patients with select T3 and T4 disease.

[a] Department of Head & Neck Surgery, David Geffen School of Medicine at UCLA, 10833 Le Conte Avenue, CHS 62-235, Los Angeles, CA 90095, USA; [b] Department of Head & Neck Surgery, David Geffen School of Medicine at UCLA, UCLA Head and Neck Cancer Program, 10833 Le Conte Avenue, CHS 62-235, Los Angeles, CA 90095, USA
* Corresponding author.
E-mail address: mstjohn@mednet.ucla.edu

Hematol Oncol Clin N Am 35 (2021) 933–947
https://doi.org/10.1016/j.hoc.2021.05.005
0889-8588/21/© 2021 Elsevier Inc. All rights reserved.

hemonc.theclinics.com

The complexity of cancer care in the twenty-first century mandates the input of a spectrum of health care providers to achieve the best possible outcome. Laryngeal and hypopharyngeal cancers occur in an anatomic region unmatched in the number of physiologic functions affected by disease and treatment including respiration, vocalization, alimentation, and physical appearance. This chapter highlights the multi-disciplinary approaches to laryngeal and hypopharyngeal cancer care. As anyone who cares for patients with cancer can attest, "If you take care of cancer, sometimes you win and sometimes you lose; if you take care of the patient, you always win."[3]

EPIDEMIOLOGY

Laryngeal carcinoma is the second most common type of head and neck cancer worldwide, affecting an estimated 12,370 patients in the United States in 2020 alone and resulting in an estimated 3,750 deaths.[4] Of these malignancies, squamous cell carcinoma (SCCa) comprises greater than 95% of laryngeal and hypopharyngeal cancers.[5] Although the incidence of laryngeal malignancy in the United States has decreased over the past decades, from 5.39 per 100,000 in 1979 to 2.55 per 100,000 in 2017, 5-year survival has declined at a less rapid pace, from 66% to 62%.[4,6] Men are affected at a ratio of greater than 4:1, with adults aged 75 to 79 years having the highest incidence.[6] Within the larynx, the most affected subsite is the glottis[7] (**Fig. 1**).

Risk Factors

Tobacco and alcohol use predispose patients to developing laryngeal and hypopharyngeal SCCa.[4] Human papillomavirus (HPV) has also been implicated as a causal factor, particularly in malignant transformation of 1-7% of all recurrent respiratory papillomatosis cases, most often caused by "low-risk" HPV subtypes 6 and 11.[8] HPV positivity has an impact on prognosis, with recent studies noting improved overall survival in HPV subtype 16 positive laryngeal SCCa.[9] Gastroesophageal reflux diseases and/or laryngopharyngeal reflux have been associated with laryngeal and hypopharyngeal malignancies, as studies have demonstrated increased amounts of pepsin in malignant, when compared with benign, neoplasms in these areas.[10] Additional risk factors for laryngeal and hypopharyngeal SCCa include exposures to hazardous materials such as wood dust, asbestos, and polycyclic hydrocarbons. Hypopharyngeal SCCa has been strongly associated with alcohol, tobacco use, and Plummer-Vinson syndrome.[11]

Survival outcomes in laryngeal cancer are affected by clinicopathologic and demographic factors, including tumor subsite, stage, treatment modality, comorbidities,

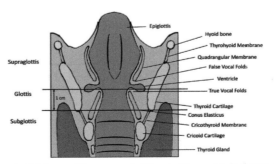

Fig. 1. Larynx with subdivisions of the supraglottis, glottis, and subglottis. (*Courtesy of* Austin Shinagawa, MD).

age at diagnosis, sex, race, marital status, income, education, and insurance status.[12] A study by Shin and colleagues from 2015 identified race as an independent predictor of overall mortality from laryngeal SCCa in the United States.[13]

PROGNOSIS BASED ON SUBSITE

It is well known that differences in survival of patients with head and neck cancer are related to tumor subsite, stage, and the presence of metastasis (**Table 1**). These differences are even more pronounced when examining survival in patients with cancer

Table 1
Tumor staging of laryngeal squamous cell carcinoma

Subsite	Tumor (T) Stage	Tumor Description
Supraglottis	T1	Limited to 1 subsite, normal VC mobility
	T2	Invades mucosa of >1 adjacent subsite of supraglottis or glottis or region(s) outside the supraglottis without fixation of larynx *(T2 is 2 or more)*
	T3	Limited to larynx with VC fixation and/or invasion of the postcricoid, preepiglottic, paraglottic space, and/or erosion of the inner laminae of thyroid cartilage
	T4a	Invades through thyroid cartilage and/or tissues beyond larynx
	T4b	Invades prevertebral space, encases carotid artery, or invades mediastinum
Glottis	T1a	Limited to 1 VC
	T1b	Involves both VCs
	T2	Extends to supraglottis and/or subglottis, and/or with impaired VC mobility
	T3	Limited to larynx with VC fixation or involvement of the inner layer of cartilage
	T4a	Invades thru thyroid cartilage and/or tissues beyond larynx
	T4b	Invades prevertebral space, encases carotid artery, or invades mediastinum
Subglottis	T1	Limited to subglottis
	T2	Extends to VC with normal/impaired mobility
	T3	Limited to larynx with VC fixation
	T4a	Invades cricoid or thyroid cartilage and/or tissues beyond larynx
	T4b	Invades prevertebral space, encases carotid artery, or invades mediastinum
Hypopharynx	T1	Limited to 1 subsite and ≤2 cm
	T2	Extends into adjacent subsite of hypopharynx or into larynx, oropharynx; 2-4 cm without fixation of hemilarynx
	T3	Tumor >4 cm or fixation of hemilarynx or extension into esophageal mucosa
	T4a	Invades ≥1: thyroid cartilage, cricoid cartilage, hyoid bone, thyroid gland, esophageal muscle, central compartment soft tissue
	T4b	Encases carotid artery or invades mediastinum or prevertebral fascia

Abbreviation: VC, vocal cord or true vocal fold.
Data from Amin MB, Edge S, Greene F, et al., eds. *AJCC Cancer Staging Manual.* 8th ed. Springer International Publishing; 2017. Accessed February 1, 2021. https://www.springer.com/gp/book/9783319406176.

16000

of the larynx and hypopharynx. Despite being anatomically adjacent, hypopharyngeal carcinoma carries a far worse prognosis when compared with laryngeal carcinoma. In fact, hypopharyngeal SCCa is associated with the worst survival of any head and neck mucosal malignancy which has has been attributed to the propensity for hypopharyngeal cancer to present at a more advanced stage due to lack of early specific symptoms in an anatomic area that is more difficult to visualize. The hypopharynx has a rich, vascular supply and increased lymphatic drainage when compared with the larynx and as such, cancers in this area are more likely to metastasize. A study by Liu and colleagues reported that patients with hypopharyngeal cancer have a worse prognosis than their age, T-stage, gender, and neck node status laryngeal counterparts, suggesting a more aggressive tumor biology and differences in molecular expression.[14] The investigators further characterized global protein expression in clinically matched samples and found that hypopharyngeal cancer displays an altered immune response with decreased immune checkpoint proteins that may be responsible for differences in survival.[14] Further research is warranted into the investigation of these altered pathways.

Subsite Involvement

The larynx itself may be divided into subsites, namely the supraglottis, glottis, and subglottis, based on embryologic origins and distinct anatomic configurations (see **Fig. 1**). Because of distinct embryologic origins, lymphatic drainage is found to differ between subsites and can predict tumor spread.[15] Metastasis from glottic tumors is rare due to paucity of lymphatic drainage at this level, however, when present, is most often unilateral. The subglottis also drains unilaterally, and regional cervical metastases predictably occur unilaterally. The supraglottis, on the contrary, forms from a distinctly separate embryologic structure, with bilateral lymphatic drainage and subsequent propensity for bilateral cervical metastases. Overall, laryngeal malignancy is most commonly confined to the larynx at the time of diagnosis due to anatomic barriers such as the quadrangular membrane and conus elasticus (see **Fig. 1**). Because of

Table 2
Laryngeal subsite survival and metastasis rates

Laryngeal Subsite	Present with Local Metastasis (%)	Present with Distant Metastasis (%)	5-y OS (%)	5-y DSS (%)
Supraglottic	40	<1	39	62
Glottic	4	<1	64	87
Subglottic	54	12	42	54

Abbreviations: 5-y, 5 year; DSS, disease-specific survival; OS, overall survival.
Data from Brandstorp-Boesen J, Falk RS, Boysen M, Brøndbo K. Impact of stage, management and recurrence on survival rates in laryngeal cancer. PLOS ONE. 2017;12(7):e0179371. https://doi.org/10.1371/journal.pone.0179371; Laryngeal Cancer Survival Rate | Throat Cancer Survival Rate. Accessed December 27, 2020.https://www.cancer.org/cancer/laryngeal-and-hypopharyngeal-cancer/detection-diagnosis-staging/survival-rates.html; Redaelli de Zinis LO, Nicolai P, Tomenzoli D, et al. The distribution of lymph node metastases in supraglottic squamous cell carcinoma: therapeutic implications. Head Neck. 2002;24(10):913-920. https://doi.org/10.1002/hed.10152; Coskun H, Mendenhall WM, Rinaldo A, et al. Prognosis of subglottic carcinoma: Is it really worse? Head Neck. 2019;41(2):511-521. https://doi.org/10.1002/hed.25172; Marchiano E, Patel DM, Patel TD, et al. Subglottic Squamous Cell Carcinoma: A Population-Based Study of 889 Cases. Otolaryngol Head Neck Surg. 2016;154(2):315-321. https://doi.org/10.1177/0194599815618190.

these differences, the oncologic outcomes when stratified by subsite differ as one might predict (**Table 2**).

The hypopharynx is immediately posterior to larynx, extending from the hyoid bone to the cricoid cartilage. Lymphatic drainage of the hypopharynx is often bilateral, extensive, and multidirectional, with high potential for widespread regional and distant metastases.[16] Unlike its laryngeal counterpart, hypopharyngeal carcinomas often present at later stages and without specific early symptoms.[14] Thus, hypopharyngeal SCCa is usually diagnosed in later stages with extensive locoregional tumor spread. As such, the relative 5-year survival is reported as 32%.[17]

PREMALIGNANT LESIONS AND PROGRESSION

Not all laryngeal lesions are malignant, and several premalignant lesions exist, including leukoplakia, erythroplakia, dysplasia, and papillomas. A recent study by Kostev and colleagues demonstrated 19% of patients diagnosed with leukoplakia went on to develop laryngeal carcinoma, although reported malignant transformation rates range from 3% to 20% in the literature.[18,19] Although dysplasia classification can be difficult and many systems have been suggested over the years, the most widely accepted classification scheme is currently that of the 2017 World Health Organization system, which stratifies leukoplakia into 1 of 3 risk categories: low-grade dysplasia, high-grade dysplasia, and carcinoma in situ.[8,20] Biopsy and histopathological examination will ultimately determine the grade of dysplasia in a premalignant lesion, although new noninvasive tools such as narrowband imaging can indicate high-risk versus low-risk dysplasia with a sensitivity and specificity of 85% and 95% respectively, without invasive biopsy.[20]

Stem cell master regulators including NANOG have been implicated in the transition from leukoplakia to malignant degeneration among patients with laryngeal cancer.[21,22] Systematic analyses of these biomarkers and related pathways will provide new insights into disease mechanisms and identify potential novel therapeutic targets, especially for patients with premalignant lesions.

The precise mechanisms underlying progression of dysplasia to carcinoma remain unclear. Although histologic dysplasia grade has been found to predict malignant transformation, mutation accumulation does not seem to be stepwise as with other malignancies.[8] Biomarkers in the biopsied specimen, such as p53 and Ki67, have been shown to correlate with dysplasia and malignancy and may serve as adjuncts to histologic examination of suspected dysplastic laryngeal lesions.[23] Primary management of leukoplakia first begins with surgical biopsy to attain a tissue diagnosis. Those with premalignant laryngeal lesions can undergo preventative treatment via phonosurgical technique with preservation of the underlying lamina propria, when appropriate, or laser excision, stripping, or ablation.[24,25] Close surveillance is vital, with protocols calling for follow-up every 6 months with differing surveillance protocols found by practice setting.[26] The authors of this chapter advocate for even closer follow-up at 3 to 4 month intervals.

TUMOR BIOLOGY AND CARCINOGENESIS

The overall steps of laryngeal/hypopharyngeal carcinogenesis and its progression mirror those of other malignancies in the aerodigestive tract. The multistep theory of carcinogenesis, first observed in colorectal adenocarcinomas, describes the accumulation of genetic changes from repeated insult that disrupts normal cellular processes resulting in dysplasia, carcinoma in situ, and invasive carcinoma.[27] Indeed, histologic sections of laryngeal cancer reveal the process of "field cancerization" involving continuous histologic changes in areas adjacent to the carcinoma.[28,29]

The key steps in carcinogenesis—namely proliferation, disruption in cell cycle regulation, and epithelial-mesenchymal transformation and invasion—have been characterized using molecular techniques. The exact number of genetic changes required for invasive laryngeal and hypopharyngeal carcinoma is unknown. However, the accumulation of genetic and epigenetic alterations affects proto-oncogenes, tumor suppressor genes, and other genes responsible for DNA repair.[30] Allelic loss and other genetic changes of classic tumor suppressor genes such as p16 (9p21) and p53 (17p) have been found in precancerous lesions.[31,32] Additional genetic breakpoints such as 11q13 amplification were frequently found in laryngeal and pharyngeal cancers.[33] Furthermore, MDM2 (an inhibitor of p53),[34] the E6 region of the HPV,[35] and other alternate cellular pathways that modulate classic tumor suppressor genes have been characterized.

In recent decades, epigenetic and transcriptomic changes have been analyzed for potential clues into the malignant transformation of precancerous lesions. However, global transcriptome and microRNA (miRNA) analyses have not yielded definitive targets.[36] The use of miRNA and other small molecules have been an area of active research involving comprehensive expression profiling in tissue[37-40] and blood.[41] Epigenetic changes such as the promoter hypermethylation of p16-associated and MLH1-associated pathways have been correlated with cancer migration, tumor invasiveness, and aggressive phenotype.[42] Our understanding of laryngeal/hypopharyngeal carcinogenesis is more complete than ever before. New targets are being uncovered with innovative hypotheses and unprecedented high-throughput techniques.

DIAGNOSIS, MANAGEMENT, AND SURGICAL TREATMENT
Presentation and Diagnosis

Initial patient presentation depends on the anatomic location in the larynx or hypopharynx that harbors the malignancy, although generally these tumors may cause hoarseness, respiratory distress, dysphagia, referred ear pain, weight loss, neck mass, globus sensation, or hemoptysis. Early hoarseness is commonly seen in glottic malignancy, with airway obstruction and hemoptysis presenting as late manifestations of glottic disease. Dysphagia and odynophagia are common in supraglottic and hypopharyngeal tumors. Subglottic tumors most often present with biphasic stridor.

Early Glottic Cancer

Surgical treatment of early laryngeal SCCa can be achieved through larynx-sparing (and therefore voice-sparing) techniques such as transoral microlaryngoscopy with laser excision of tumor. This type of surgery is often used when SCCa is confined to the glottis, an area portending an optimal prognosis. Shen and colleagues demonstrated equivalent oncologic outcomes for glottic T1N0 and T2N0 tumors with primary radiotherapy or primary surgical excision.[43] Subjective self-assessment of voice function via the Voice Handicap Index was more favorable in the group receiving surgery when compared with the radiotherapy group, although objective voice outcomes in another study by Huang and colleagues were shown to be more favorable in the radiotherapy group; therefore, discussion remains in the field as to the optimal approach in each patient.[44,45]

Advanced Laryngeal/Hyphopharyngeal Cancer

For locally advanced laryngeal and hypopharyngeal malignancies, complete surgical removal of the larynx by total laryngectomy (TL) may be warranted. Oncologic indications include extensive laryngeal SCCa (T3-T4) with bilateral extension and invasion of surrounding structures such as the esophagus, thyroid cartilage, pharynx, and aggressive non-SCCa laryngeal malignancies.[45]

Five-year survival in patients undergoing TL has been reported to be 41% in laryngeal SCCa and 29% in hypopharyngeal SCCa.[46] Woodard and colleagues showed poorer long-term survival after TL on univariate analysis with higher locoregional advanced staging, presence of comorbidities, especially cardiovascular, and location in the hypopharynx when compared with larynx. However, on multivariate analysis, only locally advanced tumor remained significant.[46] Complications such as pharyngocutaneous fistula formation, flap complication, or wound dehiscence can occur in up to one-third of patients with TL, with greater risk in those with a larger extent of resection, prior radiation, and tobacco use.[47]

Compared with primary TL, salvage TL after failed primary radiotherapy has been shown to portend similar 5-year survival rates and functional voice outcomes, although the aforementioned perioperative complications remain significantly higher in those undergoing salvage TL.[48] Interestingly, when directly comparing postoperative complications with overall survival after TL, a significant correlation has been found for perioperative complications predicting poorer oncologic outcomes and survival.[49]

ADJUVANT TREATMENT STRATEGIES IN LARYNGEAL AND HYPOPHARYNGEAL CARCINOMAS

Current management for advanced laryngeal cancers is the result of a large multiinstitutional, randomized clinical trial from the US Department of Veterans Affairs that investigated the utility of induction chemotherapy followed by definitive radiation, with laryngectomy reserved only for salvage for patients with stage III or IV carcinoma of the larynx. This model of "laryngeal preservation" spared patients with advanced stage laryngeal cancers from TL and was found to save 64% of patients from TL.[2] A study by the RTOG 91-11 instead advocated for concurrent chemotherapy and radiation as opposed to induction chemotherapy and argued for this to become the standard of care.[50] The GORTEC trial examined the feasibility of organ preservation in laryngeal cancer; it reported 3-year larynx preservation to be improved in the group receiving docetaxel in addition to cisplatin + fluorouracil compared with cisplatin + fluorouracil alone (70.3% vs 57.5%) who displayed a good response before receiving radiation with or without chemotherapy.[51] Future studies have gone on to investigate whether primary laryngectomy has superior results to salvage laryngectomy. Contrary to popular belief, a paper by Sullivan and colleagues found no difference in speech and swallowing rehabilitation outcomes and reported good outcomes after salvage total laryngectomy.[48] This study further examined outcomes between triple therapy versus doublet chemotherapy, as prior studies noted statistical differences in progression-free survival and overall survival between TPF (docetaxel, cisplatin, and 5-fluorouracil) and PF (cisplatin and 5-fluorouracil) or TP (docetaxel and cisplatin) regimens but did not corroborate those prior reports.[48,50]

The epidermal growth factor receptor (EGFR) is activated abnormally in laryngeal/pharyngeal cancers. This in turn results in uncontrolled cell division, radioresistance, and ultimately poor clinical outcomes.[52–54] These findings led to the development and approval of cetuximab (anti-EGFR monoclonal antibody).[55] The EXTREME trial demonstrated its benefits in cases of recurrent/metastatic head and neck cancer.[56] Based on these studies, cetuximab has now become a cornerstone in current treatment of head and neck cancer.

The decision to use adjuvant therapy depends on the extent of disease and final pathology. An estimated 12% to 43% of patients with laryngeal or hypopharyngeal carcinoma will be diagnosed with thyroid cartilage invasion, thereby resulting in upstaging and requiring TL with or without radiation for definitive therapy.[57] Thyroid invasion may be diagnosed by computed tomography (CT) or MRI, but neither are perfect. The utility of CT in diagnosis has a sensitivity of 49% to 71%, with an MRI sensitivity of 64% to 96%.[57] Current techniques are being developed to better identify patients with cartilage invasion, thereby preventing unnecessary TL. A recent study by Guo and colleagues describes the use of CT-based radiomics as a noninvasive imaging marker for accurate prediction of thyroid cartilage invasion.[57]

ROLE OF IMMUNE SYSTEM IN CARCINOGENESIS

Head and neck SCCa has been proven an immunosuppressive disease characterized by impaired tumor-infiltrating T lymphocytes (TIL), altered natural killer cell function, and low absolute lymphocyte count. In addition, suppressive regulatory T cells have been found to secrete cytokines such as transforming growth factor-beta and interleukin-10 and to express cytotoxic T-lymphocyte–associated protein 4 that has been linked to tumor progression. The native immune system remains vital in the eventual remission of a patient's laryngeal malignancy. TIL have been shown to be decreased in patients with recurrent laryngeal SCCa, demonstrating a role for the presence of these cells for effective eradication of malignancy.[58] Elevated levels of one specific TIL, CD103+, have been associated with improved overall survival, disease-specific survival, and disease-free survival.[59]

Similarly, elevated tumor-associated macrophages and high neutrophil to lymphocyte ratios indicate a systemic inflammatory response, which is associated with poor prognosis in head and neck malignancies.[60] The systemic inflammation response index (SIRI) is calculated via neutrophils times monocytes divided by lymphocytes and represents an overall inflammatory state in the patient with cancer. Pretreatment SIRI less than 3.26 predictably prognosticates improved response to laryngeal SCCa treatment and improved overall survival.[60]

Recent studies have highlighted numerous immune genes and their implication in the prognosis of patients with laryngeal cancer. A study by Xaio and colleagues identified 15 specific immune genes to independently predict prognosis in patients with laryngeal cancer, with more genes interestingly being upregulated than downregulated.[61] Some of these included notable genes that are also associated with prognosis in other malignancies including CRBP1 and FPR2. CRBP1 expression correlated significantly with survival, presenting a potential novel marker of long-term prognosis in laryngeal SCCa. In addition, FPR2 was also identified, which is also found overexpressed in colon cancer, melanoma, and ovarian cancer.[61]

USE OF IMMUNOMODULATORS/CELLULAR THERAPIES IN TREATMENT

Because head and neck SCCa has been found to be an immunosuppressive disease, immune checkpoint pathways have been exploited in drug delivery, as they play a major role in tumor microenvironments and are an integral component of tumor immune escape. One such studied checkpoint inhibitor in laryngeal SCC includes pembrolizumab, which is a monoclonal antibody that targets programmed cell death receptor 1 (PD-1).[62] In general, this pathway is regulated by ligand and receptor interactions between PD-1 and programmed death ligand 1 (PD-L1) and PD-L2. Recent studies have shown that PD-L1 is present in 50% to 60% of head and neck SCCa. Pembrolizumab, a highly selective monoclonal antibody that binds PD-1 and prevents binding of PD-1 and its ligands, exploits this pathway.

Checkpoint inhibitors have been used with variable success in the treatment of SCCa in the head and neck region, especially with advanced disease, recurrence, and metastases. One ongoing clinical trial (NCT02759575) is currently assessing the effectiveness of pembrolizumab + cisplatin + radiotherapy on locally advanced laryngeal SCCa that has not received prior treatment, with plans to complete the trial in 2021.[62] Additional therapeutics, including nivolumab, also work by binding PD-L1 and preventing T-cell inactivation by tumor cells.[63] The CheckMate 141 trial investigated the long-term efficacy of nivolumab in patients with recurrent or metastatic head and neck SCCa that was refractory to platinum-based therapeutics. They reported improved median overall survival in the arm receiving nivolumab, with a 1-year survival rate of 36% compared with 15% in the chemotherapy arm. The Keynote-012 trial used pembrolizumab in patients with recurrent or metastatic head and neck SCCa, with a 14% response rate and median overall survival for all patients noted to be 8 months.[64]

MUTATIONAL PROFILES OF RECURRENT LARYNGEAL CARCINOMA

Although organ preservation radiotherapy and chemotherapy have become the standard of care for many primary tumors of the larynx, recurrence still occurs. In patients with advanced stage laryngeal SCCa, recurrence rates in those treated with primary radiation or chemoradiation are as high as 50%.[59] Patients undergoing this primary treatment strategy are found to have 5-year disease-free survival ranging from 30% to 60%, with a poor prognosis in patients who experience persistent or recurrent carcinoma following treatment.[65] The behavior between primary and recurrent/persistent laryngeal carcinoma is found to differ and is hypothesized as attributable to unique mutational profiles between primary and recurrent laryngeal carcinoma.

Cancer recurrence is a complex process, propagated by subclonal populations of the primary tumor that evade apoptosis from primary treatment and gain additional deleterious mutations. A study by Hedberg and colleagues that examined paired recurrent head and neck SCCa identified 40% of new somatic variations in recurrent specimens to be absent from the initial primary tumor. Most notable were the amplification of CCND1 and mutation of DDR2, which are known to promote cellular migration, invasion, and metastasis while simultaneously promoting sensitivity to dasatinib. As such, it is suggested the recurrent tumors undergo scrutiny to identify novel therapeutic options.[65] More recent studies have further explored this theory, with Smith and colleagues identifying unique mutational profiles in fatal, recurrent laryngeal SCCa. Perhaps most notable from their work was the identification of higher rates of deleterious alterations in CDKN2a, PIK3CA, and TP53 in primary untreated tumors when compared with recurrent/persistent tumors implying that recurrent laryngeal SCCa may rely on more complex patterns of dysregulation when compared to primary laryngeal SCCa. In addition, the investigators identified histone modifier BAP1 and the DNA mismatch repair gene MSH2 to be more frequently mutated in persistent and recurrent laryngeal SCCa, hypothesizing a role for these central DNA repair pathways in the pathogenesis of recurrence or persistent disease.[65]

In addition to these genetic mutations, changes in the immunologic signatures in patients with recurrent or persistent laryngeal SCCa have been proven to be prognostic. A study by Mann and colleagues demonstrated that a higher percentage of CD4+ and CD8+ TIL correlated with improved disease-specific and disease-free survival.[59,66] The investigators went on to further characterize the role of CD103+ TIL content and found it to be a valuable predictive marker for survival in recurrent laryngeal carcinoma following primary radiation or chemoradiation.[59]

Recent advancements in prognosis include the identification of novel metabolism-gene signature profiles that may be used as biomarkers to predict prognosis. A study by Li and colleagues[67] investigated 232 patients with laryngeal carcinoma and analyzed transcriptional levels of metabolic genes. This study led to the discovery of 13 gene signatures that stratified laryngeal carcinomas into low-risk and high-risk, as well as identified those that significantly associated with overall survival and disease-free survival ($P<.05$). Further investigation into these signatures is warranted.

SURVEILLANCE

Despite advancements in oncologic agents and improvements in surgical techniques, mortality rates for head and neck malignancies such as oral cavity and pharynx have increased. Further, posttreatment surveillance is an ongoing discussion.[68] One consistent guideline across all advanced stage pathologies of head and neck carcinoma recommended by the National Comprehensive Cancer Network is "repeat of pretreatment baseline imaging within 6 months of completion therapy,"[69] with preferred modality of whole-body [8F]fludeoxyglucose PET and CT on all patients 3 to 6 months after completion of definitive therapy.[70]

A recent study by Morgan and colleagues hypothesized that a PET scan within 6 months of definitive laryngeal cancer treatment may improve cancer-specific survival, because direct visualization is often clouded by posttreatment edema and may not reveal the full extent tumor spread due to the propensity for submucosal and multicentric growth seen in recurrent tumors.[68] The investigators went on to investigate this clinical question using the Survival, Epidemiology, and End Results database and noted wide variation in posttreatment imaging despite recommendations. Despite this, their study went on to reveal that patients with stage III and IVa laryngeal carcinoma had improved cancer-specific survival when PET posttreatment imaging was used.[68]

SURVIVORSHIP

The care of the patients with laryngeal and hypopharyngeal cancer is complex. Because tumors in these regions affect many vital functions such as speaking, eating, and breathing, a multidisciplinary approach is essential to complete and thorough care. Multidisciplinary tumor boards are essential, as is care from speech and swallow therapists even before definitive treatment is sought. The team approach in head and neck cancer care functions to unite a wide range of medical specialties into one unified voice. When all members participate in generating and executing a plan of therapy, patients stand the best chance of overcoming a potentially devastating disease. If we take care of our patients, everything else takes care of itself. A multidisciplinary team is essential for all patients with laryngeal and hypopharyngeal cancer.

SUMMARY

Despite their close anatomic proximity to one another, laryngeal and hypopharyngeal SCCa have very different outcomes. Although mechanisms that drive premalignant lesions such as dysplasia to become malignant are unclear, biomarkers such as p53 and Ki67 in tumor specimens have been found to correlate with progression. Landmark trials including the RTOG-91-11 trial and US Veterans Affairs trial have revolutionized the way we treat locally advanced laryngeal cancers, sparing patients from TL. Adjuvant therapies investigating laryngeal preservation protocols using docetaxel, cisplatin, and fluorouracil have proved the addition of docetaxel beneficial. In addition, the role of EGFR in laryngeal and hypopharyngeal cancers has made cetuximab a cornerstone of treatment. The immune system has been recognized as vital in the prevention of recurrence, and as such, various immunomodulators against PD-1 are being investigated. Care of the patient with laryngeal and hypopharyngeal is complex, and a team approach should be used to ensure comprehensive and compassionate care of these patients occurs.

CLINICS CARE POINTS

- The larynx may be divided into subsites which include the supraglottis, glottis, and subglottis. Malignancy at each site portends unique prognoses and patterns of spread, with hypopharyngeal cancer carrying the worst survival of any head and neck mucosal malignancy.
- Risk factors for developing laryngeal SCCa include alcohol, tobacco use, HPV infection, acid reflux, and hazardous materials such as wood dust, asbestos, and polycyclic hydrocarbons. Hypopharyngeal SCCa has been strongly associated with alcohol, tobacco use, and Plummer Vinson syndrome.
- Although many systems have been suggested over the years for laryngeal dysplasia classification, the most widely accepted classification scheme is currently that of the 2017 World Health Organization system, which stratifies leukoplakia into 1 of 3 risk categories: low-grade dysplasia, high-grade dysplasia, and carcinoma in situ.
- A large randomized clinical trial from the US Department of Veterans Affairs demonstrated the utility of induction chemotherapy followed by definitive radiation for advanced cancers of the larynx and proposes larynx preservation as a primary treatment stategy in select patients.
- PD-L1 is present in 50% to 60% of head and neck SCCa; Inhibitors such as pembrolizumab and nivolumab are under study, with results demonstrating tumor response and improved survival, respectively.
- CD4+ and CD8+ tumor-infiltrating T lymphocytes correlate with improved disease-specific and disease-free survival in laryngeal cancer; recurrent and high-risk tumors demonstrate unique genetic profiles, with higher mutation rates in histone modifier BAP1 and DNA mismatch repair gene MSH2.
- Surveillance of advanced laryngeal and hypopharyngeal cancer follows the National Comprehensive Cancer Network guideline: "repeat of pretreatment baseline imaging within 6 months of completion therapy," with preferred modality of whole-body PET and CT on all patients 3 to 6 months after completion of definitive therapy.
- Because tumors in the larynx and hypopharynx affect many vital functions such as speaking, eating, and breathing, a multidisciplinary approach is essential, including a multidisciplinary tumor board and involvement of speech and swallow therapists before and after definitive treatment.

DISCLOSURE

The authors declare no conflicts of interest or funding sources in the writing of this manuscript.

REFERENCES

1. Forastiere AA, Zhang Q, Weber RS, et al. Long-term results of RTOG 91-11: a comparison of three nonsurgical treatment strategies to preserve the larynx in patients with locally advanced larynx cancer. J Clin Oncol 2013;31(7):845–52.
2. Department of Veterans Affairs Laryngeal Cancer Study Group, Wolf GT, Fisher SG, et al. Induction chemotherapy plus radiation compared with surgery

plus radiation in patients with advanced laryngeal cancer. N Engl J Med 1991; 324(24):1685–90.

3. St John MA. Multidisciplinary Approach to Head and Neck Cancer. Otolaryngol Clin North Am 2017;50(4):xvii–xviii.

4. American Cancer Society. American Cancer Society: Cancer Facts and Figures 2020. 2020. https://www.cancer.org/content/dam/cancer-org/research/cancer-facts-and-statistics/annual-cancer-facts-and-figures/2020/cancer-facts-and-figures-2020.pdf. [Accessed 22 November 2020].

5. Lin HW, Bhattacharyya N. Staging and survival analysis for nonsquamous cell carcinomas of the larynx. Laryngoscope 2008;118(6):1003–13.

6. United States Department of Health and Human Services Centers for Disease Control and Prevention. Centers for Disease Control National Program of Cancer Registries SEER*Stat Database: U.S. Cancer Statistics Incidence Analytic File 1998–2015. Atlanta: Centers for Disease Control and Prevention; 2018.

7. Chapter 123: Early laryngeal cancer. In: Johnson J, editor. Bailey's head and neck surgery: otolaryngology. 5th ed. Lippincott Williams & Wilkins (LWW); 2013. p. 1940–60. http://ebookcentral.proquest.com/lib/knowledgecenter/detail.action?docID=2031636. [Accessed 20 July 2020].

8. Odell E, Eckel HE, Simo R, et al. European Laryngological Society position paper on laryngeal dysplasia Part I: aetiology and pathological c assification. Eur Arch Otorhinolaryngol 2020. https://doi.org/10.1007/s00405-020-06403-y.

9. Panuganti BA, Finegersh A, Flagg M, et al. Prognostic significance of HPV status in laryngeal squamous cell carcinoma: a large-population database study. Otolaryngol Head Neck Surg 2020. https://doi.org/10.1177/0194599820976178. 194599820976178.

10. Zubčić Ž, Mendeš T, Včeva A, et al. Presence of pepsin in laryngeal tissue and saliva in benign and malignant neoplasms. Biosci Rep 2020;40(11). BSR20200216.

11. Chapter 122: Hypopharyngeal and cervical esophageal carcinoma. In: Johnson J, editor. Bailey's head and neck surgery: otolaryngology. 5th ed. Lippincott Williams & Wilkins (LWW); 2013. p. 1917–39. http://ebookcentral.proquest.com/lib/knowledgecenter/detail.action?docID=2031636. [Accessed 20 July 2020].

12. Chen S, Dee EC, Muralidhar V, et al. Disparities in mortality from larynx cancer: implications for reducing racial differences. Laryngoscope 2020. https://doi.org/10.1002/lary.29046.

13. Shin JY, Truong MT. Racial disparities in laryngeal cancer treatment and outcome: a population-based analysis of 24,069 patients. Laryngoscope 2015;125(7): 1667–74.

14. Liu J, Zhu W, Li Z, et al. Proteomic analysis of hypopharyngeal and laryngeal squamous cell carcinoma sheds light on differences in survival. Sci Rep 2020;10.

15. Wadie M, Adam SI, Sasaki CT. Development, anatomy, and physiology of the larynx. In: Shaker R, Belafsky PC, Postma GN, et al, editors. Principles of deglutition: a multidisciplinary text for swallowing and its disorders. New York: Springer; 2013. p. 175–97.

16. Saito H, Sato T, Yamashita Y, et al. Topographical analysis of lymphatic pathways from the meso- and hypopharynx based on minute cadaveric dissections: possible application to neck dissection in pharyngeal cancer surgery. Surg Radiol Anat SRA 2002;24(1):38–49.

17. Laryngeal Cancer Survival Rate|Throat Cancer Survival Rate. https://www.cancer. org/cancer/laryngeal-and-hypopharyngeal-cancer/detection-diagnosis-staging/ survival-rates.html. [Accessed 27 December 2020].
18. Kostev K, Jacob LEC, Kalder M, et al. Association of laryngeal cancer with vocal cord leukoplakia and associated risk factors in 1,184 patients diagnosed in otorhinolaryngology practices in Germany. Mol Clin Oncol 2018;8(5):689–93.
19. Isenberg JS, Crozier DL, Dailey SH. Institutional and comprehensive review of laryngeal leukoplakia. Ann Otol Rhinol Laryngol 2008;117(1):74–9.
20. Ahmadzada S, Vasan K, Sritharan N, et al. Utility of narrowband imaging in the diagnosis of laryngeal leukoplakia: Systematic review and meta-analysis. Head Neck 2020;42(11):3427–37.
21. Rodrigo JP, Villaronga MÁ, Menéndez ST, et al. A novel role for Nanog as an early cancer risk marker in patients with laryngeal precancerous lesions. Sci Rep 2017; 7(1):11110.
22. Wan P, Ongkasuwan J, Martinez J, et al. Biomarkers for malignant potential in vocal fold leukoplakia: a state of the art review. Otolaryngol Head Neck Surg 2020. https://doi.org/10.1177/0194599820957251. 194599820957251.
23. Cui W, Xu W, Yang Q, et al. Clinicopathological parameters associated with his-tological background and recurrence after surgical intervention of vocal cord leu-koplakia. Medicine (Baltimore) 2017;96(22):e7033.
24. Park JC, Altman KW, Prasad VMN, et al. Laryngeal Leukoplakia: State of the Art Review. Otolaryngol Head Neck Surg 2020. https://doi.org/10.1177/ 0194599820965910. 194599820965910.
25. Karatayli-Ozgursoy S, Bishop JA, Hillel AT, et al. Malignant salivary gland tumours of the larynx: a single institution review. Acta Otorhinolaryngol Ital 2016;36(4): 289–94.
26. Fleskens SAJHM, van der Laak JAWM, Slootweg PJ, et al. Management of laryn-geal premalignant lesions in the Netherlands. Laryngoscope 2010;120(7): 1326–35.
27. Fearon ER, Vogelstein B. A genetic model for colorectal tumorigenesis. Cell 1990; 61(5):759–67.
28. Slaughter DP, Southwick HW, Smejkal W. Field cancerization in oral stratified squamous epithelium; clinical implications of multicentric origin. Cancer 1953; 6(5):963–8.
29. Califano J, van der Riet P, Westra W, et al. Genetic progression model for head and neck cancer: implications for field cancerization. Cancer Res 1996;56(11): 2488–92.
30. Hahn WC, Weinberg RA. Rules for making human tumor cells. N Engl J Med 2002;347(20):1593–603.
31. Boyle JO, Hakim J, Koch W, et al. The incidence of p53 mutations increases with progression of head and neck cancer. Cancer Res 1993;53(19):4477–80.
32. Kamb A, Gruis NA, Weaver-Feldhaus J, et al. A cell cycle regulator potentially involved in genesis of many tumor types. Science 1994;264(5157):436–40.
33. Gibcus JH, Menkema L, Mastik MF, et al. Amplicon mapping and expression profiling identify the Fas-associated death domain gene as a new driver in the 11q13.3 amplicon in laryngeal/pharyngeal cancer. Clin Cancer Res 2007; 13(21):6257–66.
34. Osman I, Sherman E, Singh B, et al. Alteration of p53 pathway in squamous cell carcinoma of the head and neck: impact on treatment outcome in patients treated with larynx preservation intent. J Clin Oncol 2002;20(13):2980–7.

35. Scheffner M, Huibregtse JM, Vierstra RD, et al. The HPV-16 E6 and E6-AP complex functions as a ubiquitin-protein ligase in the ubiquitination of p53. Cell. 1993; 75(3):495–505.

36. Carinci F, Arcelli D, Lo Muzio L, et al. Molecular classification of nodal metastasis in primary larynx squamous cell carcinoma. Transl Res J Lab Clin Med 2007; 150(4):233–45.

37. Mirisola V, Mora R, Esposito AI, et al. A prognostic multigene classifier for squamous cell carcinomas of the larynx. Cancer Lett 2011;307(1):37–46.

38. Yu X, Li Z. The role of microRNAs expression in laryngeal cancer. Oncotarget 2015;6(27):23297–305.

39. Wang Y, Chen M, Tao Z, et al. Identification of predictive biomarkers for early diagnosis of larynx carcinoma based on microRNA expression data. Cancer Genet 2013;206(9–10):340–6.

40. Karatas OF, Yuceturk B, Suer I, et al. Role of miR-145 in human laryngeal squamous cell carcinoma. Head Neck 2016;38(2):260–6.

41. Powrózek T, Porgador A, Małecka-Massalska T. Detection, prediction, and prognosis: blood circulating microRNA as novel molecular markers of head and neck cancer patients. Expert Rev Mol Diagn 2020;20(1):31–9.

42. Pierini S, Jordanov SH, Mitkova AV, et al. Promoter hypermethylation of CDKN2A, MGMT, MLH1, and DAPK genes in laryngeal squamous cell carcinoma and their associations with clinical profiles of the patients. Head Neck 2014;36(8):1103–8.

43. Shen J, Hu K, Ma J, et al. Clinical analysis of EBRT vs TLM in the treatment of early (T1-T2N0) glottic laryngeal cancer. J Cancer 2020;11(22):6686–94.

44. Huang G, Luo M, Zhang J, et al. The voice quality after laser surgery versus radiotherapy of T1a glottic carcinoma: systematic review and meta-analysis. Oncotargets Ther 2017;10:2403–10.

45. Ceachir O, Hainarosie R, Zainea V. Total laryngectomy – past, present, future. Mædica 2014;9(2):210–6.

46. Woodard TD, Oplatek A, Petruzzelli GJ. Life after total laryngectomy: a measure of long-term survival, function, and quality of life. Arch Otolaryngol Head Neck Surg 2007;133(6):526–32.

47. Goepfert RP, Hutcheson KA, Lewin JS, et al. Complications, hospital length of stay, and readmission after total laryngectomy. Cancer 2017;123(10):1760–7.

48. Sullivan CB, Ostedgaard KL, Al-Qurayshi Z, et al. Primary laryngectomy versus salvage laryngectomy: a comparison of outcomes in the chemoradiation era. Laryngoscope 2020;130(9):2179–85.

49. Boukovalas S, Goepfert RP, Smith JM, et al. Association between postoperative complications and long-term oncologic outcomes following total laryngectomy: 10-year experience at MD Anderson Cancer Center. Cancer 2020;126(22): 4905–16.

50. Su X, He H-C, Ye Z-L, et al. A 10-year study on larynx preservation compared with surgical resection in patients with locally advanced laryngeal and hypopharyngeal cancers. Front Oncol 2020;10. https://doi.org/10.3389/fonc.2020.535893.

51. Shetty AV, Wong DJ. Systemic treatment for squamous cell carcinoma of the head and neck. Otolaryngol Clin North Am 2017;50(4):775–82.

52. Liang K, Ang KK, Milas L, et al. The epidermal growth factor receptor mediates radioresistance. Int J Radiat Oncol Biol Phys 2003;57(1):246–54.

53. Temam S, Kawaguchi H, El-Naggar AK, et al. Epidermal growth factor receptor copy number alterations correlate with poor clinical outcome in patients with head and neck squamous cancer. J Clin Oncol 2007;25(16):2164–70.

54. Kalyankrishna S, Grandis JR. Epidermal growth factor receptor biology in head and neck cancer. J Clin Oncol 2006;24(17):2666–72.
55. Bonner JA, Harari PM, Giralt J, et al. Radiotherapy plus cetuximab for squamous-cell carcinoma of the head and neck. N Engl J Med 2006;354(6):567–78.
56. Vermorken JB, Mesia R, Rivera F, et al. Platinum-based chemotherapy plus cetuximab in head and neck cancer. N Engl J Med 2008;359(11):1116–27.
57. Guo R, Guo J, Zhang L, et al. CT-based radiomics features in the prediction of thyroid cartilage invasion from laryngeal and hypopharyngeal squamous cell carcinoma. Cancer Imaging 2020;20(1):81.
58. Tagliabue M, Maffini F, Fumagalli C, et al. A role for the immune system in advanced laryngeal cancer. Sci Rep 2020;10(1):18327.
59. Mann JE, Smith JD, Birkeland AC, et al. Analysis of tumor-infiltrating CD103 resident memory T-cell content in recurrent laryngeal squamous cell carcinoma. Cancer Immunol Immunother CII 2019;68(2):213–20.
60. Chuang H-C, Tsai M-H, Lin Y-T, et al. The clinical impacts of pretreatment peripheral blood ratio on lymphocytes, monocytes, and neutrophils among patients with laryngeal/hypopharyngeal cancer treated by chemoradiation/radiation. Cancer Manag Res 2020;12:9013–21.
61. Xiao H, Su Q, Li C. Identification of prognostic immune genes in laryngeal cancer. J Int Med Res 2020;48(11).
62. Saleh K, Eid R, Haddad FG, et al. New developments in the management of head and neck cancer – impact of pembrolizumab. Ther Clin Risk Manag 2018;14: 295–303.
63. Ferris RL, Blumenschein G, Fayette J, et al. Nivolumab vs investigator's choice in recurrent or metastatic squamous cell carcinoma of the head and neck: 2-year long-term survival update of CheckMate 141 with analyses by tumor PD-L1 expression. Oral Oncol 2018;81:45–51.
64. Seiwert TY, Burtness B, Mehra R, et al. Safety and clinical activity of pembrolizumab for treatment of recurrent or metastatic squamous cell carcinoma of the head and neck (KEYNOTE-012): an open-label, multicentre, phase 1b trial. Lancet Oncol 2016;17(7):956–65.
65. Smith JD, Birkeland AC, Rosko AJ, et al. Mutational profiles of persistent/recurrent laryngeal squamous cell carcinoma. Head Neck 2019;41(2):423–8.
66. Hoesli R, Birkeland AC, Rosko AJ, et al. Proportion of CD4 and CD8 tumor infiltrating lymphocytes predicts survival in persistent/recurrent laryngeal squamous cell carcinoma. Oral Oncol 2018;77:83–9.
67. Li W, Fu M, Zhao K, et al. Development and validation of a novel metabolic signature for predicting prognosis in patients with laryngeal cancer. Eur Arch Otorhino-laryngol 2020. https://doi.org/10.1007/s00405-020-06444-3.
68. Morgan RL, Eguchi MM, McDermott J, et al. Comparative effectiveness of post-treatment imaging modalities for Medicare patients with advanced head and neck cancer. Cancer 2020. https://doi.org/10.1002/cncr.33244.
69. Colevas AD, Yom SS, Pfister DG, et al. NCCN guidelines insights: head and neck cancers, version 1.2018. J Natl Compr Cancer Netw JNCCN 2018;16(5):479–90.
70. Heineman TE, Kuan EC, St John MA. When should surveillance imaging be performed after treatment for head and neck cancer? Laryngoscope 2017;127(3): 533–4.

Cancer of the Paranasal Sinuses

Melissa A. Taylor, MD, MPH[a], Nabil F. Saba, MD, FACP[b],*

KEYWORDS

- Sinonasal cancer • Epidemiology • Treatment • Chemotherapy • Surgery
- Radiation • Clinical outcomes

KEY POINTS

- Sinonasal cancers are a rare and diverse subtype of malignancies and comprise only 0.2% of all malignancies.
- They often present at later stages due to their anatomic location and have significant associated morbidity due to critical surrounding structures.
- Sinonasal cancers are treated with a multimodal approach, with surgery and radiation therapy being the mainstay of treatment and chemotherapy frequently used in the neoadjuvant setting.
- Because of their rarity, there are limited randomized clinical trials to establish the most appropriate treatment regimens.
- Outcomes are poor with 5-year overall survival of 32%; however, this varies greatly by histologic subtype.

INTRODUCTION

Malignancies of the nasal cavity and paranasal sinuses are rare and make up only around 0.2% of all cancers and only 3% to 5% of cancers in the upper respiratory tract (**Table 1**).[1] The overall incidence is only 0.556/100,000 per year, with men almost twice as likely to be affected as women. The incidence rate has remained relatively stable over time. Sinonasal cancers are made up of a histologically diverse group of pathologies, with the most common being squamous cell carcinoma followed by adenocarcinoma. Most of the tumors occur in the nasal cavity (43.9%) followed by the maxillary sinuses (35.9%).[2] There are a variety of environmental, occupational, and genetic risk factors including exposure to wood or leather dust, nickel, Epstein-Barr virus, salted fish diet, and exposure to high-risk human papillomavirus (HPV).[3] Because of the anatomic location of these tumors, they often have an insidious onset of symptoms

[a] Department of Internal Medicine, Emory University, 49 Jesse Hill Jr. Drive, Atlanta, GA 30303, USA; [b] Hematology Medical Oncology and Otolaryngology, Head and Neck Oncology Program, Winship Cancer Institute of Emory University, 1365 Clifton Road # C2110, Atlanta, GA 30322, USA
* Corresponding author.
E-mail address: nfsaba@emory.edu

Hematol Oncol Clin N Am 35 (2021) 949–962
https://doi.org/10.1016/j.hoc.2021.05.006
0889-8588/21/© 2021 Elsevier Inc. All rights reserved.

and present at a late stage of diagnosis. Sinonasal tumors can cause significant morbidity due to involvement or invasion of surrounding structures including the orbits, olfactory nerve, facial nerves, and intracranial space. Only 12% of paranasal sinus tumors have lymph node involvement and only 6% have metastatic involvement at the time of diagnosis.[4]

The main treatment modalities are surgical resection and radiation therapy with chemotherapy in the neoadjuvant or adjuvant setting. Historically, open craniofacial resection was the gold-standard surgical treatment until the 1990s when endoscopic surgical techniques were more widely used with improvements in cosmetic outcomes.[5,6] Radiation therapy is another mainstay of treatment of sinonasal tumors and can be used alone in the case of specific early stage tumors for improved cosmetic outcomes or more frequently in combination with surgical resection.[7] Systemic therapy is also a critical treatment modality in the neoadjuvant and adjuvant setting with success depending on stage and histologic subtype. Because of the rarity of these types of tumors, there are relatively few randomized control trials examining specific chemotherapy regimens. Overall outcomes of sinonasal cancers are poor. When combining all subtypes, collectively, the 5-, 10-, and 20-year survival is 45.7%, 32.2%, and 16.4%, respectively; however, outcomes vary when specific histologic subtype is taken into consideration.[8]

EPIDEMIOLOGY

The most common histologic subtype of paranasal sinus malignancies is squamous cell carcinoma, comprising 60% to 75% of cases.[9] The next most common histologic subtypes are adenocarcinoma followed by adenoid cystic carcinoma, representing approximately 15% and 10% of paranasal sinus malignancies, respectively. The remaining paranasal sinus malignancies are made up of extremely rare but diverse histologic subtypes including mucoepidermoid carcinoma, acinic cell carcinoma, sinonasal undifferentiated carcinoma, melanoma, olfactory neuroblastoma, and sinonasal neuroendocrine tumors. In addition, there are extremely rare subsets of sarcomas including rhabdomyosarcoma, chondrosarcoma, Ewing sarcoma, and lymphomas such as natural killer (NK)/T-cell lymphomas and diffuse large B-cell lymphomas.[10] Overall, the incidence of sinonasal malignancies is rare, with 0.556 cases per 100,000 people per year or about 2000 new diagnoses per year. The incidence has remained relatively stable over the last 30 years. Sinonasal cancer occurs more frequently in older adults and the elderly, with 80% of those being diagnosed at 55 years of age or older. Sinonasal malignancies affect men 1.8 times more frequently than women (58.3% vs 41.7%) and occur 9 times more frequently among white compared with black populations (82.2% vs 9%). Almost half of these malignancies originate in the nasal cavities with just more than one-third originating in the maxillary sinuses and around one-tenth in the ethmoid sinuses. Malignancies originating in the frontal and sphenoid sinuses occur less frequently, each comprising less than 3% of all sinonasal tumor sites, respectively.[2]

Certain occupational, environmental, and biological risk factors increase the risk of developing sinonasal malignancy. The relationship between specific occupations and the development of sinonasal cancer has been well documented.[11-19] Squamous cell carcinoma of the nasal cavity has been shown to occur more frequently in nickel workers compared with the general population, with nickel compounds being a known carcinogen.[18,19] Adenocarcinoma has been associated with wood dust exposure, with occupations such as carpenters and sawmill workers having higher incidence compared with the general population.[11,12] The International Agency for

Table 1
Treatment and outcomes for various sinonasal malignancies

Tumor Type	Treatment Modality	5-y Overall Survival
Sinonasal squamous cell carcinoma	Surgical resection, adjuvant radiation, chemotherapy (platinum + taxane alone ± 5-FU)[55]	30%
Adenocarcinoma	Surgery, radiation, chemotherapy (cisplatin, 5-FU, and leucovorin if mutation in p-53)[61]	72.7% intestinal type 95.2% nonintestinal type
Adenoid cystic carcinoma	Surgery, radiation, chemotherapy (cisplatin, doxorubicin, and cyclophosphamide)[76]	61%
Olfactory neuroblastoma	Surgery, radiation, chemotherapy (cisplatin + etoposide, or cyclophosphamide + vincristine ± Adriamycin)[77]	69%
Sinonasal neuroendocrine carcinoma	Surgery, chemotherapy (platinum + etoposide)[78]	50.8%
Sinonasal undifferentiated carcinoma	Radiation, surgery, chemotherapy (platinum regimens + cyclophosphamide, doxorubicin, vincristine, 5-FU)[79-81]	34.9%
Sinonasal mucosal melanoma	Surgery, radiation, checkpoint inhibitor therapy, chemotherapy (cisplatin, vinblastine, dacarbazine)[82]	33%
Rhabdomyosarcoma	Surgery, chemoradiation (vincristine, Adriamycin, cyclophosphamide)[83]	28.4%
NK/T-cell lymphoma	Radiation, chemotherapy (dexamethasone, methotrexate, ifosfamide, L-asparaginase, etoposide), pembrolizumab[84]	54.8%
Diffuse large B-cell lymphoma	Anthracycline-based chemotherapy + rituximab[85]	68%

Research on Cancer has identified wood dust exposure, especially dust from hard and exotic woods, as a known carcinogen to humans.[19] Specific chemical compounds in industry, such as chromium, isopropyl alcohol, and radium, have been shown to increase the risk of sinonasal cancer.[13] Social habits such as cigarette smoking and alcohol use have also been shown to increase risk of developing sinonasal cancer.[16]

The incidence of sinonasal cancer varies greatly between regions of the world. Adenocarcinoma is more common than squamous cell carcinoma in Europe with most cases localized to the ethmoid sinuses.[20–22] Although HPV is more frequently associated with malignancies arising in the oropharynx, a study at Johns Hopkins found that of 161 identified sinonasal carcinomas, 21% were positive for high-risk HPV DNA, specifically type 16 (82%) and mostly squamous cell carcinoma histologic subtype (82%).[23] Another study from the National Cancer Database revealed that 31.7% of sinonasal squamous cell carcinoma cases were associated with HPV.[24] Sinonasal cancers associated with high-risk HPV have also been shown to have more favorable outcomes and are more likely to be found in a younger population.[25,26]

CLINICAL EVALUATION AND DIAGNOSIS

Cancer of the paranasal sinuses has an insidious onset and is often diagnosed late in disease. The locations of origin are often hidden, being empty airspaces, and they are often asymptomatic. If symptoms do occur, they are often nonspecific and underestimated by patients, such as nasal obstruction, epistaxis, chronic rhinitis or sinusitis, and difficulty swallowing.[27] Up to 60% to 70% of cancers of the paranasal sinuses arise in the maxillary sinuses, followed by 20% to 30% arising in the nasal cavity, 10% to 15% in the ethmoid sinuses, and 1% to 2% in the sphenoid sinuses. Symptoms vary based on invasion of surrounding structures. Tumors arising in the maxillary sinuses can invade the orbit causing changes in vision such as proptosis and diplopia. Invasion to the infratemporal fossa, pterygopalatine fossae, and the masseteric space can cause trismus, facial swelling, tooth or jaw pain, and numbness of the midface. Tumors arising from the nasal cavity should be distinguished from skin cancers that can arise in a similar site, particularly those originating in the septum. Nasal cavity tumors can invade the ethmoid sinuses, anterior cranial fossa, and orbit superiorly; the maxillary sinuses and the palate inferiorly; and the subcutaneous tissue and skin anteriorly. Tumors originating in the ethmoid sinuses can affect surrounding structures relatively easily; the orbit can be invaded via lateral or posterior extension causing visual symptoms, the olfactory nerves can be affected by superior extension, and invasion into the intracranial space can also occur. Tumors arising in the sphenoid sinuses can extend into the intracranial space, orbital apex, or cavernous sinuses.[28]

When a patient presents with symptoms concerning for cancer of the paranasal sinuses, the next step toward establishing a diagnosis is imaging. CT is more sensitive and specific to determine osseous margins and involvement, whereas MRI is superior at identifying soft tissue resolution and perineural, orbital, or intracranial spread. Imaging is essential to differentiating tumor from secretions, infection, or granulation. It is also essential to determine stage and prognosis as well as treatment such as ability to be surgically resected, approach, and radiation therapy fields.[29,30] Definitive diagnosis requires histologic evaluation by biopsy, which is generally obtained by endoscopic evaluation for direct visualization of the tumor. Thorough examination of the oral cavity as well as visual and neurologic examination is also essential for initial diagnostic workup.[31]

NECK INVOLVEMENT AND MANAGEMENT

Lymph node metastasis at diagnosis is relatively rare for paranasal sinus cancer, with an overall incidence of 12%. The rate of lymph node involvement for maxillary sinus tumors at presentation is 8.3% and even lower for ethmoid sinus tumors at 1.6%. Early or late lymph node metastasis is a poor prognostic factor. For tumors of the ethmoid sinuses, the 5-year survival rate was 45.3% for those without lymph node involvement compared with 0% for lymph node involvement at presentation. For maxillary sinus tumors, the 5-year survival rate was 50.6% for those without lymph node involvement compared with 16.8% with lymph node involvement.[4] Treatment of the neck with radiation and/or surgery is indicated for tumors with lymph node involvement at presentation; however there is not conclusive evidence for prophylactic neck dissection or radiation for cases without lymph node involvement at diagnosis.[32] For tumors of the nasal cavity and ethmoid sinuses, prophylactic neck radiation is usually not recommended except for specific circumstances (capillary involvement or poorly differentiated tumors) because lymph node involvement is rare. Undifferentiated carcinoma cases have been shown to have a high rate of regional recurrence (25%), and in these cases there is indication for prophylactic irritation of the neck.[33] When lymph node involvement occurs, the most common sites of involvement include the retropharyngeal nodes and the periparotid nodes.[34]

STAGING

Because of the unique staging system of maxillary sinus cancer, as discussed later, there is a higher incidence of lymph node involvement with stage T2 compared with T3 or T4 due to the involvement of the hard palate or nasal cavity in T2 tumors.[4] Metastasis of tumors of the paranasal sinuses is extremely rare but when it does occur the most commonly associated sites are the lung, liver, and bone.[35] Staging for paranasal sinus cancer is based on the eighth TNM system developed by the American Joint Committee on Cancer and the Union for International Cancer Control in 2017. In this system there is separate T staging for maxillary sinus tumors and ethmoid sinus tumors, and there is not a standard staging system for tumors of the frontal or sphenoid sinuses.[36]

THERAPEUTIC OPTIONS

Because of the rarity of paranasal sinus malignancies, there are limited clinical trial data for multimodal therapy approaches. Surgery and radiation remain the mainstay of treatment; however, more advanced stages of paranasal sinus malignancies require systemic therapy.

SURGICAL TECHNIQUES

Surgical resection is the primary treatment of paranasal sinus malignancies; however, because of their physical location, surgery can be technically challenging. Surrounding structures include the brain, orbit, carotid arteries, and cranial nerves, which lead to high risk of morbidity following surgery. Open craniofacial resection was historically the gold-standard surgical procedure and improved 5-year survival from 28% in the mid twentieth century to 51% in the 1990s. Survival data for open craniofacial resection techniques are based on case reports and meta-analyses.[37] A study spanning 20 years looked at outcomes for 220 patients undergoing craniofacial resection at 2 institutions and found a 5-year disease-free survival rate of 54.5%. Histology, location, stage, and treatment modality also played a role in 5-year survival rate.[5]

In the late 1990s, research reporting on endoscopic approaches to resection began to appear; however, most of these studies targeted early stage cancers for endoscopic resection and a combined surgical and endoscopic approach for more advanced stage disease. A study looking at 184 patients between 1996 and 2006 treated with endoscopic surgery or assisted by endoscopic surgery found a 5-year disease-free survival of 94.4% for adenocarcinoma and 60.7% for squamous cell carcinoma. In contrast, a similar cohort treated with cranioendoscopic approach reported 5-year disease-free survival of 57.9% for adenocarcinoma and 53.5% for squamous cell carcinoma. Although the results of this study seem drastically different than craniofacial resection, the study had tumor cohorts with similar histology and staging, which makes drawing definite conclusions comparing the 2 techniques difficult.[6] A pooled analysis of 1400 cases from retrospective studies stratified by surgical approach and stage found an increase in local recurrence in the surgical group (open or endoscopic assisted) of 38.5% compared with 17.8% in the endoscopic group. However, an important consideration is that smaller tumors were more likely to be resected via endoscopic approach, and tumors with more extensive involvement of surrounding structures, as seen in higher stages, were more likely to be resected with surgical approach.[38]

Patient factors are also important to consider when evaluating surgical approaches. A study looking at the effects of age and surgical technique found that for elderly patients aged 70 years and older, open craniofacial resection was associated with a significant increase in mortality, complications, and worse outcomes regardless of location or stage of tumor.[39] The most important predictor of survival regardless of technique is obtaining negative margins, which is similar between endoscopic and open craniofacial resection.[40] The selection of surgical approach should take into account the approach that is most likely to achieve negative margins.

Resection can result in a high degree of morbidity due to the importance of surrounding structures. Complications of both open craniofacial and endoscopic resection include cerebrospinal fluids leaks, infection, cranial nerve injuries, and hemorrhage.[37] Endoscopic approach is associated with less morbidity related to cosmetic issues compared with open craniofacial resection and is also associated with shorter hospital length of stay. In a study by Nicolai and colleagues, a cohort of 184 patients underwent either cranioendoscopic resection or endoscopic resection alone. The complication rate was 6% in the endoscopic group and 16% in the cranioendoscopic group, with cerebrospinal fluid leak being the most common complication in both groups. The average length of stay was shorter in the endoscopic group at 3.7 days compared with 15.4 days for cranioendoscopic resection.[6] Location of the tumor is an important consideration when determining the role of primary surgical resection, given the cosmetic morbidity and the addition of radiotherapy in the role of primary treatment of paranasal sinus malignancies.

RADIATION THERAPY

In addition to surgery, radiation therapy is a critical modality of treatment of paranasal sinus malignancies. Depending on the size and location of the tumor, radiotherapy alone or with surgical resection can result in similar survival outcomes without devastating cosmetic morbidity.[41] Primary therapy with radiation can yield favorable cosmetic outcomes in the nasal vestibule region, such as stage I tumors of the nasal cavity, anterior nasal septal lesions, and lateral wall nasal regions.[42] These regions can be treated with external beam radiation therapy, brachytherapy, or both.[43] Primary radiation therapy is also indicated for patients who cannot undergo surgery but have locally advanced lesions. Postsurgical radiation is indicated in cases where surgical resection identified tumors of high grade, high-risk histologic features, positive margins, or the tumor has invaded perineural or lymphovascular spaces.[7] A study by Jansen and colleagues examined the features of patients who were selected for radiotherapy alone and found that the 6 most common parameters included likelihood of successful complete surgical removal; age greater than 65 years; advanced stage; and evidence of invasion of the nasopharynx, palate, or skull base.

Complications associated with radiation therapy included panhypopituitarism and visual complications.[35] Postoperative radiation therapy is widely used for paranasal sinus cancer. Patients with cancer of the maxillary sinuses in particular experienced significant reduction in local occurrence when the ipsilateral side of the neck was treated with postoperative radiation therapy, likely due to treating areas of undetectable disease.[44]

Advancements in radiation therapy techniques have improved the role of radiation in treatment of sinonasal tumors. The delivery of intensity-modulated radiation therapy (IMRT) as either a primary therapy or in adjuvant with chemotherapy or surgery has shown comparable effectiveness but improved toxicity profiles, such as lower rates of radiation-induced blindness, when compared with conventional 2-dimensional radiation therapy across multiple studies.[45–47] In instances where the radiation field involves optic structures, a technique called hyperfractionation has been preferred over IMRT due to decreased concentration of radiation over the optic structures resulting in decreased visual complications.[48] Proton beam radiation therapy reduces the radiation dose significantly by using protons instead of photons and provides similar rates of local control without toxicity from high-dose photon therapy or traditional radiation therapy. These new techniques provide a decrease in radiation-related toxicities while having equivalent rates of local control; however, they have not been shown to improve overall survival rates of paranasal sinus cancer compared with traditional radiation therapy.[49]

SYSTEMIC THERAPY

Because of the rarity of cancer of the nasal cavity and paranasal sinuses compared with other cancers of the head and neck, it is difficult to rely on randomized control trials to determine the role of systemic treatment. The importance of systemic therapy in targeting distant metastasis as well as achieving local control is becoming more recognized as a critical treatment modality in head and neck cancer and is hoped that it will begin to be applied to sinonasal cancers. Systemic therapy can be used as either neoadjuvant or adjuvant therapy, and there are also special considerations regarding the role of systemic therapy with specific subtypes of sinonasal cancer.

NEOADJUVANT THERAPY

The first studies to examine the role of systemic neoadjuvant therapy when combined with surgery and/or radiation showed encouraging results. A 1988 study by LoRusso and colleagues examined 16 patients with advanced, stage III or stage IV sinonasal cancer who were treated with platinum-based chemotherapy followed by surgery and/or radiation and found an overall response rate of 82%, complete response rate of 44%, and partial response rate of 38%.[50] In 1992, a study by Eriksson and colleagues examined the role of neoadjuvant cisplatin + 5-fluorouracil (FU) followed by definitive treatment with surgery and/or radiation in local control and organ preservation. The study looked at 12 patients with advanced nonadenocarcinoma sinonasal cancer and found that 11 patients achieved local control and 10 patients had no evidence of disease at 27-month follow-up.[51] An Italian study in 2003 by Licitra and colleagues looked at 49 patients with resectable paranasal sinus tumors treated with cisplatin + 5-FU + leucovorin followed by definitive surgery and/or radiation therapy and found an overall survival at 3 years of 69%.[52] A more recent study in 2011 by Hanna and colleagues examined 46 patients with advanced sinonasal cancer treated with induction chemotherapy with a regimen of platinum and taxanes followed by surgery and/or radiation. The results indicated a 2-year overall survival of 67%, and 87% of patients were able to have orbital preservation.[53]

Although these studies showed promising results, there are important limitations to consider. The studies were all retrospective, single-institution studies with no randomization or stratification by histopathology. The advantages to neoadjuvant chemotherapy include optimization of drug delivery, ability to give higher chemotherapy doses compared with the adjuvant setting, and toxicities being more transient in the induction setting. The major disadvantage, however, is potential delay in definitive surgical or radiation therapy, which is the mainstay of treatment.[54] More studies are needed to be able to more accurately evaluate the role of neoadjuvant therapy in sinonasal cancer. A current randomized phase II clinical trial sponsored by the ECOG-ACRIN Cancer Research Group (EA3163, NCT03493425) is examining the role of neoadjuvant chemotherapy with carboplatin or cisplatin ± docetaxel before surgery and/or radiation in patients with stage III and stage IVA nasal cavity and paranasal sinus cancer, which will provide more information regarding the role of neoadjuvant therapy.

ADJUVANT THERAPY

Although surgery remains the primary method of definitive treatment of sinonasal cancers, there is a role for chemotherapy in the adjuvant setting. Adjuvant chemotherapy is occasionally used in combination with radiation therapy, specifically when high-risk pathologic features exist due to the radiosensitive properties of certain chemotherapy regimens.[55] Data regarding the role of adjuvant or concurrent chemotherapy with radiation following surgery are scarce for sinonasal cancers. A study by Robin and colleagues using the National Cancer Database found that when compared with surgery alone, patients treated with adjuvant therapy (HR 0.658, $P<.001$), adjuvant chemoradiation therapy (HR 0.696, $P = .002$), or neoadjuvant therapy (HR 0.656, $P = .007$) had improved overall survival.[56] Another study by Farrell and colleagues found that patients treated with surgery with or without adjuvant therapy had a lower 24-month and 60-month mortality risk compared to definitive RT or chemoradiation (HR 1.97, $P<.001$).[57] At present, there is not enough data to support adjuvant chemotherapy as a standard treatment in the setting of sinonasal cancers, and more research is needed to determine any possible role of adjuvant chemotherapy for sinonasal cancer.

SPECIAL CONSIDERATIONS BASED ON HISTOLOGIC SUBTYPE

Specific histotypes have different responses to treatment modalities. Small cohort studies show that squamous cell carcinoma of the sinonasal tract is responsive to platinum-based doublet therapy, specifically cisplatin or carboplatin and 5-FU for neoadjuvant therapy.[58,59] Adenocarcinomas of the sinonasal tract are usually treated with surgery and adjuvant radiation therapy; tumors expressing functional p53 have been shown to have some response with the neoadjuvant use of cisplatin, 5-FU, and leucovorin.[60,61] The most aggressive subtype of sinonasal cancer, sinonasal undifferentiated carcinoma, has been shown to be chemosensitive with improved survival with addition of systemic chemotherapy to surgical treatment.[62] There is, however, lack of consensus on a specific preoperative regimen, as a variety of induction regimens have been used, including platinum-based regimens as well as combination of cyclophosphamide, doxorubicin, and vincristine.[63] As far as sinonasal neuroendocrine carcinoma is concerned, the data on preoperative chemotherapy are extremely limited; however, the existing data suggest improvement in overall survival and disease-free survival with cisplatin + 5-FU, docetaxel, or etoposide in the neoadjuvant setting.[64] Sinonasal primary mucosal melanomas have shown promising results with the use of targeted therapies such as c-KIT inhibitors and immune checkpoint blockade therapies such as cytotoxic T-lymphocyte–associated protein 4 monoclonal antibodies and anti-PD1 antibodies.[65] Olfactory neuroblastomas have been shown to respond to neoadjuvant vincristine + cyclophosphamide or etoposide + ifosfamide + platinum in limited studies.[66,67] There are a large number of various subtypes of sarcomas of the sinonasal tract. Sarcomas are treated with systemic therapy along with surgery and radiation with specific chemotherapy regimens usually based on the sarcoma subtype.[68] Lymphomas also comprise a subset of sinonasal tumors, with B-cell lymphomas showing response to anthracycline-based chemotherapy plus rituximab and NK/T lymphomas showing response to pembrolizumab.[69]

CLINICAL OUTCOMES

Overall outcomes of sinonasal cancers are poor. When combining all subtypes, collectively, the 5-, 10-, and 20-year survival is 45.7%, 32.2%, and 16.4%, respectively.[8] About half of all patients with sinonasal cancer present at an advanced stage and 6% show metastatic disease at the time of presentation; however, because sinonasal cancer comprises a large variation of histologic subtypes, it is essential to take into account these specific subtypes when estimating a patient's outcome.[21]

Squamous cell carcinomas carry a poor prognosis with a 5-year and 10-year survival of 30% and 21%; prognosis is particularly poor for patients older than 50 years, black patients, and those who present with advanced stage at diagnosis.[70] Adenocarcinoma has a more favorable prognosis, with a 5-year disease-free survival of 71.2% for nonintestinal type and 69.3% for intestinal type. Worse prognoses have been associated with age 75 years or older, being African American, a paranasal sinus primary, high histologic grade, and locally advanced disease at diagnosis.[71] Adenoid cystic carcinoma has a 5-year survival of 61%, and factors associated with unfavorable outcomes include location in the frontal sinus, perineural or lymphovascular invasion, urban residency, and high-grade and advanced stage at the time of diagnosis.[72] Sinonasal mucosal melanoma has 3-, 5-, and 15-year overall survival rates of 50%, 33%, and 14.3%, with nasal cavity origin and T3 stage at diagnosis associated with a relatively better outcome.[73] Olfactory neuroblastoma has a 5-year overall survival of 69% with older age and higher grade at diagnosis associated with worse overall survival.[74] Sinonasal undifferentiated carcinomas are the most aggressive, with an overall survival at 3, 5, and 10 years of 44.3%, 34.9%, and 31.3%, respectively, and median survival of 22.1 months.[75]

SUMMARY

Sinonasal malignancies are a rare and pathologically diverse subset of head and neck cancer. Because of their anatomic location, the associated significant morbidity with involvement of surrounding critical structures and cosmetic complications, and the late-stage presentation with insidious onset of symptoms, sinonasal malignancies remain one of the most challenging malignancies to treat. They often require a multimodality approach with surgery, radiation, and chemotherapy; randomized clinical trial data are scarce and desperately needed to improve the outcomes of patients with this disease.

CLINICS CARE POINTS

- Sinonasal malignancies make up a diverse and rare subset of cancers comprising less than 1% of all malignancies.
- Risk factors include environmental and occupation exposures, living in endemic regions, and certain genetic factors.
- Sinonasal malignancies generally present at an advanced stage and have significant associated morbidity due to their anatomic location.
- Surgical resection and radiation therapy are the mainstays of treatment, but chemotherapy is often used in the neoadjuvant setting.
- Because of their rarity, there is scarce randomized clinical trial data examining specific chemotherapy regimens and timing of treatment.
- Outcomes are generally poor with 5-year overall survival of around 32%; however, this varies by histologic subtype.

DISCLOSURE

The authors have nothing to disclose.

REFERENCES

1. Lund VJ, Stammberger H, Nicolai P. European position paper on endoscopic management of tumours of the nose, paranasal sinuses and skull base. Rhinol Suppl 2010;1:1–143.
2. Turner JH, Reh DD. Incidence and survival in patients with sinonasal cancer: a historical analysis of population-based data. Head Neck 2012;34:877–85.
3. International Agency for Research on Cancer. IARC monographs on the evaluation of carcinogenic risk to humans. Arsenic, metals, fibres and dusts, Volume 100-C. Lyon, France: International Agency for Research on Cancer; 2012.
4. Cantù G, Bimbi G, Miceli R. Lymph node metastases in malignant tumors of the paranasal sinuses. Arch Otolaryngol Neck Surg 2008;134(2):170.
5. Dulguerov P, Jacobsen MS, Allal AS, et al. Nasal and paranasal sinus carcinoma: are we making progress? Cancer 2001;92:3012–29.
6. Nicolai P, Battaglia P, Bignami M. Endoscopic surgery for malignant tumors of the sinonasal tract and adjacent skull base: a 10-year experience. Am J Rhinol 2008; 22(3):308–16.
7. Wang K, Zanation AM, Chera BS. The role of radiation therapy in the management of sinonasal and ventral skull base malignancies. Otolaryngol Clin North Am 2017;50(2):419–32.
8. Gore MR. Survival in sinonasal and middle ear malignancies: a population-based study using the SEER 1973-2015 database. BMC Ear Nose Throat Disord 2018; 18:13.
9. Sanghvi S, Khan MN, Patel NR, et al. Epidemiology of sinonasal squamous cell carcinoma: A comprehensive analysis of 4994 patients. Laryngoscope 2014; 124(1):76–83.

10. Haerle SK, Gullane PJ, Witterick IJ, et al. Sinonasal carcinomas. epidemiology, pathology, and management. Neurosurg Clin N Am 2013;24(1):39–49.
11. Acheson ED. Nasal cancer in woodworkers in the furniture industry. Br Med J 1968;2(5605):587–96.
12. Acheson ED, Hadfield EH, Macbeth RG. Carcinoma of the nasal cavity and accessory sinuses in woodworkers. Lancet 1967;1(7485):311–2.
13. Roush GC. Epidemiology of cancer of the nose and paranasal sinuses: current concepts. Head Neck Surg 1979;2(1):3–11.
14. Schwaab G, Julieron M, Janot F. Epidemiology of cancers of the nasal cavities and paranasal sinuses. Neurochirurgie 1997;43(2):61–3.
15. Torjussen W, Solberg LA, Hogetveit AC. Histopathologic changes of nasal mucosa in nickel workers: a pilot study. Cancer 1979;44(3):963–74.
16. Zheng W, McLaughlin JK, Chow WH, et al. Risk factors for cancers of the nasal cavity and paranasal sinuses among white men in the United States. Am J Epidemiol 1993;138(11):965–72.
17. Luce D, Leclerc A, Morcet JF, et al. Occupational risk factors for sinonasal cancer: a case-control study in France. Am J Ind Med 1992;21(2):163–75.
18. Torjussen W. Occupational nasal cancer caused by nickel and nickel compounds. Rhinology 1985;23(2):101–5.
19. D'Errico A, Pasian S, Baratti A. A case-control study on occupational risk factors for sinonasal cancer. Occup Environ Med 2009;66(7):448–55.
20. D'Aguillo C, Kanumuri V, Khan M, et al. Demographics and survival trends in sinonasal adenocarcinoma from 1973 to 2009. IFAR 2014;4:771–6.
21. Kilic S, Samarrai R, Kilic SS, et al. Incidence and survival of sinonasal adenocarcinoma by site and histologic subtype. Acta Otolaryngol 2018;138:415–21.
22. Kuijpens J, Louwman M, Takes R, et al. Sinonasal cancer in The Netherlands: Follow-up of a population based study 1989-2014 and incidence of occupation-related adenocarcinoma. Head Neck 2018;40:2462–8.
23. Bishop JA, Guo TW, Smith DF, et al. Human papillomavirus-related carcinomas of the sinonasal tract. Am J Surg Pathol 2013;37(2):185–92.
24. Kilic S, Kilic SS, Kim ES, et al. Significance of human papillomavirus positivity in sinonasal squamous cell carcinoma. Int Forum Allergy Rhinol 2017;7:980–9.
25. Lewis JS. Sinonasal squamous cell carcinoma: a review with emphasis on emerging histologic subtypes and the role of human papillomavirus. Head Neck Pathol 2016;10:60–7.
26. Lewis JS, Westra WH, Thompson ID, et al. The sinonasal tract: another potential "hot spot" for carcinomas with transcriptionally-active human papillomavirus. Head Neck Pathol 2014;8:241–9.
27. Mayr SI, Hafizovic K, Waldfahrer F, et al. Characterization of initial clinical symptoms and risk factors for sinonasal adenocarcinomas: results of a case-control study. Int Arch Occup Environ Health 2010;83(6):631–8.
28. Siddiqui F, Smith RV, Yom SS, et al. Expert Panel on Radiation Oncology - Head and Neck Cancer. ACR appropriateness criteria® nasal cavity and paranasal sinus cancers. Head Neck 2017;39(3):407–18.
29. Das S, Kirsch CFE. Imaging of lumps and bumps in the nose: A review of sinonasal tumours. Cancer Imaging 2005;5(1):167–77.
30. Loevner LA, Sonners AI. Imaging of neoplasms of the paranasal sinuses. Neuroimaging Clin N Am 2004;14(4):625–46.
31. Jégoux F, Métreau A, Louvel G, et al. Paranasal sinus cancer. Eur Ann Otorhinolaryngol Head Neck Dis 2013;130(6):327–35.

32. Stern SJ, Goepfert H, Clayman G. Squamous cell carcinoma of the maxillary sinus. Arch Otolaryngol Head Neck Surg 1993;119(9):964–9.
33. Katz TS, Mendenhall WM, Morris CG, et al. Malignant tumors of the nasal cavity and paranasal sinuses. Head Neck 2002;24(9):821–9.
34. Cummings CW, Haughey BH, Thomas JR. Otolaryngology-head and neck surgery. 4th. St. Louis: Mosby; 2004.
35. Jansen EP, Keus RB, Hilgers FJ, et al. Does the combination of radiotherapy and debulking surgery favor survival in paranasal sinus carcinoma? Int J Radiat Oncol Biol Phys 2000;48(1):27.
36. Kraus DH, Lydiatt WM, Patel SG. In: Amin MB, editor. Nasal cavity and paranasal sinuses. American Joint Committee on Cancer. 8th. New York: Springer; 2017. p. 137.
37. Carlton DA, David Beahm D, Chiu AG. Sinonasal malignancies: Endoscopic treatment outcomes. Laryngoscope Investig Otolaryngol 2019;4(2):259–63.
38. Meccariello G, Deganello A, Choussy O. Endoscopic nasal versus open approach for the management of sinonasal adenocarcinoma: a pooled-analysis of 1826 patients. Head Neck 2016;38(S1):E2267–74.
39. Ganly I, Patel SG, Singh B. Craniofacial resection for malignant tumors involving the skull base in the elderly. Cancer 2011;117(3):563–71.
40. Higgins TS, Thorp B, Rawlings BA, et al. Outcome results of endoscopic vs craniofacial resection of sinonasal malignancies: a systematic review and pooled-data analysis. Int Forum Allergy Rhinol 2011;1(4):255–61.
41. Thorup C, Sebbesen L, Dano H, et al. Carcinoma of the nasal cavity and paranasal sinuses in Denmark 1995-2004. Acta Oncol 2010;49(3):389–94.
42. Goepfert H. The vex and fuss about nasal vestibule cancer. Head Neck 1999; 21(5):383–4.
43. Wallace A, Morris CG, Kirwan J, et al. Radiotherapy for squamous cell carcinoma of the nasal vestibule. Am J Clin Oncol 2007;30(6):612–6.
44. Bristol IJ, Ahamad A, Garden AS. Postoperative radiotherapy for maxillary sinus cancer: long-term outcomes and toxicities of treatment. Int J Radiat Oncol Biol Phys 2007;68(3):719–30.
45. Madani I, Bonte K, Vakaet L, et al. Intensity-modulated radiotherapy for sinonasal tumors: Ghent University Hospital update. Int J Radiat Oncol Biol Phys 2009;73: 424–32.
46. Daly ME, Chen AM, Bucci MK. Intensity-modulated radiation therapy for malignancies of the nasal cavity and paranasal sinuses. Int J Radiat Oncol Biol Phys 2007;67:151–7.
47. Chen AM, Daly ME, Bucci MK. Carcinomas of the paranasal sinuses and nasal cavity treated with radiotherapy at a single institution over five decades: are we making improvement? Int J Radiat Oncol Biol Phys 2007;69:141–7.
48. Monroe AT, Bhandare N, Morris CG, et al. Preventing radiation retinopathy with hyperfractionation. Int J Radiat Oncol Biol Phys 2005;61:856–64.
49. Chera BS, Malyapa R, Louis D. Proton therapy for maxillary sinus carcinoma. Am J Clin Oncol 2009;32:296–303.
50. LoRusso P, Tapazoglu E, Kish JA, et al. Chemotherapy for paranasal sinus carcinoma. A 10-year experience at Wayne state university. Cancer 1988;62:1–5.
51. Bjork-Eriksson T, Mercke C, Petruson B, et al. Potential impact on tumor control and organ preservation with cisplatin and 5-fluorouracil for patients with advanced tumors of the paranasal sinuses and nasal fossa. A prospective pilot study. Cancer 1992;70(11):2615–20.

52. Licitra L, Locati LD, Cavina R, et al. Primary chemotherapy followed by anterior craniofacial resection and radiotherapy for paranasal cancer. Ann Oncol 2003; 14(3):367–72.
53. Hanna EY, Cardenas AD, DeMonte F, et al. Induction chemotherapy for advanced squamous cell carcinoma of the paranasal sinuses. Arch Otolaryngol Head Neck Surg 2011;137(1):78.
54. Hoffmann TK. Systemic therapy strategies for head-neck carcinomas: current Status. Curr Top Otorhinolaryngol Head Neck Surg 2012;11.
55. Mierzwa ML, Nyati MK, Morgan MA, et al. Recent advances in combined modality therapy. Oncologist 2010;15(4):372–81.
56. Robin TP, Jones BL, Gordon OM, et al. A comprehensive comparative analysis of treatment modalities for sinonasal malignancies. Cancer 2017;123(16):3040–9.
57. Farrell NF, Mace JC, Detwiller KY, et al. Predictors of survival outcomes in sinonasal squamous cell carcinoma: an analysis of the National Cancer Database. Int Forum Allergy Rhinol 2021;11(6):1001–11.
58. Rosen A, Vokes EE, Scher N, et al. Locoregionally advanced paranasal sinus carcinoma. Favorable survival with multimodality therapy. Arch Otolaryngol Head Neck Surg 1993;119(7):743–6.
59. Pare A, Blanchard P, Rosellini S, et al. Outcomes of multimodal management for sinonasal squamous cell carcinoma. J Craniomaxillofac Surg 2017;45(8): 1124–32.
60. Bossi P, Perrone F, Miceli R, et al. Tp53 status as guide for the management of ethmoid sinus intestinal-type adenocarcinoma. Oral Oncol 2013;49(5):413–9.
61. Licitra L, Suardi S, Bossi P, et al. Prediction of TP53 status for primary cisplatin, fluorouracil, and leucovorin chemotherapy in ethmoid sinus intestinal-type adenocarcinoma. J Clin Oncol 2004;22(24):4901–6.
62. Reiersen DA, Pahilan ME, Devaiah AK. Meta-analysis of treatment outcomes for sinonasal undifferentiated carcinoma. Otolaryngol Head Neck Surg 2012; 147(1):7–14.
63. Musy PY, Reibel JF, Levine PA. Sinonasal undifferentiated carcinoma: the search for a better outcome. Laryngoscope 2002;112(8):1450–5.
64. Rosenthal DI, Barker JL, El-Naggar AK, et al. Sinonasal malignancies with neuroendocrine differentiation: Patterns of failure according to histologic phenotype. Cancer 2004;101(11):2567–73.
65. Ganti A, Raman A, Shay A, et al. Treatment modalities in sinonasal mucosal melanoma: A national cancer database analysis. Laryngoscope 2019;130(2): 272–82.
66. Loy AH, Reibel JF, Read PW, et al. Esthesioneuroblastoma: continued follow-up of a Single Institution's Experience. Arch Otolaryngol Head Neck Surg 2006; 132(2):134.
67. Kim BS, Vongtama R, Juillard G. Sinonasal undifferentiated carcinoma: case series and literature review. Am J Otolaryngol 2004;25(3):162–6.
68. Edmonson JH. Chemotherapeutic approaches to soft tissue sarcomas. Semin Surg Oncol 1994;10(5):357–63.
69. Peng KA, Kita AE, Suh JD, et al. Sinonasal lymphoma: case series and review of the literature: Sinonasal lymphoma. Int Forum Allergy Rhinol 2014;4:670.
70. Ansa B, Goodman M, Ward K, et al. Paranasal sinus squamous cell carcinoma incidence and survival based on surveillance, epidemiology, and end results data, 1973 to 2009. Cancer 2013;119(14):2602–10.
71. Chen MM, Roman SA, Sosa JA, et al. Predictors of survival in sinonasal adenocarcinoma. J Neurol Surg B Skull Base 2015;76(3):208–13.

72. Trope M, Triantafillou V, Kohanski MA, et al. Adenoid cystic carcinoma of the si-nonasal tract: a review of the national cancer database. Int Forum Allergy Rhinol 2019;9(4):427–34.
73. Dreno M, Georges M, Espitalier F, et al. Sinonasal mucosal melanoma: A 44-case study and literature analysis. Eur Ann Otorhinolaryngol Head Neck Dis 2017; 134(4):237–42.
74. Yin Z, Wang Y, WU Y, et al. Age distribution and age-related outcomes of olfactory neuroblastoma: a population-based analysis. Cancer Management Res 2018;10: 1359–64.
75. Chambers KJ, Lehmann AE, Remenschneider A, et al. Incidence and survival patterns of sinonasal undifferentiated carcinoma in the United States. J Neurol Surg B Skull Base 2015;76(2):94–100.
76. Papaspyrou G, Hoch S, Rinaldo A, et al. Chemotherapy and targeted therapy in adenoid cystic carcinoma of the head and neck: a review. Head Neck 2011;33(6): 905–11.
77. Eden BV, Debo RF, Larner JM, et al. Esthesioneuroblastoma. Long-term outcome and patterns of failure—the University of Virginia experience. Cancer 1994;73: 2556–62.
78. Patil VM, Joshi A, Noronha V, et al. Neoadjuvant chemotherapy in locally advanced and borderline resectable nonsquamous sinonasal tumors (esthesio-neuroblastoma and sinonasal tumor with neuroendocrine differentiation). Int J Surg Oncol 2016;2016.
79. Morand GB, Anderegg N, Vital D, et al. Outcome by treatment modality in sino-nasal undifferentiated carcinoma (SNUC): A case-series, systematic review and meta-analysis. Oral Oncol 2017;75:28–34.
80. Amit M, Abdelmeguid AS, Watcherporn T, et al. Induction chemotherapy response as a guide for treatment optimization in sinonasal undifferentiated car-cinoma. J Clin Oncol 2019;37:504–12.
81. Tyler MA, Holmes B, Patel ZM. Oncologic management of sinonasal undifferenti-ated carcinoma. Curr Opin Otolaryngol Head Neck Surg 2019;27:59–66.
82. Amit M, Tam S, Abdelmeguid AS, et al. Role of adjuvant treatment in sinonasal mucosal melanoma. J Neurol Surg B Skull Base 2017;78:512–8.
83. Kobayashi K, Matsumoto F, Miyakita Y, et al. Impact of surgical margin in skull base surgery for head and neck sarcomas. J Neurol Surg B Skull Base 2018; 79:437–44.
84. Au WY. Current management of nasal NK/T-cell lymphoma. Oncology 2010;24:4.
85. Varelas AN, Eggerstedt M, Ganti A, et al. Epidemiologic, prognostic, and treat-ment factors in sinonasal diffuse large B -cell lymphoma. Laryngoscope 2019; 129(6):1259–64.

Nasopharyngeal Carcinoma and Its Association with Epstein-Barr Virus

Harish N. Vasudevan, MD, PhD[a], Sue S. Yom, MD, PhD, MAS[b],*

KEYWORDS

- Nasopharyngeal carcinoma • Epstein-Barr virus • Cell-free DNA • Chemotherapy
- Radiation therapy

KEY POINTS

- Epstein-Barr virus is the etiologic agent responsible for endemic forms of nasopharyngeal carcinoma (NPC) and serves as a key diagnostic marker.
- In patients with NPC, the best correlations of circulating EBV DNA levels to disease burden have been found using plasma-based quantitative real-time PCR methods.
- The lack of EBV detection assay standardization has impeded progress in developing EBV DNA as a plasma biomarker in cancer.

INTRODUCTION

Nasopharyngeal carcinoma (NPC) is considered rare in most Western countries, with an overall incidence of less than 1 per 100,000 person-years, but it is an endemic disease in many other regions of the world where incidence rates can be more than 20 per 100,000 person-years.[1] In 2018, there were 129,079 new cases worldwide resulting in 72,987 deaths.[2] Countries with some of the highest incidence rates of NPC include Malaysia, Singapore, Indonesia, Vietnam, and Brunei, and regions of southern China such as Guangzhou and Hong Kong have a similar incidence. Other affected populations are found in the Middle East, Mediterranean, North Africa, and the circumpolar indigenous populations. In these higher risk populations, there can be notable ethnic and familial clustering, and numerous studies have mapped the genetic susceptibility to NPC to the HLA locus and adjacent genes in the major histocompatibility complex region of chromosome 6p21.[3] However, although this shared genetic susceptibility is responsible for the clustered incidence of this disease among endemic populations, which is likely conditioned by environmental or

[a] Department of Radiation Oncology, University of California San Francisco, Helen Diller Cancer Research Building, 1450 3rd street, HD403, San Francisco, CA 94158, USA; [b] Department of Radiation Oncology, University of California San Francisco, Precision Cancer Medicine Building, 1825 4th Street, Suite L1101, San Francisco, CA 94158, USA
* Corresponding author.
E-mail address: Sue.Yom@ucsf.edu

Hematol Oncol Clin N Am 35 (2021) 963–971
https://doi.org/10.1016/j.hoc.2021.05.007
0889-8588/21/© 2021 Elsevier Inc. All rights reserved.

other cultural factors such as diet (preserved foods containing carcinogenic nitrosamines),[4] the underlying etiologic cause of endemic-type NPC is the herpesvirus Epstein-Barr virus (EBV).

Epstein-Barr Virus and Nasopharyngeal Carcinoma

EBV is one of the world's most disseminated viruses with more than 90% individuals worldwide showing antibodies indicating prior infection. Prevention of infection, which usually occurs through transmitted bodily secretions, is not considered feasible.[5] EBV is best known as the cause of infectious mononucleosis but is also associated with several lymphoid and epithelial human cancers such as Burkitt and Hodgkin lymphomas, posttransplant lymphoproliferative disorder (PTLD), natural killer T cell lymphoma, gastric adenocarcinoma, and NPC, among others.[6] EBV is also associated with several major autoimmune and immune deficiency-related conditions.[7]

The closest association of EBV with a human malignancy is with NPC. EBV episomes are found in virtually all NPC cells with demonstration of monoclonal EBV in tumor cells, and elevated anti-EBV antibodies and free viral DNA in plasma correlate to diagnosis and tumor burden. After an initial infection, the virus establishes a latent reservoir in resting memory B lymphocytes and induces their continuous proliferation.[8] However, in contrast to the known ability of EBV to transform primary B cells and immortalize them, EBV does not transform nasopharyngeal epithelial cells into proliferative clones. Rather, latent EBV infection is a key feature of premalignant nasopharyngeal epithelial cells.[9] The latency program specific to epithelial cells results in the expression of viral genes such as EBER and EBNA1, LMP1, and LMP2A, which initiate the transformation of premalignant nasopharyngeal epithelial cells that is critical for the development of NPC. Observations of high expression of BART-microRNAs suggest their role in promoting epithelial cell survival.[10] This process is also supported by an accumulation of acquired genetic alterations in precancerous lesions. The latent and lytic gene products drive clonal expansion and are supported by stromal inflammation of the nasopharyngeal mucosa. Further genetic alterations are acquired during tumor progression and may drive growth in subclones with clinically relevant implications for recurrence or metastasis, although such relationships have yet to be fully explored.

Given the close relationship of EBV infection to the development of NPC, EBV DNA is a natural candidate to be a disease biomarker with possibilities for screening, diagnosis, and monitoring of therapeutic efficacy and minimal residual disease. EBV DNA can be found in brush biopsy samples, saliva, and the blood. However, the optimally tested specimen type and copy number thresholds that should be used as a cutoff for diagnosis have been somewhat controversial. Considering the options available using blood collection, it seems that cell-free specimens are superior to cellular specimens when using EBV DNA as a tumor marker. For instance, in a study of 57 patients with EBV-associated cancers or cancers of a type related to EBV but not EBV+, quantitative polymerase chain reaction (qPCR) from whole blood was occasionally positive when there was not EBV in the index cancer. Patients undergoing chemotherapy or with suppressed immune systems might manifest increased levels of circulating B cells with latent EBV, and thus testing including the cellular (peripheral blood mononuclear cell [PBMCs]) component could result in detectable findings that are not related to the tumor. Therefore, when collecting peripheral blood specimens, EBV DNA detected from the plasma, or what is called cell-free DNA (cfDNA), has been deemed by many to be the biomarker of choice in patients with EBV+ malignancies.[11]

DISCUSSION
Cell-Free DNA Comprises a Plasma Biomarker in Cancer

cfDNA, defined as fragmented DNA found in plasma outside a cellular compartment, offers promise for both diagnosis and surveillance in cancer. In the context of NPC, these are short viral DNA fragments that are released by the NPC tumor cells during apoptosis. In numerous settings, the potential of cfDNA to directly impact patient care and inform novel mechanistic insights into tumor evolution have been recognized.[12] Although cfDNA is observed in healthy patients and nononcologic contexts,[13] the existence of elevated cfDNA levels in patients with cancer, which can serve as a clinically significant biomarker, has been appreciated for decades.[14] Numerous technical innovations and large-scale translational studies have expanded on these early observations to define the clinical utility of cfDNA, overcoming many challenges of measuring cfDNA from primary patient samples such as low absolute cfDNA levels, short half-life in circulation, and differentiation of cancer-associated from normal cfDNA. Although absolute cfDNA levels can vary significantly between patients, levels within a patient are quite robust.

Thus cfDNA monitoring has demonstrated utility for treatment response and assessment of residual disease after definitive therapies across many disease sites. For example, cfDNA allows for monitoring of tumor dynamics in colorectal cancer,[15] breast cancer,[16] and localized lung cancer,[17] providing an alternative approach to assess residual disease status and risk stratify patients for additional therapy. In the case of virally mediated malignancies, the unique molecular signature of viral particles provides an additional layer of specificity to facilitate cfDNA analysis. As another example, in the case of human papilloma virus (HPV)-associated oropharyngeal cancer, plasma HPV levels measured via digital droplet PCR show potential value for both strain-specific diagnosis and assessment of treatment response.[18,19] Taken together, there exists a mounting preponderance of evidence supporting the use of cfDNA for clinical cancer applications particularly in the setting of virally mediated malignancies wherein tumor-associated viral sequences can generate a robust cfDNA signature.

For NPC, several studies support the use of plasma EBV DNA levels as both a prognostic and predictive biomarker.[20] However, it is critical to distinguish cancer-associated EBV from alternate causes for a detectable plasma EBV level. In that regard, it should be understood that the EBV viral load, whether tested in PBMCs or serum/plasma, is transiently elevated at the time of infection, but as a rule, healthy infected individuals have a low frequency of EBV-positive B cells in the circulation and a low viral load. On the other hand, in conditions such as PTLD, increased numbers of EBV-infected B cells and an increased number of EBV genomes in some portion of the infected B cells will result in a high viral load. EBV viremia in the plasma or serum is detected in patients with NPC or PTLD but is rarely detected in healthy infected individuals. Although the first harbinger of EBV-related PTLD is often increasing EBV DNA copies in PBMCs, EBV DNA in plasma is more specific and correlates better to disease activity.

As a tumor marker for NPC, the best evidence supports qPCR-based detection of cell-free EBV DNA in plasma as having the strongest correlation to response and prognosis.[21] This technique was first reported in 1999[22] and was subsequently confirmed as being correlated to clinical stage and, when EBV DNA values were found to be persistent or recurrent, as a biomarker of disease relapse in patients with treated disease.[23,24] This feature offers the possibility that EBV DNA assays could be used for prognostic determination at diagnosis or for minimal residual disease monitoring in the posttreatment NPC population after receiving curative intent chemoradiation.

Furthermore, recent studies have shown that levels of EBV DNA detection correlate with response to induction chemotherapy and that rapid clearance of detectable levels is associated with a favorable prognosis.[25,26] When induction is used before a curative intent program, the response to the initial chemotherapy may be important in tailoring subsequent therapy. In a study of patients with metastatic/recurrent NPC, the investigators proposed a switch of chemotherapy regimen if early clearance was not achieved.[27] Finally, EBV DNA may also have applications in decision making for surgically treated patients. In a study of patients with local recurrence of tumor, high EBV DNA levels before salvage tumor resection predicted the development of distant metastases.[28] EBV DNA thus has myriad promising clinical applications in enhancing prognostication and decision making for patients with NPC at all stages of disease.

In the following sections, we review established and novel approaches for plasma EBV DNA measurement in NPC with an emphasis on comparing next-generation sequencing to conventional PCR assays from both technical and translational perspectives. We then summarize published efforts to evaluate the utility of plasma EBV levels in NPC patient management and conclude by looking forward to the incorporation of EBV cfDNA monitoring into current clinical trial protocols and the application for NPC screening, highlighting the broader paradigm of cfDNA as a tool for cancer screening and prevention.[29]

Multiple Complementary Methods Exist to Measure Plasma Epstein-Barr Virus DNA in Patients with Nasopharyngeal Cancer

Broadly, approaches to measure plasma EBV DNA in patients with NPC comprise either PCR-based strategies to estimate viral load or leveraging of next-generation sequencing platforms to directly count viral nucleic acid fragments. Initial efforts identifying elevated plasma EBV DNA levels in patients with NPC assayed for specific EBV viral genome fragments such as the EBV nuclear antigen I (EBNA1)[30] and the *BAMHI*-W repeat region.[22] Further work confirmed that these EBV DNA fragments are indeed naked viral DNA fragments released from NPC cells consistent with cancer-associated cfDNA harboring distinct size and fragmentation characteristics.[31] The success of these PCR-based approaches led to the development of numerous parallel assays targeting additional EBV-specific viral genome regions such as the *Pol-1* and *LM-2* genes, motivating efforts to systematically compare different PCR-based assays and establish a consensus approach to EBV plasma DNA measurement.[32] Although such a consensus remains elusive, direct comparisons of these different PCR assays revealed concordance across methods. Evaluation of *Pol-1*, *BAMHI*-W, and *LMP2* assays suggested that all 3 assays reliably detect plasma EBV DNA levels with highest concentrations from the *BAMHI*-W assay,[33] and additional work showed increased sensitivity with *BAMHI*-W PCR compared with *LMP2* measurement likely due to variable amplification of the *BAMHI*-W repetitive domain.[34]

Nevertheless, in clinical practice, the lack of a standardized EBV DNA assay is a continuing barrier to use. The sensitivity of detection depends on the performance characteristics of the specific test, which may depend on the assay design, procedures, extraction method, and cutoff values. For example, in a survey of 15 tests, sensitivities were reported ranging from 53% to 96%.[35] At present, in Asia, many of the centers that have used EBV DNA assessment in their clinical processes tend to favor qPCR targeting the *BAMHI*-W region of the EBV genome.[24] A large-scale harmonization effort carried out by the NRG Oncology cooperative group was thus developed around a *BAMHI*-W assay to be used at laboratories in Asia and the United States for the purposes of the clinical trial NRG-HN001.[36] Nonetheless, it remains the case that there are numerous other qPCR methods in use for EBV DNA detection, and these vary widely in their target and test characteristics.[37] In sum, PCR-based measurement of plasma EBV DNA remains the standard of care for patients with NPC, and future efforts will likely require continued multi-institutional collaboration to establish a common approach within the prospective clinical trial framework.

Although PCR-based EBV assays remain the standard of care at many institutions, such approaches suffer from numerous shortcomings, motivating emerging development of novel methods leveraging high-throughput sequencing.[38] As noted earlier, high technical variability both across and between PCR assays remains a challenge, including differences between assays based on amplicon size, relative quantification estimates (which inform delineation of a threshold for a positive result), and variability in standards used for PCR calibration, all of which affect key assay characteristics such as sensitivity, specificity, and limit of detection.

In that regard, next-generation sequencing offers numerous advantages for detection of tumor-associated viral DNA. First, sequencing-based approaches provide information regarding the EBV DNA sequence itself, which would help both better differentiate EBV of NPC origin and identify viral DNA motifs with prognostic or predictive significance. Second, sequencing provides a measure of DNA size, which provides another method to stratify tumor-derived EBV fragments from nontumor EBV DNA. Third, PCR-based assays depend on an intact target amplicon region within the viral genome, whereas sequencing-based approaches permit quantification of any EBV DNA fragments mapping to the viral genome. Finally, whereas the lower detection limit of the *BAM*HI-W assay is 20 EBV genomes per milliliter of plasma,[22,39] sequencing-based assays can theoretically lower this detection limit both by more sensitive detection of absolute EBV DNA abundance and integrating information regarding sequence content and fragment size, providing a greater dynamic range to improve target sensitivity and specificity.

Indeed, an early report applying a targeted next-generation sequencing approach to plasma EBV detection in NPC demonstrated distinct molecular characteristics and size profiles for NPC-associated EBV DNA when compared with non-NPC EBV DNA.[38] Building on this approach, identification of specific EBV single-nucleotide variants (SNVs) in patients with NPC led to the construction of a sequence-based NPC risk score associated with clinical outcomes,[40] underscoring the potential for novel biological insights from sequencing-based methods. In addition to DNA sequencing, whole-genome methylation analysis demonstrated disease-specific EBV epigenetic profiles between patients with NPC, lymphoma, and mononucleosis, and integration of both DNA sequencing and methylation profiling improved the positive predictive value of plasma EBV DNA-based NPC screening in an endemic population.[41] Future efforts to expand this analysis to larger cohorts, incorporate additional genomic methods, and develop novel, complementary approaches to plasma EBV DNA detection remain areas of needed investigation.

Serum Epstein-Barr Virus DNA Monitoring in Nasopharyngeal Carcinoma Demonstrates Predictive and Prognostic Utility Leveraged in Ongoing Clinical Trial Design

Technical innovation and standardization of plasma EBV DNA detection in NPC is motivated by its now well-established prognostic significance and clinical utility. Early studies demonstrated the utility of plasma EBV DNA to risk stratify patients with additional precision beyond traditional clinical staging criteria.[42,43] Building on these findings, investigation of the relationship between posttreatment plasma EBV and clinical outcome showed that postchemoradiation plasma EBV DNA levels stratify patients with NPC into clinically significant prognostic subgroups,[44] and moreover, plasma EBV DNA levels also carry prognostic significance after induction chemotherapy,[26] thus providing an additional tool to guide patient management within this treatment paradigm. More recently, posttreatment plasma EBV DNA has been associated with metastatic progression,[45] and there is support for the utility of plasma EBV DNA levels for prognostication in the metastatic setting.[46] In summary, despite continually evolving prospective data evaluating the relationship between plasma EBV DNA levels and NPC prognosis for various complex clinical scenarios, postchemoradiation plasma EBV DNA levels appear to be a robust prognostic biomarker to guide clinical decision making following upfront therapy for patients with NPC.

Given these observations, ongoing clinical trials are now directly incorporating plasma EBV DNA levels into study design. One example, NRG-HN001 (https://clinicaltrials.gov/ct2/show/NCT02135042), incorporates the testing of plasma EBV DNA levels to risk stratify patients following definitive chemoradiation. The trial simultaneously explores the merits of both treatment intensification in patients with detectable postchemoradiation EBV levels randomized to gemcitabine and paclitaxel versus cisplatin and 5-fluorouracil (5-FU) versus treatment deintensification in patients with undetectable postchemoradiation EBV levels randomized to cisplatin and 5-FU versus observation in this lower-risk subgroup. The primary outcome in the treatment ceintensification comparison is noninferior overall survival, whereas that in the treatment intensification subgroup is superior progression-free survival, again highlighting the dual prognostic utility of plasma EBV DNA levels. However, it should be noted that another previous randomized controlled trial in Hong Kong, NPC-0502, found no survival differences or decreases in distant metastasis resulting from additional gemcitabine-cisplatin chemotherapy for high-risk patients having detectable EBV DNA after conclusion of chemoradiation.[44]

SUMMARY
Future Directions for Epstein-Barr Virus as a Biomarker in Nasopharyngeal Carcinoma

Despite considerable technical and translational progress in establishing the utility of EBV DNA as a clinically significant biomarker in NPC, numerous additional areas remain ripe for investigation. First, does next-generation sequencing yield clinically actionable insights beyond conventional PCR? The question of whether certain EBV strains are preferentially selected in malignancies has not easily been resolved.[47] Such a query could be approached both from the perspective of population-level screening, which is of particular public health importance in regions with high NPC prevalence, and with regard to prognostic and predictive utility for patients with confirmed NPC. Indeed, as discussed earlier, early returns suggest that multiplatform genomic approaches do indeed improve diagnostic parameters and provide additional translational information such as prognostic SNVs, methylation profiles, and EBV genomic size/fragmentation patterns. Second, is plasma the uniquely preferred biospecimen for determination of EBV in NPC? Numerous studies suggest that transoral brush biopsies provide sufficient material for EBV detection for certain clinical scenarios,[48,49] underscoring parallels to HPV-associated oropharyngeal cancer where genomic analysis of saliva and plasma both seem to represent viable diagnostic avenues.[50] In any case and perhaps most importantly, despite admirable advancements in the scientific understanding of EBV pathogenesis in NPC and numerous large-scale clinical-translational efforts, a continuing lack of standardized methods for EBV DNA measurement procedures in NPC precludes the type of prospective multi-institutional efforts needed to both validate published PCR-based findings or rapidly translate novel next-generation sequencing-based approaches to the clinic to impact the maximal number of patients.

CLINICS CARE POINTS

- EBV testing should be considered in patients with a diagnosis of nasopharyngeal carcinoma.
- Longitudinal tracking of plasma EBV in patients with NPC pre- and post-treatment can guide evaluation of treatment response.
- PCR-based EBV testing remains the standard of care for plasma-based diagnostic evaluation.

DISCLOSURE

H.N. Vasudevan: none; S.S. Yom: research grants from Genentech, Merck, Bristol-Myers Squibb, and BioMimetix.

REFERENCES

1. Mahdavifar N, Ghoncheh M, Mohammadian-Hafshejani A, et al. Epidemiology and inequality in the incidence and mortality of nasopharynx cancer in Asia. Osong Public Heal Res Perspect 2016;7(6):360–72.
2. Bray F, Ferlay J, Soerjomataram I, et al. Global cancer statistics 2018: GLOBO-CAN estimates of incidence and mortality worldwide for 36 cancers in 185 countries. CA Cancer J Clin 2018;68(6):394–424.
3. Ning L, Ko JMY, Yu VZ, et al. Nasopharyngeal carcinoma MHC region deep sequencing identifies HLA and novel non-HLA TRIM31 and TRIM39 loci. Commun Biol 2020;3(1):1–13.
4. Zheng YM, Tuppin P, Hubert A, et al. Environmental and dietary risk factors for nasopharyngeal carcinoma: A case-control study in Zangwu County, Guangxi, China. Br J Cancer 1994;69(3):508–14.
5. Niedobitek G, Meruand N, Delecluse HJ. Epstein-Barr virus infection and human malignancies. Int J Exp Pathol 2001;82(3):149–70.
6. Young LS, Rickinson AB. Epstein-Barr virus: 40 Years on. Nat Rev Cancer 2004; 4(10):757–68.
7. Capone G, Fasano C, Lucchese G, et al. EBV-associated cancer and autoimmunity: Searching for therapies. Vaccines 2015;3(1):74–89.
8. Mrozek-Gorska P, Buschle A, Pich D, et al. Epstein–Barr virus reprograms human B lymphocytes immediately in the prelatent phase of infection. Proc Natl Acad Sci U S A 2019;116(32):16046–55.
9. Tsao SW, Tsang CM, Lo KW. Epstein-barr virus infection and nasopharyngeal carcinoma. Philos Trans R Soc B Biol Sci 2017;372(1732). https://doi.org/10.1098/rstb.2016.0270.
10. Kang D, Skalsky RL, Cullen BR. EBV BART MicroRNAs target multiple pro-apoptotic cellular genes to promote epithelial cell survival. PLoS Pathog 2015; 11(6):e1004979.
11. Tsai DE, Luskin MR, Kremer BE, et al. A pilot trial of quantitative Epstein-Barr virus polymerase chain reaction in patients undergoing treatment for their malignancy: Potential use of Epstein-Barr virus polymerase chain reaction in multiple cancer types. Leuk Lymphoma 2015;56(5):1530–2.
12. Corcoran RB, Chabner BA. Application of Cell-free DNA Analysis to Cancer Treatment. N Engl J Med 2018;379(18):1754–65.
13. Madnel P, Metais P. Nuclear acids in human blood plasma. C R Seances Soc Biol Fil 1948;142(3–4):241–3.

14. Leon SA, Shapiro B, Sklaroff DM, et al. Free DNA in the serum of cancer patients and the effect of therapy - PubMed. Cancer Res 1977;37(3):646–50.
15. Diehl F, Schmidt K, Choti MA, et al. Circulating mutant DNA to assess tumor dynamics. Nat Med 2008;14(9):985–90.
16. Garcia-Murillas I, Schiavon G, Weigelt B, et al. Mutation tracking in circulating tumor DNA predicts relapse in early breast cancer. Sci Transl Med 2015;7(302):302ra133.
17. Chaudhuri AA, Chabon JJ, Lovejoy AF, et al. Early detection of molecular residual disease in localized lung cancer by circulating tumor DNA profiling. Cancer Discov 2017;7(12):1394–403.
18. Chera BS, Kumar S, Beaty BT, et al. Rapid clearance profile of plasma circulating tumor HPV type 16 DNA during chemoradiotherapy correlates with disease control in HPV-associated oropharyngeal cancer. Clin Cancer Res 2019;25(15):4682–90.
19. Hanna GJ, Supplee JG, Kuang Y, et al. Plasma HPV cell-free DNA monitoring in advanced HPV-associated oropharyngeal cancer. Ann Oncol 2018;29(9):1980–6.
20. Chua MLK, Wee JTS, Hui EP, et al. Nasopharyngeal carcinoma. Lancet 2016; 387(10022):1012–24.
21. Abusalah MAH, Gan SH, Al-hatamleh MAI, et al. Recent advances in diagnostic approaches for epstein–barr virus. Pathogens 2020;9(3). https://doi.org/10.3390/pathogens9030226.
22. Lo YM, Chan LY, Lo KW, et al. Quantitative analysis of cell-free Epstein-Barr virus DNA in plasma of patients with nasopharyngeal carcinoma. Cancer Res 1999; 59(6):1188–91.
23. Allen Chan KC. Plasma Epstein-Barr virus DNA as a biomarker for nasopharyngeal carcinoma. Chin J Cancer 2014;33(12):598–603.
24. Lin J-C, Wang W-Y, Chen KY, et al. Quantification of plasma epstein–barr virus dna in patients with advanced nasopharyngeal carcinoma. N Engl J Med 2004; 350(24):2461–70.
25. Liu LT, Tang LQ, Chen QY, et al. The prognostic value of plasma Epstein-Barr viral DNA and tumor response to neoadjuvant chemotherapy in advanced-stage nasopharyngeal carcinoma. Int J Radiat Oncol Biol Phys 2015;93(4):862–9.
26. Huang CL, Sun ZQ, Guo R, et al. Plasma Epstein-Barr Virus DNA Load After Induction Chemotherapy Predicts Outcome in Locoregionally Advanced Nasopharyngeal Carcinoma. Int J Radiat Oncol Biol Phys 2019;104(2):355–61.
27. Wang WY, Twu CW, Chen HH, et al. Plasma EBV DNA clearance rate as a novel prognostic marker for metastatic/recurrent nasopharyngeal carcinoma. Clin Cancer Res 2010;16(3):1016–24.
28. Chan JYW, Wong STS. The role of plasma Epstein-Barr virus DNA in the management of recurrent nasopharyngeal carcinoma. Laryngoscope 2014;124(1):126–30.
29. Cohen JD, Li L, Wang Y, et al. Detection and localization of surgically resectable cancers with a multi-analyte blood test. Science 2018;359(6378):926–30.
30. Mutirangura A, Pornthanakasem W, Theamboonlers A, et al. Epstein-Barr viral DNA in serum of patients with nasopharyngeal carcinoma. Clin Cancer Res 1998;4(3):665–9.
31. Chan KCA, Zhang J, Chan ATC, et al. Molecular characterization of circulating EBV DNA in the plasma of nasopharyngeal carcinoma and lymphoma patients. Cancer Res 2003;63(9):2028–32.
32. Kim KY, Le QT, Yom SS, et al. Current state of PCR-based Epstein-barr virus DNA testing for nasopharyngeal cancer. J Natl Cancer Inst 2017;109(4):1–7.
33. Le QT, Jones CD, Yau TK, et al. A comparison study of different PCR assays in measuring circulating plasma Epstein-Barr virus DNA levels in patients with nasopharyngeal carcinoma. Clin Cancer Res 2005;11(16):5700–7.

34. Sanosyan A, Fayd'herbe de Maudave A, Bollore K, et al. The impact of targeting repetitive BamHI-W sequences on the sensitivity and precision of EBV DNA quantification. PLoS One 2017;12(8):e0183856.

35. Fung SYH, Lam JWK, Chan KCA. Clinical utility of circulating Epstein-Barr virus DNA analysis for the management of nasopharyngeal carcinoma. Chin Clin Oncol 2016;5(2). https://doi.org/10.21037/cco.2016.03.07.

36. Le QT, Zhang Q, Cao H, et al. An international collaboration to harmonize the quantitative plasma Epstein-Barr virus DNA assay for future biomarker-guided trials in nasopharyngeal carcinoma. Clin Cancer Res 2013;19(8):2208–15.

37. Hayden RT, Hokanson KM, Pounds SB, et al. Multicenter comparison of different real-time PCR assays for quantitative detection of Epstein-Barr virus. J Clin Microbiol 2008;46(1):157–63.

38. Lam WKJ, Jiang P, Chan KCA, et al. Sequencing-based counting and size profiling of plasma Epstein–Barr virus DNA enhance population screening of nasopharyngeal carcinoma. Proc Natl Acad Sci U S A 2018;115(22):E5115–24.

39. Chan KCA, Woo JKS, King A, et al. Analysis of plasma Epstein–Barr virus DNA to screen for nasopharyngeal cancer. N Engl J Med 2017;377(6):513–22.

40. Lam WKJ, Ji L, Tse OYO, et al. Sequencing analysis of plasma epstein-barr virus dna reveals nasopharyngeal carcinoma-associated single nucleotide variant profiles. Clin Chem 2020;66(4):598–605.

41. Lam WKJ, Jiang P, Chan KCA, et al. Methylation analysis of plasma DNA informs etiologies of Epstein-Barr virus-associated diseases. Nat Commun 2019; 10(1):1–11.

42. Hui EP, Li WF, Ma BB, et al. Integrating postradiotherapy plasma Epstein–Barr virus DNA and TNM stage for risk stratification of nasopharyngeal carcinoma to adjuvant therapy. Ann Oncol 2020;31(6):769–79.

43. Leung SF, Zee B, Ma BB, et al. Plasma Epstein-Barr viral deoxyribonucleic acid quantitation complements tumor-node-metastasis staging prognostication in nasopharyngeal carcinoma. J Clin Oncol 2006;24(34):5414–8.

44. Chan ATC, Hui EP, Ngan RKC, et al. Analysis of plasma Epstein-Barr virus DNA in nasopharyngeal cancer after chemoradiation to identify high-risk patients for adjuvant chemotherapy: A randomized controlled trial. J Clin Oncol 2018; 36(31):3091–100.

45. Chen FP, Huang XD, Lv JW, et al. Prognostic potential of liquid biopsy tracking in the posttreatment surveillance of patients with nonmetastatic nasopharyngeal carcinoma. Cancer 2020;126(10):2163–73.

46. An X, Wang FH, Ding PR, et al. Plasma Epstein-Barr virus DNA level strongly predicts survival in metastatic/recurrent nasopharyngeal carcinoma treated with palliative chemotherapy. Cancer 2011;117(16):3750–7.

47. Chang CM, Yu KJ, Mbulaiteye SM, et al. The extent of genetic diversity of Epstein-Barr virus and its geographic and disease patterns: A need for reappraisal. Virus Res 2009;143(2):209–21.

48. Lam JWK, Chan JYW, Ho WK, et al. Use of transoral nasopharyngeal brush biopsy for Epstein-Barr virus DNA detection of local recurrence of nasopharyngeal carcinoma after radiotherapy. Head Neck 2016;38:E1301–4.

49. Ng RHW, Ngan R, Wei WI, et al. Trans-oral brush biopsies and quantitative PCR for EBV DNA detection and screening of nasopharyngeal carcinoma. Otolaryngol Head Neck Surg 2014;150(4):602–9.

50. Wang Y, Springer S, Mulvey CL, et al. Detection of somatic mutations and HPV in the saliva and plasma of patients with head and neck squamous cell carcinomas. Sci Transl Med 2015;7(293):293ra104.

Salivary Gland Cancers

Vatche Tchekmedyian, MD, MEd

KEYWORDS

- Acinic cell carcinoma • Adenoid cystic carcinoma • Mucoepidermoid carcinoma
- Salivary duct carcinoma • Salivary gland carcinoma

KEY POINTS

- Salivary gland tumors are a heterogeneous group of malignancies with variable underlying biology and clinical behavior.
- Surgery is the cornerstone of management in the early stage setting. While the role of adjuvant radiation is well delineated, the addition of chemotherapy to radiation remains an unanswered clinical question.
- Biologically rationale systemic therapies targeting androgen signaling, HER2, and TRK have become an important component of treatment of salivary gland tumors in the recurrent/metastatic setting.

INTRODUCTION

Salivary gland tumors arise from the major (parotid, submandibular, sublingual glands) and minor salivary glands scattered through the upper aerodigestive tract. These malignancies are heterogeneous with variable underlying biology and clinical behavior. Given the rarity and heterogeneity of these tumors, therapeutic trials are challenging to perform and interpret. Many clinical trials in salivary gland cancers include all histologic subtypes, making efficacy in specific tumor types difficult to delineate.[1] Despite these difficulties, there have been significant steps forward in recent years in the biological understanding, molecular characterization, and therapeutic implications for several salivary gland cancers.

In this review, the author summarize a general approach to the definitive management of salivary cancers and reviews the distinct biology and treatment implications for the major histologic subtypes in recurrent/metastatic settings.

SALIVARY GLAND HISTOLOGY AND CELL OF ORIGIN

Salivary glands are exocrine glands comprising microscopic units called acini. Acini are the secretory units that produce serous fluid or mucous. Fluid is secreted into intercalated ducts leading to striated ducts, propelled by surrounding myoepithelial cells. Each component of this cellular machinery and architecture had malignant potential, including

Tufts University School of Medicine, MaineHealth Cancer Care, 265 Western Avenue, Suite 2, South Portland, ME 04106, USA
E-mail address: vtchekmedy@mmc.org

Hematol Oncol Clin N Am 35 (2021) 973–990
https://doi.org/10.1016/j.hoc.2021.05.011
0889-8588/21/© 2021 Elsevier Inc. All rights reserved.

the luminal (acinar and ductal) and the abluminal (myoepithelial and basal) components, thus making up the heterogeneous nature of salivary gland cancers.

There are over 20 distinct histopathologic malignant salivary gland tumors, according to the World Health Organization Classification of Salivary Gland Malignancies (**Box 1**).[2] Careful pathologic assessment is extremely important in establishing the correct histologic diagnosis and informing additional molecular testing.

EPIDEMIOLOGY

There has been an increase in the incidence of salivary gland tumors in the United States over time.[3] In the United States, salivary gland cancers made up 6.3% of head and neck cancers from 1974 to 1975 and 8.1% of all head and neck cancers from 1998 to 1999.[4] An analysis of the Surveillance, Epidemiology, and End Results (SEER) Database revealed the incidence of major salivary gland cancer increased from 10.4 per million in 1973 to 16 per million in 2009.[3] This increase was largely driven by increased detection of small (<2 cm) tumors, possibly due to widespread use and improvements in diagnostic imaging technology.[3,5]

Population-based studies demonstrate that approximately 65% to 86% of all salivary gland tumors are benign.[6–9] The most common site for salivary gland tumors is the parotid, followed by the submandibular gland and then the sublingual gland.

Box 1
WHO classification of malignant salivary gland tumors

Mucoepidermoid Carcinoma

Adenoid Cystic Carcinoma

Acinic Cell Carcinoma

Adenocarcinoma, Not Otherwise Specified (NOS)

Salivary Duct Carcinoma

Carcinoma ex Pleomorphic Adenoma

Secretory Carcinoma

Intraductal Carcinoma

Myoepithelial Carcinoma

Epithelial-Myoepithelial Carcinoma

Polymorphous Adenocarcinoma

Clear Cell Carcinoma

Basal Cell Carcinoma

Sebaceous Adenocarcinoma

Carcinosarcoma

Poorly Differentiated Carcinoma (undifferentiated carcinoma, large cell, and small cell neuroendocrine carcinoma)

Lymphoepithelial Carcinoma

Squamous Cell Carcinoma

Oncocytic Carcinoma

From El-Naggar AK, Chan JKC, Grandis JR et al. (eds). No Title. In: Tumours of Salivary Glands. WHO Classification of Head and Neck Tumours (Ed 4). Lyon, France; 2017:159.

Generally, the potential for malignancy increases as the size of the gland decreases—approximately 15% to 25% of parotid tumors are malignant, a rate that rises to 40% of submandibular tumors and 90% of sublingual tumors. Approximately 40% of minor salivary gland tumors are malignant.[10] Despite this, given its size, the parotid gland is still the most common site to develop a malignant salivary tumor.

The most common malignant tumor is mucoepidermoid carcinoma, accounting for greater than 50% of malignant salivary gland tumors, followed by adenoid cystic carcinoma (ACC) and by adenocarcinoma not otherwise specified (NOS).[9,11,12] True primary squamous cell carcinomas of the salivary glands are rare and more often represent intraparotid metastases from other primary sites, including skin or the upper aerodigestive tract. ACC is the most common distant metastatic tumor, accounting for 37% of cases, followed by adenocarcinoma NOS (14%), mucoepidermoid carcinoma (12%), salivary duct carcinoma (12%), and carcinoma ex pleomorphic adenoma (11%).[13]

While clear epidemiologic risk factors for salivary malignancies do not exist, it was recently demonstrated that approximately one-third of patients with recurrent/metastatic ACC were found to carry at least 1 pathogenic germline mutation, highlighting the importance of accurate family history and considering genetic counseling and germline testing in this patient population.[14]

APPROACH TO LOCAL/REGIONAL DISEASE FOR SALIVARY TUMORS

Clinics care points

- Surgery is the cornerstone of curative management, and radiation can be considered based on pathologic risk factors.
- The utility of adjuvant chemotherapy plus radiation is of uncertain benefit.
- Adjuvant androgen deprivation and human epidermal growth factor receptor 2 (HER2)-targeted therapies are active research areas in non-ACC subtypes.

Definitive Management

Surgical resection is widely favored for initial management of locally or regionally advanced salivary gland cancer irrespective of histologic subtype. Neck dissection is recommended for clinical nodal positivity, though elective neck dissection for a clinically node-negative neck is more controversial. There is a relatively high rate of occult nodal involvement in a clinically node-negative neck (ranging from 12%-45%), and occult nodal involvement is associated with large ($\geq$ 4 cm) and high-grade primary tumors.[15,16] If radiation is planned, there is less benefit to elective node dissection.[17] In the inoperable setting, definitive radiation or concurrent chemotherapy and radiation may be offered.[18–20]

Adjuvant Therapy

Adjuvant radiation therapy is typically offered in the setting of high-grade lesions, advanced T and N stages, positive margins, and perineural invasion or lymphovascular invasion. Data supporting the use of adjuvant therapy is primarily retrospective, showing an association with improved survival in these high-risk patients.[21]

In the absence of definitive data, combined modality adjuvant therapy with chemotherapy and radiation is an area of controversy, and management is extrapolated from the larger body of evidence from head and neck squamous cell carcinoma.

Retrospective studies of adjuvant therapies in salivary gland malignancies have provided mixed data. An analysis of 2210 patients from the National Cancer Database found inferior 2-year and 5-year overall survival with combined adjuvant chemotherapy plus radiotherapy versus radiotherapy alone, even when controlling for age, comorbidities, T and N stage, margin status, and histologic type.[22] Similar results were seen in an analysis of 741 elderly patients with salivary cancers from the SEER database.[23]

While these data suggest no benefit and possibly a detriment to the addition of chemotherapy to radiotherapy in the adjuvant setting for malignant salivary gland cancers, there are several caveats. Only a small fraction of patients in each study received concurrent adjuvant chemotherapy and radiation, indicating an inherent selection bias toward the highest-risk patients. This risk may not be completely controlled for by statistical means. Additionally, no information is provided about the choice of agent, dosing, or the number of cycles of chemotherapy received. Smaller single-institution studies have shown both feasibility and efficacy of adjuvant concurrent chemotherapy and radiation.[20,24] The National Comprehensive Cancer Network (NCCN) guidelines list a category 2B recommendation for systemic therapy plus radiation in the adjuvant setting.[25] It is clear that prospective study is needed to address this question.

The Radiation Therapy Oncology Group (RTOG) 1008 trial is a multi-institutional randomized phase III trial of radiation alone (60–66 Gy in 2-Gy daily fractions) versus radiation with concurrent weekly cisplatin in high-risk resected salivary tumors, including pathologic T3–T4 or N1–N3, or T1–2N0 with a close ($\leq$1 mm) or positive margin (NCT01220583). This trial recently reached accrual, and the results are eagerly anticipated to guide decision-making in the adjuvant setting.

Role of Neutrons

A previous collaborative trial between the RTOG and Medical Research Council in Great Britain randomized patients with inoperable or recurrent major or minor salivary tumors to receive either conventional photon and/or electron radiotherapy versus fast neutron radiotherapy.[26] Thirty-two patients were randomized, and the study showed improved local/regional control in the neutron arm (85% vs 33% complete response rate). Criticisms of this study include the small sample size and imbalance of major clinical factors (unresectable vs recurrent) between trial arms. The two-year survival rate was 62% for neutrons and 25% for photons without a statistically significant difference at 10 years.[27] Given concerns over greater long-term toxicity as well as for practical reasons (there is currently only a single neutron site in the United States), neutrons have largely fallen out of favor.

Proton beam radiation therapy is a promising avenue for reducing radiation toxicity in the primary or adjuvant treatment of salivary gland cancers, though further prospective data are needed.[28]

Special Considerations

Some specific adjuvant therapy circumstances warrant further elaboration. Given the predilection of ACC for neurotropic spread and local recurrence, adjuvant radiation is routinely recommended. With surgery alone, local failure rates of parotid ACCs approximate 50%.[29] The addition of adjuvant radiation improves local control in over 90% of cases.[30] This practice is supported by several retrospective studies of postoperative radiotherapy demonstrating an improvement in local recurrence-free survival for ACC, although the effect on overall survival has not been as clearly elucidated.[31-33] The radiation field often includes the neural pathways to the skull base, which can lead to radiographic findings that are difficult to distinguish from recurrent perineural disease.

Salivary duct carcinomas are characterized by a near-universal expression of the androgen receptor (AR). Adjuvant endocrine therapy with androgen deprivation therapy (ADT) using a luteinizing hormone-releasing hormone agonist or bicalutamide is an active area of research. In one retrospective cohort study of patients with high-risk (stage IVa) resected AR expressing salivary duct carcinomas, 22 patients received adjuvant ADT (ranging from 1–5 years) and were compared with 111 patients in the control arm. ADT use was associated with a longer 3-year disease-free survival, at 48.2% and 27.7%, respectively (P = .037).[34] Case reports have evaluated the use of external beam radiotherapy with ADT in the definitive treatment setting along a paradigm similar to high-risk prostate cancer.[35] While not standard of care, these avenues provide consideration for oncologists treating high-risk salivary duct carcinomas or other AR-positive salivary gland cancers.

Approximately another one-third of salivary duct carcinomas have amplification of HER2.[36,37] Retrospective data of small cohorts and case series have examined the use of trastuzumab in the adjuvant setting.[38,39] In one such study, 8 patients were treated with adjuvant carboplatin, paclitaxel, and trastuzumab with concurrent radiation in the adjuvant setting followed by 1 year of adjuvant trastuzumab.[38] In this analysis, 63% of patients (5/8) were disease-free more than 2 years after treatment.[38] An ongoing clinical trial is evaluating postoperative adjuvant ado-trastuzumab emtansine (T-DM1) in HER2-positive salivary gland cancer (NCT04620187).

APPROACH TO RECURRENT/METASTATIC DISEASE

Clinics care points

- Low-grade, asymptomatic recurrent/metastatic salivary gland tumors such as ACC, mucoepidermoid carcinoma, and acinic cell carcinoma (AciCC) may undergo surveillance.

- Lenvatinib can be considered for patients with progressive ACC requiring therapy.

- Salivary duct carcinoma and other high-grade tumors require immediate therapy.

- Evaluation for AR expression and HER2 amplification and other potentially actionable genetic alterations (ALK, RET, BRAF) is important in determining systemic therapy options for non-ACC salivary gland carcinoma.

- Salivary secretory carcinoma is characterized by a translocation involving ETV6 and NTRK3, which is highly sensitive to TRK inhibition.

- There is currently no standard role for immunotherapy in the treatment of recurrent salivary gland cancers.

ADENOID CYSTIC CARCINOMA

ACCs account for the largest share of salivary gland cancers leading to distant metastatic disease. Treatment failures occur in 36% to 62% of cases, with a distant failure rate of 29% to 38%.[40,41] Risk of failure increases with perineural invasion of large nerves as well as solid histology at more advanced initial stages.[41,42]

In the setting of metastatic disease, the median duration of survival is approximately 3 years, though 10% of patients have survival of more than 10 years.[40] Lung-only metastatic disease (accounting for 67% of metastases) portends an improved prognosis compared with other distant metastatic sites such as liver and bone.[41–43]

Approximately 50% of ACCs are characterized by a t(6;9)(q22-23;p23-24) translocation that conjoins the transcription factors MYB and NFIB.[44–46] MYB overexpression is thought to play a key oncogenic role in the pathogenesis of ACC through the dysregulation of several target genes mediating apoptosis, cell cycle control, and cell growth/angiogenesis but is not directly actionable.[44]

For local/regional recurrences or solitary sites of symptomatic disease, local therapies including radiation, surgery, or ablative therapies can be considered.[47] Systemic therapy is indicated for symptomatic locally recurrent or metastatic disease that is no longer amenable to local therapies and for multifocal progressive ACC.[47] Most patients with metastatic ACC can undergo surveillance imaging without requiring upfront systemic therapy.

Chemotherapy

ACC is traditionally thought of as a chemo-resistant disease; however, in patients with progressive disease not amenable to surgery or radiation, there is a role for traditional cytotoxic chemotherapy. Vinorelbine and mitoxantrone have favorable toxicity profiles with disease stabilization and objective responses measured on prospective clinical trials and are reasonable therapeutic options.[48,49] Epirubicin and cisplatin also have single-agent activity but with greater toxicity.[50–52] Combination regimens including cisplatin/vinorelbine and cyclophosphamide, doxorubicin, and cisplatin have increased activity, albeit at the cost of increased toxicity, and can be considered in fit, symptomatic patients.[53–56] Paclitaxel and gemcitabine have limited activity based on prospective study and are not recommended.[56,57]

Tyrosine Kinase Inhibitors

Several tyrosine kinase inhibitors have been trialed singly in trials for ACC, including sunitinib,[58] sorafenib,[59,60] axitinib,[61] dasatinib,[62] regorafenib,[63] and dovitinib,[64,65] with mostly disappointing results, with response rates ranging from 0% to 11%. Given that greater than 90% of ACCs have c-kit expression,[66] the c-kit inhibitor imatinib was trialed without any objective responses.[67]

Lenvatinib is an oral multitargeted TKI with significant inhibitory activity against the vascular endothelial growth factor receptors 1 to 3, fibroblast growth factor receptors (FGFRs) 1 to 3, KIT, platelet-derived growth factor receptors alpha and beta, and RET.[68–72] Lenvatinib was shown in 2 studies to have activity in ACC, with response rates of 12% to 15%, with a larger fraction of patients who had significant reductions in tumor size that did not meet criteria for a major response.[73,74] In the context of this data, lenvatinib has an NCCN grade 2b recommendation for progressive, recurrent, or metastatic ACC.[25] Toxicities can be significant, with a 63% rate of grade III or IV toxicity, most commonly hypertension, and less commonly hemorrhage, cardiac dysfunction, fistula formation, acute coronary syndrome, and posterior reversible leukoencephalopathy syndrome.[73] In a carefully selected patient population, lenvatinib may have a role in the palliative management of ACC.

NOTCH

Activating *NOTCH* mutations are present in approximately 20% of ACC and are associated with a more aggressive disease course.[75] This population has high rates of bone and liver metastases and a poorer prognosis.[75] In preliminary results from the ACCURACY trial, an open-label, multicenter study of AL101—a small molecule selective gamma-secretase inhibitor—showed early disease activity with a response rate of 15% in this patient population.[76] This represents the first recurring targetable genetic alteration in ACC.

Epigenetic Modifiers

Recurrent mutations in genes regulating chromatin remodeling, including those involved in histone acetyltransferase/deacetylase activity and histone methyltransferase/

demethylase function, have been identified in sequencing studies of ACC.[45] A phase 2 study of the oral small molecule histone deacetylase inhibitor vorinostat showed a partial response rate of 7% (2/30) by RECIST, though 66% (20/30) had a decrease in the size of tumors suggesting clinical activity.[77] In a subsequent phase II study of pembrolizumab and vorinostat in recurrent/metastatic head and neck squamous cell cancer and salivary cancers, objective response was seen in one-twelfth of patients with ACC, suggesting the combination did not add significant antitumor activity.[78]

Immunotherapy

Immunotherapy in ACC has had limited success. The NISCAHN trial evaluated the programmed cell-death receptor 1 (PD1) monoclonal antibody nivolumab (3 mg/kg every 2 weeks) in 46 recurrent/metastatic ACC patients.[79] The primary end-point was the 6-month nonprogression rate, with 33% of ACC reaching this target, and a response rate of 8.8%.[79] A single-arm phase II trial of the CTLA4 monoclonal antibody ipilimumab (1 mg/kg every 6 weeks) and the PD1 monoclonal antibody nivolumab (3 mg/kg every 2 weeks) showed a response rate of only 6%, although the responses seen were substantial, with reductions of 73.1% and 58.4% by RECIST.[80]

Future Directions

Several interesting therapeutic avenues are currently being investigated for ACC. The Peter MacCallum Cancer Center (Melbourne, Australia) engineered a DNA vaccine against the *MYB* gene that is currently in a clinical study (NCT03287427). Retinoic acid was shown to suppress *c-myb* expression in preclinical models,[81] thus informing a study of all-trans retinoic acid in advanced ACC (NCT03999684). The first-in-class protein arginine methyltransferase inhibitor (PRMT5) GSK3326595 has shown an early signal of activity with a response rate of 21% (3/14) in a basket trial that included 14 subjects with ACC, which will likely inform further trials.[82] Given that over 90% of ACC express the prostate-specific membrane antigen (PSMA) with positive uptake on PSMA-PET, the radiolabeled PSMA-binding small molecule lutetium-177 (^{177}Lu) is being investigated in this population (NCT04291300).[83–85] The combination of lenvatinib and pembrolizumab is currently also being investigated for augmenting the tumor microenvironment and allowing for improved efficacy over single-agent immunotherapy (NCT04209660). For a rare disease, this certainly is an exciting and diverse array of biologically rational investigative approaches.

SALIVARY DUCT CARCINOMA, ADENOCARCINOMA NOT OTHERWISE SPECIFIED, AND CARCINOMA EX PLEOMORPHIC ADENOMA

Salivary duct carcinoma is an aggressive malignant salivary cancer with a propensity for nodal involvement and distant metastatic disease. Treatment with standard aggressive curative therapy with surgery with or without adjuvant radiation leaves disappointing results. Approximately 50% of patients will develop distant metastatic disease after such therapy.[86,87] A remarkable 60% to 79% of salivary duct carcinomas have potentially actionable genetic alterations, including *ERBB2*, *PIK3CA*, *HRAS*, *ALK*, and *BRAF*.[37,88]

There is near-uniform expression of the AR in salivary duct carcinoma, which has important therapeutic implications.[89] A prospective phase II trial of combined androgen blockade with leuprorelin acetate and bicalutamide in AR-positive salivary gland carcinoma demonstrated a best overall response of 41.7% and progression-free survival of 8.8 months.[90]

Second-generation hormonal therapy has shown mixed results. A phase II cooperative group trial (Alliance A091404) of the antiandrogen enzalutamide demonstrated 2/46 confirmed responses and 5 additional unconfirmed responses (3 of whom developed progressive disease after the initial response).[91] This suggests that while there is activity in this population, the responses are not durable.[91]

Salivary duct carcinoma is typically a chemo-sensitive disease. Retrospectively, carboplatin and paclitaxel showed a response rate of 39% in an analysis of 18 patients with salivary duct carcinoma.[92] A frontline trial through the European Organization for Research and Treatment of Cancer is evaluating the efficacy and safety of chemotherapy (cisplatin plus doxorubicin or carboplatin plus paclitaxel) versus ADT (leuprolide and bicalutamide) in the treatment of patients with recurrent or metastatic AR expressing salivary gland carcinomas (NCT01969578). ADT alone can be considered a firstline option in patients with low burden, asymptomatic, HER2-negative disease.

Approximately 31% to 44% of salivary duct carcinomas have amplification of HER2.[36,37] A phase II single-arm trial of trastuzumab 8 mg/kg loading, followed by 6 mg/kg every 3 weeks with docetaxel 70 mg/m2 every 3 weeks, showed an impressive response rate of 70.2% and median PFS of 8.9 months.[93] A phase II basket trial evaluating pertuzumab plus trastuzumab included 15 patients with HER2-positive salivary gland cancer with a response rate of 60%.[94] T-DM1 has shown disease activity even after progression through trastuzumab.[95,96] Ten patients with salivary gland cancer were included in a phase II basket trial of T-DM1 in HER2-amplified cancers assessed by next-generation sequencing. This trial demonstrated remarkable activity, including an overall response rate of 90%, including 5 complete responses, even after prior therapy with antiandrogens, trastuzumab, and pertuzumab.[96]

In a phase II basket trial of vemurafenib, a selective oral inhibitor of BRAF V600, in multiple nonmelanoma cancers with *BRAF* V600E mutations, a patient with salivary duct carcinoma had a complete response to therapy.[97]

AR positivity is also noted on 90% of carcinoma ex pleomorphic adenoma and about 26% of patients with adenocarcinoma NOS, suggesting enhanced response to androgen deprivation in these patient populations.[98] HER2 amplifications are also present at a lower rate in adenocarcinoma NOS (13.5%) and carcinoma ex pleomorphic adenoma (29%), in addition to other potentially actionable alterations including RET-rearrangements.[99] Treatment can be pursued along a similar paradigm to salivary duct carcinoma in these other histologies.[100]

SALIVARY SECRETORY CARCINOMA

Salivary secretory carcinoma, formerly known as mammary analog secretory carcinoma (MASC), is a rare salivary tumor, initially described in 2010, with features similar to secretory carcinoma of the breast and previously mischaracterized as AciCC.[101,102] The tumor is defined by the t(12;15) (q13;q25) translocation, creating a fusion of the *ETV6* and *NTRK3* genes.[101] This translocation leads to activation of various signaling pathways, including the mitogen-activating protein kinase and the phosphoinositide 3-kinase pathways.[103] Clinical behavior of MASC is typically indolent, though more aggressive disease can be seen in a subset of patients.[102]

The advent of selective TRK inhibitors has led to dramatic responses in this rare patient population.[104] A basket trial of the selective TRK inhibitor larotrectinib included 12 patients with salivary secretory carcinoma.[105] The study demonstrated a response rate of 75% in the entire cohort, with excellent duration of responses, leading to the tumor agnostic approval of this agent.[105] The response rate was enriched in patients with salivary tumors, rising to 90%, as confirmed in a pooled analysis of 3 early phase studies.[106]

MUCOEPIDERMOID CARCINOMA

Mucoepidermoid carcinoma (MEC) is the most common salivary malignancy, though it accounts for a smaller share of metastatic cases. Approximately 56% to 66% of cases are characterized by the t(11,19) (q14–21;p12–13) translocation that results in the fusion gene *CRTC1-3-MAML2*, a key oncogenic driver in this malignancy.[107–111] This translocation leads to both CREB-dependent and CREB independent changes in gene expression.[112] Some studies have found the fusion to be associated with low-grade/intermediate-grade disease occurring in younger patients and associated with improved prognosis, whereas other studies have failed to identify an association with prognosis.[110,111,113] Grade of tumor is consistently associated with survival, with high-grade tumors associated with higher nodal stage and poorer outcomes and low-grade or intermediate-grade tumors associated with more favorable outcomes.[114]

While not yet a targetable alteration, preclinical models evaluating the functional impact of *CRTC1-MAML2* fusion have shown aberrant p16-CKD4/6-RB pathway activity.[108] The CRTC1-MAML2 oncoprotein also causes upregulation of the epidermal growth factor receptor (EGFR) ligand amphiregulin, causing an autocrine loop promoting growth and survival in MEC.[115] Case studies have reported responses to EGFR directed therapy in MEC of the lung, even in the absence of sensitizing EGFR mutations, though a phase II trial of the EGFR inhibitor gefitinib that included 2 patients with MEC did not show any responses[116–119] Preclinical models have suggested that combined inhibition with CDK4/6 inhibitors and EGFR inhibition may have a synergistic antitumor effect, perhaps informing future clinical trials.[108]

In a study of comprehensive genomic profiling of 48 MECs, the most common genetic alterations in MEC involve *CDKN2A* (42%) and *TP53* (40%).[120] Additional potentially actionable genetic alterations exist at lower levels including *BAP1* (21%) *PIK3CA* (21%), *FGFR* (13%), *BRCA* (11%), *HRAS* (10%), *ERBB2* amplification (8%).[120] Mutations in *PIK3CA* and *TP53* were enriched in higher grade MECs.[120]

ACINIC CELL CARCINOMA

AciCC is typically a low-grade tumor with an excellent long-term prognosis when treated in the early stage, with a 5-year disease-specific survival of 91%.[121] Distant metastases develop in approximately 12% of cases based on early series.[122] A small fraction of patients may have a more aggressive course, and high-grade tumors are associated with poorer overall survival.[121,123] As in ACC, low-grade AciCC with lung-only metastases can undergo active surveillance before requiring systemic therapy.

Only recently has a recurrent interchromosomal rearrangement [t(4;9) (q13;q31)] been identified in AciCC.[124] This rearrangement causes approximation of active enhancer regions from the secretory Ca-binding phosphoprotein gene cluster at 4q13 with the nuclear receptor subfamily 4 group 4 member 3 (NR4A3) at 9q31. This translocation leads to upregulation of NR4A3 and is a likely oncogenic driver in this condition.[124] This advance in understanding the underlying biology is an important step forward in developing targeted therapeutic strategies.

IMMUNOTHERAPY

In the phase 1b KEYNOTE-028 trial, 26 patients with PDL1-positive (≥1% membranous tumor staining) recurrent/metastatic salivary gland tumors were treated with single-agent pembrolizumab (10 mg/kg every 2 weeks).[125] All histologic subtypes were included, and the overall response rate was 12% (3/26), with responses seen in 2 patients with adenocarcinoma and 1 with high-grade serous carcinoma.

The NISCAHN trial evaluated the single-agent PD1 monoclonal antibody nivolumab (3 mg/kg every 2 weeks) in 52 recurrent/metastatic non-ACC salivary gland patients.[79] The 6-month nonprogression rate was only 14% (7/50) and a partial response rate of only 4% (2/50) in this cohort.[79]

In the phase II KEYNOTE-158 trial, tumor mutational burden was prospectively evaluated as a predictive biomarker for response to single-agent pembrolizumab, using a cutoff of ≥10 mutations per megabase (Mut/Mb) and leading to the tumor-agnostic approval of pembrolizumab for this indication.[126] Three patients with salivary gland carcinoma met the criteria, one of whom had a partial response.[126] It should be noted that one of the three patients with salivary gland carcinoma also had high microsatellite instability, and it is unclear whether this is the patient who responded to therapy.[126] Approximately 13% of patients with salivary gland carcinoma (not divided by histologic subtype) have a tumor mutational burden of ≥10 Mut/Mb.[127]

Future directions of immunotherapy in salivary gland cancers include evaluating combined checkpoint blockade with nivolumab plus ipilimumab (NCT03172624 and NCT03146650) and other combinations such as pembrolizumab and lenvatinib (NCT0409660).

DISCLOSURE

Stock ownership in Infinity Pharmaceuticals, Hookipa Pharma, and Aprea Therapeutics, Inc.

REFERENCES

1. Ho AL, Pfister DG. Challenges and Opportunities for Developing New Therapeutics for Salivary Gland Cancers. J Oncol Pract 2018;14(2):109–10.
2. Seethala R, Stenman G. Update from the 4th Edition of the World Health Organization Classification of Head and Neck Tumours: Tumors of the Salivary Gland. Head Neck Pathol 2017;11(1):55–67.
3. Del Signore AG, Megwalu UC. The rising incidence of major salivary gland cancer in the United States. Ear Nose Throat J 2017;96(3):E13–6.
4. Carvalho AL, Nishimoto IN, Califano JA, et al. Trends in incidence and prognosis for head and neck cancer in the United States: a site-specific analysis of the SEER database. Int J Cancer 2005;114(5):806–16.
5. Davies L, Welch HG. Increasing Incidence of Thyroid Cancer in the United States, 1973-2002. JAMA 2006;295(18):2164–7.
6. Araya J, Martinez R, Niklander S, et al. Incidence and prevalence of salivary gland tumours in Valparaiso, Chile. Med Oral Patol Oral Cir Bucal 2015;20(5): e532–9.
7. Pinkston JA, Cole P. Incidence rates of salivary gland tumors: results from a population-based study. Otolaryngol Head Neck Surg 1999;120(6):834–40.
8. Jones AV, Craig GT, Speight PM, et al. The range and demographics of salivary gland tumours diagnosed in a UK population. Oral Oncol 2008;44(4): 407–17.
9. Fonseca FP, Carvalho M de V, de Almeida OP, et al. Clinicopathologic analysis of 493 cases of salivary gland tumors in a Southern Brazilian population. Oral Surg Oral Med Oral Pathol Oral Radiol 2012;114(2):230–9.

10. Loyola AM, de Araújo VC, de Sousa SO, et al. Minor salivary gland tumours. A retrospective study of 164 cases in a Brazilian population. Eur J Cancer B Oral Oncol 1995;31B(3):197–201.
11. Li L-J, Li Y, Wen Y-M, et al. Clinical analysis of salivary gland tumor cases in West China in past 50 years. Oral Oncol 2008;44(2):187–92.
12. Bradley PJ, McGurk M. Incidence of salivary gland neoplasms in a defined UK population. Br J Oral Maxillofac Surg 2013;51(5):399–403.
13. Mimica X, McGill M, Hay A, et al. Distant metastasis of salivary gland cancer: Incidence, management, and outcomes. Cancer 2020;126(10):2153–62.
14. Ho AS, Ochoa A, Jayakumaran G, et al. Genetic hallmarks of recurrent/metastatic adenoid cystic carcinoma. J Clin Invest 2019;129(10):4276–89.
15. Armstrong JG, Harrison LB, Thaler HT, et al. The indications for elective treatment of the neck in cancer of the major salivary glands. Cancer 1992;69:615–9.
16. Stennert E, Kisner D, Jungehuelsing M, et al. High Incidence of Lymph Node Metastasis in Major Salivary Gland Cancer. Arch Otolaryngol Neck Surg 2003;129(7):720–3.
17. Chen AM, Garcia J, Lee NY, et al. Patterns of nodal relapse after surgery and postoperative radiation therapy for carcinomas of the major and minor salivary glands: what is the role of elective neck irradiation? Int J Radiat Oncol Biol Phys 2007;67(4):988–94.
18. Matthiesen C, Thompson S, Steele A, et al. Radiotherapy in treatment of carcinoma of the parotid gland, an approach for the medically or technically inoperable patient. J Med Imaging Radiat Oncol 2010;54(5):490–6.
19. Ha H, Keam B, Ock CY, et al. Role of concurrent chemoradiation on locally advanced unresectable adenoid cystic carcinoma. Korean J Intern Med 2021;36(1):175–81.
20. Schoenfeld JD, Sher DJ, Norris CMJ, et al. Salivary gland tumors treated with adjuvant intensity-modulated radiotherapy with or without concurrent chemotherapy. Int J Radiat Oncol Biol Phys 2012;82(1):308–14.
21. Mahmood U, Koshy M, Goloubeva O, et al. Adjuvant Radiation Therapy for High-Grade and/or Locally Advanced Major Salivary Gland Tumors. Arch Otolaryngol Neck Surg 2011;137(10):1025–30.
22. Amini A, Waxweiler TV, Brower JV, et al. Association of Adjuvant Chemoradiotherapy vs Radiotherapy Alone With Survival in Patients With Resected Major Salivary Gland Carcinoma: Data From the National Cancer Data Base. JAMA Otolaryngol Neck Surg 2016;142(11):1100–10.
23. Tanvetyanon T, Fisher K, Caudell J, et al. Adjuvant chemoradiotherapy versus with radiotherapy alone for locally advanced salivary gland carcinoma among older patients. Head Neck 2016;38(6):863–70.
24. Tanvetyanon T, Qin D, Padhya T, et al. Outcomes of postoperative concurrent chemoradiotherapy for locally advanced major salivary gland carcinoma. Arch Otolaryngol Head Neck Surg 2009;135(7):687–92.
25. National Comprehensive Cancer Network. NCCN Clinical Practice Guidelines in Oncology. Head and Neck Cancers. Available at: https://www.nccn.org/guidelines/guidelines-detail?category=1&id=1437. Accessed May 20, 2021.
26. Laramore GE, Krall JM, Griffin TW, et al. Neutron versus photon irradiation for unresectable salivary gland tumors: final report of an RTOG-MRC randomized clinical trial. Radiation Therapy Oncology Group. Medical Research Council. Int J Radiat Oncol Biol Phys 1993;27(2):235–40.

27. Griffin TW, Pajak TF, Laramore GE, et al. Neutron vs photon irradiation of inoperable salivary gland tumors: results of an RTOG-MRC Cooperative Randomized Study. Int J Radiat Oncol Biol Phys 1988;15(5):1085–90.

28. Romesser PB, Cahlon O, Scher E, et al. Proton beam radiation therapy results in significantly reduced toxicity compared with intensity-modulated radiation therapy for head and neck tumors that require ipsilateral radiation. Radiother Oncol 2016;118(2):286–92.

29. Guillamondegui OM, Byers RM, Luna MA, et al. Aggressive surgery in treatment for parotid cancer: the role of adjunctive postoperative radiotherapy. Am J Roentgenol Radium Ther Nucl Med 1975;123(1):49–54.

30. McNaney D, McNeese MD, Guillamondegui OM, et al. Postoperative irradiation in malignant epithelial tumors of the parotid. Int J Radiat Oncol Biol Phys 1983; 9(9):1289–95.

31. Chen Y, Zheng Z-Q, Chen F-P, et al. Role of Postoperative Radiotherapy in Nonmetastatic Head and Neck Adenoid Cystic Carcinoma. J Natl Compr Canc Netw 2020;18(11):1476–84.

32. Ali S, Palmer FL, Katabi N, et al. Long-term local control rates of patients with adenoid cystic carcinoma of the head and neck managed by surgery and postoperative radiation. Laryngoscope 2017;127(10):2265–9.

33. Bjørndal K, Krogdahl A, Therkildsen MH, et al. Salivary adenoid cystic carcinoma in Denmark 1990-2005: Outcome and independent prognostic factors including the benefit of radiotherapy. Results of the Danish Head and Neck Cancer Group (DAHANCA). Oral Oncol 2015;51(12):1138–42.

34. van Boxtel W, Locati LD, van Engen-van Grunsven ACH, et al. Adjuvant androgen deprivation therapy for poor-risk, androgen receptor-positive salivary duct carcinoma. Eur J Cancer 2019;110:62–70.

35. Soper MS, Iganej S, Thompson LDR. Definitive treatment of androgen receptor-positive salivary duct carcinoma with androgen deprivation therapy and external beam radiotherapy. Head Neck 2014;36(1):E4–7.

36. Locati LD, Perrone F, Losa M, et al. Treatment relevant target immunophenotyping of 139 salivary gland carcinomas (SGCs). Oral Oncol 2009;45(11):986–90.

37. Dogan S, Ng CKY, Xu B, et al. The repertoire of genetic alterations in salivary duct carcinoma including a novel HNRNPH3-ALK rearrangement. Hum Pathol 2019;88:66–77.

38. Limaye SA, Posner MR, Krane JF, et al. Trastuzumab for the treatment of salivary duct carcinoma. Oncologist 2013;18(3):294–300.

39. Berendika J, Jungić S, Tubić B, et al. Adjuvant Treatment of the Salivary Duct Carcinoma with Her2 Overexpression. Case Rep Oncol 2021;14(1):610–5.

40. Spiro RH. Distant metastasis in adenoid cystic carcinoma of salivary origin. Am J Surg 1997;174(5):495–8.

41. Fordice J, Kershaw C, El-Naggar A, et al. Adenoid cystic carcinoma of the head and neck: predictors of morbidity and mortality. Arch Otolaryngol Head Neck Surg 1999;125(2):149–52. http://www.ncbi.nlm.nih.gov/pubmed/10037280.

42. Hanna GJ, Bae JE, Lorch JH, et al. Long-term outcomes and clinicogenomic correlates in recurrent, metastatic adenoid cystic carcinoma. Oral Oncol 2020;106:104690.

43. van der Wal JE, Becking AG, Snow GB, et al. Distant metastases of adenoid cystic carcinoma of the salivary glands and the value of diagnostic examinations during follow-up. Head Neck 2002;24(8):779–83.

44. Persson M, Andren Y, Mark J, et al. Recurrent fusion of MYB and NFIB transcription factor genes in carcinomas of the breast and head and neck. Proc Natl Acad Sci U S A 2009;106(44):18740–4.

45. Ho AS, Kannan K, Roy DM, et al. The mutational landscape of adenoid cystic carcinoma. Nat Genet 2013;45(7):791–8.

46. Chen TY, Keeney MG, Chintakuntlawar AV, et al. Adenoid cystic carcinoma of the lacrimal gland is frequently characterized by MYB rearrangement. Eye 2017;31:720. https://doi.org/10.1038/eye.2016.307.

47. Laurie SA, Ho AL, Fury MG, et al. Systemic therapy in the management of metastatic or locally recurrent adenoid cystic carcinoma of the salivary glands: a systematic review. Lancet Oncol 2011;12(8):815–24.

48. Verweij J, de Mulder PH, de Graeff A, et al. Phase II study on mitoxantrone in adenoid cystic carcinomas of the head and neck. EORTC Head and Neck Cancer Cooperative Group. Ann Oncol 1996;7(8):867–9.

49. Airoldi M, Bumma C, Bertetto O, et al. Vinorelbine treatment of recurrent salivary gland carcinomas. Bull Cancer 1998;85(10):892–4.

50. Licitra L, Marchini S, Spinazzè S, et al. Cisplatin in advanced salivary gland carcinoma. A phase II study of 25 patients. Cancer 1991;68(9):1874–7.

51. Schramm VLJ, Srodes C, Myers EN. Cisplatin therapy for adenoid cystic carcinoma. Arch Otolaryngol 1981;107(12):739–41.

52. Vermorken JB, Verweij J, de Mulder PH, et al. Epirubicin in patients with advanced or recurrent adenoid cystic carcinoma of the head and neck: a phase II study of the EORTC Head and Neck Cancer Cooperative Group. Ann Oncol 1993;4(9):785–8.

53. Airoldi M, Pedani F, Succo G, et al. Phase II randomized trial comparing vinorelbine versus vinorelbine plus cisplatin in patients with recurrent salivary gland malignancies. Cancer 2001;91(3):541–7.

54. Dreyfuss AI, Clark JR, Fallon BG, et al. Cyclophosphamide, doxorubicin, and cisplatin combination chemotherapy for advanced carcinomas of salivary gland origin. Cancer 1987;60(12):2869–72.

55. Belani CP, Eisenberger MA, Gray WC. Preliminary experience with chemotherapy in advanced salivary gland neoplasms. Med Pediatr Oncol 1988;16(3):197–202.

56. van Herpen CML, Locati LD, Buter J, et al. Phase II study on gemcitabine in recurrent and/or metastatic adenoid cystic carcinoma of the head and neck (EORTC 24982). Eur J Cancer 2008;44(17):2542–5.

57. Gilbert J, Li Y, Pinto HA, et al. Phase II trial of taxol in salivary gland malignancies (E1394): a trial of the Eastern Cooperative Oncology Group. Head Neck 2006;28(3):197–204.

58. Chau NG, Hotte SJ, Chen EX, et al. A phase II study of sunitinib in recurrent and/or metastatic adenoid cystic carcinoma (ACC) of the salivary glands: Current progress and challenges in evaluating molecularly targeted agents in ACC. Ann Oncol 2012;23(6):1562–70.

59. Thomson DJ, Silva P, Denton K, et al. Phase II trial of sorafenib in advanced salivary adenoid cystic carcinoma of the head and neck. Head Neck 2015;37(2):182–7.

60. Locati LD, Perrone F, Cortelazzi B, et al. A phase II study of sorafenib in recurrent and/or metastatic salivary gland carcinomas: Translational analyses and clinical impact. Eur J Cancer 2016;69:158–65.

61. Ho AL, Dunn L, Sherman EJ, et al. A phase II study of axitinib (AG-013736) in patients with incurable adenoid cystic carcinoma. Ann Oncol 2016;27(10): 1902–8.
62. Wong SJ, Karrison T, Hayes DN, et al. Phase II trial of dasatinib for recurrent or metastatic c-KIT expressing adenoid cystic carcinoma and for nonadenoid cystic malignant salivary tumors. Ann Oncol 2016;27(2):318–23.
63. Ho AL, Sherman EJ, Baxi SS, et al. Phase II study of regorafenib in progressive, recurrent/metastatic adenoid cystic carcinoma. J Clin Oncol 2016;34(15_suppl): 6096.
64. Dillon PM, Petroni GR, Horton BJ, et al. A phase II study of dovitinib in patients with recurrent or metastatic adenoid cystic carcinoma. Clin Cancer Res 2017; 23(15):4138–45.
65. Keam B, Kim S-B, Shin SH, et al. Phase 2 study of dovitinib in patients with metastatic or unresectable adenoid cystic carcinoma. Cancer 2015;121(15): 2612–7.
66. Holst VA, Marshall CE, Moskaluk CA, et al. KIT protein expression and analysis of c-kit gene mutation in adenoid cystic carcinoma. Mod Pathol 1999;12(10): 956–60.
67. Pfeffer MR, Talmi Y, Catane R, et al. A phase II study of Imatinib for advanced adenoid cystic carcinoma of head and neck salivary glands. Oral Oncol 2007; 43(1):33–6.
68. Matsui J, Funahashi Y, Uenaka T, et al. Multi-kinase inhibitor E7080 suppresses lymph node and lung metastases of human mammary breast tumor MDA-MB-231 via inhibition of vascular endothelial growth factor-receptor (VEGF-R) 2 and VEGF-R3 kinase. Clin Cancer Res 2008;14(17):5459–65.
69. Matsui J, Yamamoto Y, Funahashi Y, et al. E7080, a novel inhibitor that targets multiple kinases, has potent antitumor activities against stem cell factor producing human small cell lung cancer H146, based on angiogenesis inhibition. Int J Cancer 2008;122(3):664–71.
70. Okamoto K, Kodama K, Takase K, et al. Antitumor activities of the targeted multi-tyrosine kinase inhibitor lenvatinib (E7080) against RET gene fusion-driven tumor models. Cancer Lett 2013;340(1):97–103.
71. Tohyama O, Matsui J, Kodama K, et al. Antitumor Activity of Lenvatinib (E7080): An Angiogenesis Inhibitor That Targets Multiple Receptor Tyrosine Kinases in Preclinical Human Thyroid Cancer Models. J Thyroid Res 2014;2014. https://doi.org/10.1155/2014/638747.
72. Yamamoto Y, Matsui J, Matsushima T, et al. Lenvatinib, an angiogenesis inhibitor targeting VEGFR/FGFR, shows broad antitumor activity in human tumor xenograft models associated with microvessel density and pericyte coverage. Vasc Cell 2014;6(1). https://doi.org/10.1186/2045-824X-6-18.
73. Tchekmedyian V, Sherman EJ, Dunn L, et al. Phase II study of lenvatinib in patients with progressive, recurrent or metastatic adenoid cystic carcinoma. J Clin Oncol 2019;37(18). https://doi.org/10.1200/JCO.18.01859.
74. Locati LD, Galbiati D, Calareso G, et al. Patients with adenoid cystic carcinomas of the salivary glands treated with lenvatinib: Activity and quality of life. Cancer 2020;126(9):1888–94.
75. Ferrarotto R, Mitani Y, Diao L, et al. Activating NOTCH1 mutations define a distinct subgroup of patients with adenoid cystic carcinoma who have poor prognosis, propensity to bone and liver metastasis, and potential responsiveness to Notch1 inhibitors. J Clin Oncol 2017;35(3):352–60.

76. Ferrarotto R. ACCURACY a phase II trial of AL101, a selective gamma secretase inhibitor, in subjects with recurrent/metastatic (R/M) adenoid cystic carcinoma (ACC) harboring Notch activating mutations (Notchmut). Ann Oncol 2020; 31(Suppl_4):S599–628.

77. Goncalves PH, Heilbrun LK, Barrett MT, et al. A phase 2 study of vorinostat in locally advanced, recurrent, or metastatic adenoid cystic carcinoma. Oncotarget 2017;8(20):32918–29.

78. Rodriguez CP, Wu QV, Voutsinas J, et al. A Phase II Trial of Pembrolizumab and Vorinostat in Recurrent Metastatic Head and Neck Squamous Cell Carcinomas and Salivary Gland Cancer. Clin Cancer Res 2020;26(4):837–45.

79. Fayette J, Even C, Digue L, et al. NISCAHN: A phase II, multicenter nonrandomized trial aiming at evaluating nivolumab (N) in two cohorts of patients (pts) with recurrent/metastatic (R/M) salivary gland carcinoma of the head and neck (SGCHN), on behalf of the Unicancer Head & Neck Group. J Clin Oncol 2019;37(15_suppl):6083.

80. Tchekmedyian V, Sherman EJ, Dunn L, et al. A phase II trial cohort of nivolumab plus ipilimumab in patients (Pts) with recurrent/metastatic adenoid cystic carcinoma (R/M ACC). J Clin Oncol 2019;37(15_suppl):6084.

81. Mandelbaum J, Shestopalov IA, Henderson RE, et al. Zebrafish blastomere screen identifies retinoic acid suppression of MYB in adenoid cystic carcinoma. J Exp Med 2018;215(10):2673–85. https://doi.org/10.1084/jem. 20180939.

82. Siu LL, Rasco DW, Vinay SP, et al. METEOR-1: A phase I study of GSK3326595, a first-in-class protein arginine methyltransferase 5 (PRMT5) inhibitor, in advanced solid tumors. Ann Oncol 2019;30(Supplement 5):v159–93.

83. Klein Nulent TJW, van Es RJJ, Krijger GC, et al. Prostate-specific membrane antigen PET imaging and immunohistochemistry in adenoid cystic carcinoma-a preliminary analysis. Eur J Nucl Med Mol Imaging 2017;44(10): 1614–21.

84. van Boxtel W, Lütje S, van Engen-van Grunsven ICH, et al. (68)Ga-PSMA-HBED-CC PET/CT imaging for adenoid cystic carcinoma and salivary duct carcinoma: a phase 2 imaging study. Theranostics 2020;10(5):2273–83.

85. Hofman MS, Violet J, Hicks RJ, et al. [(177)Lu]-PSMA-617 radionuclide treatment in patients with metastatic castration-resistant prostate cancer (LuPSMA trial): a single-centre, single-arm, phase 2 study. Lancet Oncol 2018;19(6): 825–33.

86. Barnes L, Rao U, Krause J, et al. Salivary duct carcinoma. Part I. A clinicopathologic evaluation and DNA image analysis of 13 cases with review of the literature. Oral Surg Oral Med Oral Pathol 1994;78(1):64–73.

87. Jaehne M, Roeser K, Jaekel T, et al. Clinical and immunohistologic typing of salivary duct carcinoma: a report of 50 cases. Cancer 2005;103(12):2526–33.

88. Dalin MG, Desrichard A, Katabi N, et al. Comprehensive molecular characterization of salivary duct carcinoma reveals actionable targets and similarity to apocrine breast cancer. Clin Cancer Res 2016;22(18):4623–33.

89. Boon E, Bel M, van der Graaf WTA, et al. Salivary duct carcinoma: Clinical outcomes and prognostic factors in 157 patients and results of androgen deprivation therapy in recurrent disease (n=31)—Study of the Dutch head and neck society (DHNS). J Clin Oncol 2016;34(15_suppl):6016.

90. Fushimi C, Tada Y, Takahashi H, et al. A prospective phase II study of combined androgen blockade in patients with androgen receptor-positive metastatic or

locally advanced unresectable salivary gland carcinoma. Ann Oncol 2018; 29(4):979–84.

91. Ho AL, Foster NR, Zoroufy AJ, et al. Alliance A091404: A phase II study of enzalutamide (NSC# 766085) for patients with androgen receptor-positive salivary cancers. J Clin Oncol 2019;37(15_suppl):6020.

92. Nakano K, Sato Y, Sasaki T, et al. Combination chemotherapy of carboplatin and paclitaxel for advanced/metastatic salivary gland carcinoma patients: differences in responses by different pathological diagnoses. Acta Otolaryngol 2016;136(9):948–51.

93. Takahashi H, Tada Y, Saotome T, et al. Phase II Trial of Trastuzumab and Docetaxel in Patients With Human Epidermal Growth Factor Receptor 2-Positive Salivary Duct Carcinoma. J Clin Oncol 2019;37(2):125–34.

94. Kurzrock R, Bowles DW, Kang H, et al. Targeted therapy for advanced salivary gland carcinoma based on molecular profiling: results from MyPathway, a phase IIa multiple basket study. Ann Oncol 2020;31(3):412–21.

95. Corrêa TS, Matos GDR, Segura M, et al. Second-Line Treatment of HER2-Positive Salivary Gland Tumor: Ado-Trastuzumab Emtansine (T-DM1) after Progression on Trastuzumab. Case Rep Oncol 2018;11(2):252–7.

96. Li BT, Shen R, Offin M, et al. Ado-trastuzumab emtansine in patients with HER2 amplified salivary gland cancers (SGCs): Results from a phase II basket trial. J Clin Oncol 2019;37(15_suppl):6001.

97. Hyman DM, Puzanov I, Subbiah V, et al. Vemurafenib in Multiple Nonmelanoma Cancers with BRAF V600 Mutations. N Engl J Med 2015;373(8):726–36.

98. Dalin MG, Watson PA, Ho AL, et al. Androgen Receptor Signaling in Salivary Gland Cancer. Cancers (Basel) 2017;9(2):17.

99. Wang K, Russell JS, McDermott JD, et al. Profiling of 149 Salivary Duct Carcinomas, Carcinoma Ex Pleomorphic Adenomas, and Adenocarcinomas, Not Otherwise Specified Reveals Actionable Genomic Alterations. Clin Cancer Res 2016;22(24):6061–8.

100. Di Villeneuve L, Souza IL, Tolentino FDS, et al. Salivary Gland Carcinoma: Novel Targets to Overcome Treatment Resistance in Advanced Disease. Front Oncol 2020;10:2097. https://www.frontiersin.org/article/10.3389/fonc.2020.580141.

101. Skálová A, Vanecek T, Sima R, et al. Mammary analogue secretory carcinoma of salivary glands, containing the ETV6-NTRK3 fusion gene: a hitherto undescribed salivary gland tumor entity. Am J Surg Pathol 2010;34(5):599–608.

102. Sethi R, Kozin E, Remenschneider A, et al. Mammary analogue secretory carcinoma: update on a new diagnosis of salivary gland malignancy. Laryngoscope 2014;124(1):188–95.

103. Vaishnavi A, Le AT, Doebele RC. TRKing down an old oncogene in a new era of targeted therapy. Cancer Discov 2015;5(1):25–34.

104. Drilon A, Li G, Dogan S, et al. What hides behind the MASC: clinical response and acquired resistance to entrectinib after ETV6-NTRK3 identification in a mammary analogue secretory carcinoma (MASC). Ann Oncol 2016;27(5):920–6.

105. Drilon A, Laetsch TW, Kummar S, et al. Efficacy of Larotrectinib in TRK Fusion-Positive Cancers in Adults and Children. N Engl J Med 2018;378(8):731–9.

106. Hong DS, DuBois SG, Kummar S, et al. Larotrectinib in patients with TRK fusion-positive solid tumours: a pooled analysis of three phase 1/2 clinical trials. Lancet Oncol 2020;21(4):531–40.

107. Tonon G, Modi S, Wu L, et al. t(11;19)(q21;p13) translocation in mucoepidermoid carcinoma creates a novel fusion product that disrupts a Notch signaling pathway. Nat Genet 2003;33(2):208–13.

108. Chen Z, Ni W, Li J-L, et al. The CRTC1-MAML2 fusion is the major oncogenic driver in mucoepidermoid carcinoma. JCI Insight 2021;6(7). https://doi.org/10.1172/jci.insight.139497.

109. Birkeland AC, Foltin SK, Michmerhuizen NL, et al. Correlation of Crtc1/3-Maml2 fusion status, grade and survival in mucoepidermoid carcinoma. Oral Oncol 2017;68:5–8.

110. Seethala RR, Dacic S, Cieply K, et al. A reappraisal of the MECT1/MAML2 translocation in salivary mucoepidermoid carcinomas. Am J Surg Pathol 2010;34(8):1106–21.

111. Saade RE, Bell D, Garcia J, et al. Role of CRTC1/MAML2 Translocation in the Prognosis and Clinical Outcomes of Mucoepidermoid Carcinoma. JAMA Otolaryngol Head Neck Surg 2016;142(3):234–40.

112. Chen J, Li J-L, Chen Z, et al. Gene expression profiling analysis of CRTC1-MAML2 fusion oncogene-induced transcriptional program in human mucoepidermoid carcinoma cells. BMC Cancer 2015;15:803.

113. Nakayama T, Miyabe S, Okabe M, et al. Clinicopathological significance of the CRTC3–MAML2 fusion transcript in mucoepidermoid carcinoma. Mod Pathol 2009;22(12):1575–81.

114. Chen MM, Roman SA, Sosa JA, et al. Histologic grade as prognostic indicator for mucoepidermoid carcinoma: a population-level analysis of 2400 patients. Head Neck 2014;36(2):158–63.

115. Chen Z, Chen J, Gu Y, et al. Aberrantly activated AREG-EGFR signaling is required for the growth and survival of CRTC1-MAML2 fusion-positive mucoepidermoid carcinoma cells. Oncogene 2014;33(29):3869–77.

116. Lee KWC, Chan ABW, Lo AWI, et al. Erlotinib in metastatic bronchopulmonary mucoepidermoid carcinoma. J Thorac Oncol 2011;6(12):2140–1.

117. Rossi G, Sartori G, Cavazza A, et al. Mucoepidermoid carcinoma of the lung, response to EGFR inhibitors, EGFR and K-RAS mutations, and differential diagnosis. Lung Cancer 2009;63(1):159–60.

118. Han S-W, Kim H-P, Jeon YK, et al. Mucoepidermoid carcinoma of lung: potential target of EGFR-directed treatment. Lung Cancer 2008;61(1):30–4.

119. Jakob JA, Kies MS, Glisson BS, et al. Phase II study of gefitinib in patients with advanced salivary gland cancers. Head Neck 2015;37(5):644–9.

120. Wang K, McDermott JD, Schrock AB, et al. Comprehensive genomic profiling of salivary mucoepidermoid carcinomas reveals frequent BAP1, PIK3CA, and other actionable genomic alterations. Ann Oncol 2017;28(4):748–53.

121. Hoffman HT, Karnell LH, Robinson RA, et al. National Cancer Data Base report on cancer of the head and neck: acinic cell carcinoma. Head Neck 1999;21:297–309.

122. Spiro RH, Huvos AG, Strong EW. Acinic cell carcinoma of salivary origin. A clinicopathologic study of 67 cases. Cancer 1978;41(3):924–35.

123. Zbären P, Schreiber B, Lehmann W, et al. [Acinar cell carcinoma of the salivary glands]. Laryngol Rhinol Otol (Stuttg) 1987;66(6):320–3.

124. Haller F, Bieg M, Will R, et al. Enhancer hijacking activates oncogenic transcription factor NR4A3 in acinic cell carcinomas of the salivary glands. Nat Commun 2019;10(1):368.

125. Cohen RB, Delord JP, Doi T, et al. Pembrolizumab for the treatment of advanced salivary gland carcinoma: Findings of the Phase 1b KEYNOTE-028 Study. Am J Clin Oncol 2018. https://doi.org/10.1097/COC.0000000000000429.

126. Marabelle A, Fakih M, Lopez J, et al. Association of tumour mutational burden with outcomes in patients with advanced solid tumours treated with pembrolizumab: prospective biomarker analysis of the multicohort, open-label, phase 2 KEYNOTE-158 study. Lancet Oncol 2020;21(10):1353–65.

127. Shao C, Li G, Huang L, et al. Prevalence of High Tumor Mutational Burden and Association With Survival in Patients With Less Common Solid Tumors. JAMA Netw Open 2020;3(10):e2025109.

Cutaneous Malignancies of the Head and Neck

Gino K. In, MD, MPH[a], Jacob S. Thomas, MD[a], Ann W. Silk, MD, MS[b],*

KEYWORDS

- Melanoma • Cutaneous squamous cell carcinoma • Basal cell carcinoma
- Merkel cell carcinoma

KEY POINTS

- Aggressive cutaneous squamous cell carcinoma and basal cell carcinoma can cause high morbidity due to local destruction, warranting use of multimodal therapy including surgery, radiation therapy, and systemic therapy.
- In melanoma, systemic therapies (immune checkpoint inhibitors and MAPK pathway inhibitors) improve survival in the metastatic and recurrence-free survival in the adjuvant setting.
- In Merkel cell carcinoma, immune checkpoint blockade has replaced chemotherapy in the first-line metastatic setting and dramatically improved survival for responders.
- PD-L1 testing by immunohistochemistry is not required to select patients for immune checkpoint blockade therapy in any of the cutaneous malignancies.

INTRODUCTION

The skin of the face, ears, neck, and scalp receives small daily doses of ultraviolet radiation (UVR) throughout our lifetimes (**Fig. 1**).[1,2] UVR may induce skin carcinogenesis via multiple mechanisms, including (1) DNA damage and (2) immunosuppression. A crucial tenet of primary prevention of cutaneous malignancy (CM) is protection against UVR; sun protection behaviors include use of protective clothing, hats, sunblock with SPF 30+, and avoidance of direct sun exposure during peak hours (10 AM to 4 PM). Secondary prevention involves close follow-up with dermatology for regular total body skin examination. For patients with a history of numerous CMs, chemoprevention with nicotinamide or acitretin, may reduce the number of new primary keratinocyte carcinomas that develop each year by 25% to 40%.[3–5]

In addition to UVR, another important risk factor for CMs is immunosuppression. Patients with a history of organ transplantation, human immunodeficiency virus (HIV)/AIDS, autoimmune disorders, and hematologic malignancies, are all at significantly higher risk

[a] Norris Comprehensive Cancer Center and University of Southern California Keck School of Medicine, 1441 Eastlake Avenue, Los Angeles, CA 90033, USA; [b] Dana-Farber Cancer Institute and Harvard Medical School, 450 Brookline Avenue, LW503, Boston, MA 02215, USA
* Corresponding author.
E-mail address: ann_silk@dfci.harvard.edu

Hematol Oncol Clin N Am 35 (2021) 991–1008
https://doi.org/10.1016/j.hoc.2021.05.008
0889-8588/21/© 2021 Elsevier Inc. All rights reserved.

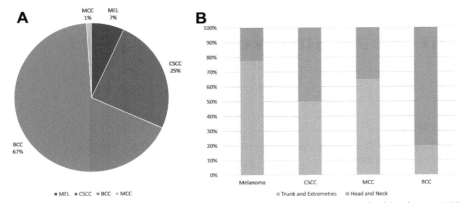

Fig. 1. (A) Percentage of the most common CMs of the head and neck, by histology. *BCC and CSCC are not reported to national cancer registries, and therefore are potentially underestimated. (B) Anatomic distribution of the most common CMs of the head and neck.

of CM. Patients with Merkel cell carcinoma (MCC) are nearly 30 times more likely to have lymphoma or leukemia as a comorbidity.[6,7] It is hypothesized that normal immunosurveillance is disrupted by quantitative or qualitative deficiencies in the immune system, and dysplastic precursor lesions are not able to be cleared by the host.

The etiologic role of UVR, with resultant high rates of somatic mutations, combined with the immunogenicity of CM, has facilitated the use of novel immune checkpoint inhibitors for patients with advanced disease, leading to improvements in survival and quality of life. Meanwhile, identification of signaling pathways unique to distinct CM (ie, hedgehog signaling in basal cell carcinoma [BCC], MAPK activation in melanoma [MEL]) has also allowed development of targeted therapies.

The management of CMs is increasingly complex, due to patient-related and tumor-related factors. Multidisciplinary management is critical, and should involve not only surgical, radiation, and medical oncology, but also other specialties, such as plastic surgery, and Mohs micrographic surgery. Patients with CM are often elderly, and may be frail, with multiple comorbidities, or other psychosocial factors. In addition, tumors that are symptomatic or located in specific anatomic sites may require specialized care to achieve optimal outcomes. To further complicate matters, the management of MEL and MCC has been extensively studied and well defined, but there has been much less progress for cutaneous squamous cell carcinoma (CSCC) and BCC, in which a lack of consensus guidelines leaves practitioners with difficult decision-making. Here, we review the current state-of-the-art in CMs as pertinent to the clinician treating disease of the head and neck.

CUTANEOUS SQUAMOUS CELL CARCINOMA

CSCC and BCC of the skin are collectively known as keratinocyte carcinomas (KCs). The exact incidence of KCs is unknown, but it was estimated in 2012 that more than 5 million cases of KC were treated in the United States.[8] Actinic keratoses are precancerous lesions that give rise to CSCC at a rate of approximately 1% per year.[9] Treatment with topical 5-fluorouracil can eliminate actinic keratoses and thus reduce the risk of CSCC.[10] Another major risk factor for CSCC is chronic inflammation from non-healing wounds. CSCCs associated with chronic wounds, known as "Marjolin ulcers," are associated with poor prognosis.[11,12] Last, immunosuppression can significantly increase the risk of CSCC. In solid organ transplant recipients, it is estimated that there is a 70-fold increase in the incidence of CSCC compared with the general population.[13]

Risk for recurrence of CSCC can be estimated by a combination of clinical and pathologic factors. The best-established clinical risk factors are location and size. CSCC in the head and neck area may be more likely to recur than CSCC involving the trunk or extremities.[14] The "mask area of the face" is considered high risk.[15] Tumors larger than 2 cm and certain pathologic features are at higher risk for metastasis and poorer survival (**Box 1**).[16]

Complete surgical excision with standard surgical excision or Mohs micrographic surgery (MMS) achieves excellent disease control in the vast majority of cases. MMS is often preferred for head and neck CSCC for improved cosmetic outcomes as well as intraoperative analysis of the excision margin.[14] Sentinel lymph node biopsy (SLNB) has been shown to have prognostic value; however, there is no proven survival benefit and therefore the role of SLNB remains unclear.[17,18] Full lymph node dissection should be performed for known or clinically suspected nodal involvement. CSCC of the head and neck may also metastasize to the parotid gland, which may lead to parotidectomy in addition to neck dissection.[19]

Adjuvant radiation therapy (RT) may be considered for patients with high-risk features. CSCC is highly sensitive to radiation. Data to support the efficacy of adjuvant RT is limited to retrospective heterogeneous studies.[20,21] Because radiation to the head and neck can have significant morbidity, patients must be selected appropriately in a multidisciplinary fashion. Radiation to the skin of the head and neck can potentially lead to nonhealing skin ulcers, cataracts, soft tissue/bone necrosis, and poor cosmetic outcomes.[22,23] There are limited data regarding the use of sensitizing systemic therapy in the adjuvant setting. One phase 3 randomized controlled study demonstrated that adding weekly carboplatin to RT was no better than RT alone.[24] However, sensitization with cisplatin and cetuximab has not been tested in a randomized controlled trial; thus, the decision to use systemic therapy concurrently in the adjuvant setting can only be based on expert opinion or extrapolation from the mucosal head and neck squamous cell literature.[25] Patients with unresectable regional disease should be carefully selected for definitive treatment using RT. Some patients may be treated with primary radiation if surgery is not feasible.[26,27] Concurrent cisplatin and concurrent cetuximab are part of national guidelines, but with limited data to support this approach, as well as the availability of other systemic treatments, patients should be counseled appropriately.

Box 1
Histopathological features that confer increased risk of recurrence

High-risk features of primary cutaneous squamous cell carcinoma

Diameter $\geq$2 cm

Poorly differentiated

Depth beyond subcutaneous fat

Perineural invasion

Ear, temple, or anogenital location

Data from Schmults CD, Karia PS, Carter JB, et al: Factors predictive of recurrence and death from cutaneous squamous cell carcinoma: a 10-year, single-institution cohort study. JAMA Dermatol 149:541-7, 2013

Locally advanced or metastatic CSCC that is not amenable to surgery or definitive RT may be treated with palliative systemic therapy. Prospective phase 2 clinical trials have led to regulatory approval of the programmed death (PD)-1 inhibiting antibodies cemiplimab and pembrolizumab. In 2018, results from a phase 1/2 study of cemiplimab in advanced/metastatic CSCC were reported. Most patients enrolled in this trial had CSCC with head or neck as the primary site (66%). The overall response rate (ORR) in the phase 2 study was 47% in the total population.[28] Subset analyses based on primary tumor site are not reported. Biomarker analysis showed no correlation between PD–ligand 1 expression or tumor mutational burden (TMB) and clinical response.[29] A 2020 report of a phase 2 trial with pembrolizumab (CARSKIN) in a similar patient population demonstrated similar efficacy with a response rate of 42%. In this trial, PD-L1 positive patients had a significantly higher ORR than PD-L1 negative patients (55% vs 17%, $P = .02$).[30] Patients with a history of allogeneic organ transplantation were not included in any of the checkpoint inhibitor studies, and in the absence of safety and efficacy data in this population, checkpoint inhibitors should be avoided. Small trials to test the safety of checkpoint inhibitors in the transplant population have begun enrollment.

Patients who are not candidates for immunotherapy or do not respond to immunotherapy are treated with epidermal growth factor receptor (EGFR)-targeted therapy with or without chemotherapy. Responses to cytotoxic chemotherapy, such as cisplatin, docetaxel, and 5-fluorouracil, and EGFR antibodies such as cetuximab have been demonstrated in several prospective and retrospective studies.[31,32] These trials were conducted before the use of checkpoint inhibitors. All patients with disease progression after checkpoint inhibitor therapy should be considered for clinical trials.

BASAL CELL CARCINOMA

BCC is the most common cancer in the United States. Sun exposure is the primary risk factor for BCC, and as such BCC of the head and neck accounts for approximately 70% of all cases.[33,34] Chronic immunosuppression increases the risk for BCC; however, not as much as for squamous cell carcinoma.[35] BCC of the head and neck is more likely to recur than BCC of the trunk or extremities.[36,37]

Both standard surgical excision and MMS are acceptable surgical options for BCC. MMS has demonstrated decreased recurrence rates for recurrent BCC, but several studies have failed to show superiority for primary BCC lesions.[38,39] BCC has a low incidence of metastatic spread, including regional lymph nodes, and as such, SLNB or lymph node dissections are not routinely performed.[40]

Adjuvant RT to the surgical bed may be considered for patients with high-risk features such as extensive perineural involvement or positive margins.[41,42] Although there are no prospective randomized studies demonstrating the benefit of adjuvant radiation, retrospective studies demonstrate good outcomes for patients who were treated with adjuvant radiation. For example, a series of 95 patients from the Netherlands reported in 2020 followed patients with BCC of the head and neck with incomplete resections managed with adjuvant radiation. Local recurrences occurred in only 3.6% of patients.[43]

Primary radiation for lesions not amenable to surgery also has excellent outcomes. Retrospective studies demonstrate 5-year recurrence rates between 4% and 16%.[26,37] A randomized controlled trial was completed in patients with head and neck BCC comparing standard surgery with primary radiation. Surgery was shown to have lower recurrence rates and superior cosmetic outcomes compared with primary radiation.[44] A long-term follow-up study confirmed improved cosmesis after surgery and stable to deteriorated cosmesis after radiotherapy.[45]

Patients with locally advanced, recurrent, or metastatic BCC may be candidates for systemic therapy. The best studied drugs in this setting are Hedgehog pathway inhibitors (HHI), such as vismodegib and sonidegib, which inhibit the cell surface receptor smoothened homolog (SMO). Efficacy of vismodegib 150 mg by mouth daily was demonstrated in a large open-label phase 2 trial, the SafeTy Events in VIsmodEgib (STEVIE) study.[46] Of the 1215 patients enrolled, 1119 had locally advanced BCC and 96 had metastatic disease. Eighty-one percent of all patients in the study had BCC of the head and neck. In the locally advanced cohort, the ORR was 69% with 33% complete response (CR). For metastatic disease, the ORR was 37% with 5% CR. Adverse events included muscle spasm, alopecia, dysgeusia, weight loss, nausea, fatigue, and arthralgias. Treatment-associated adverse events led to discontinuation of therapy in 31% of patients. After several months, the chronic low-grade side effects of vismodegib often become intolerable, and dose interruptions may be necessary to improve tolerability without limiting efficacy.[47] A phase 2 study of sonidegib showed similar efficacy and toxicity results.[48] There are no head-to-head comparisons of the 2 drugs; however, a meta-analysis demonstrated similar ORRs but more upper gastrointestinal symptoms with sonidegib.[49] Data for the use of other systemic therapies for BCC are limited only to case reports.

BCC has the highest rate of mutations per megabase among all cancers. This has led to an investigation of PD-1 immunotherapy, which has only been reported in abstract form to date (ESMO 2020). Cemiplimab was tested in a phase 2 study of 84 patients with locally advanced BCC that had progressed on first-line HHI, resulting in a response rate of 31% with 5 CR and 21 partial response (PR).[50] Based on these results, the FDA approved cemiplimab in February 2021 for patients with advanced BCC who have disease progression despite HHI or who are inappropriate for HHI therapy.

CUTANEOUS MELANOMA

The incidence of cutaneous MEL continues to rise, with an estimated 100,350 new cases of melanoma in the United States in 2020.[51] MEL is the fifth and sixth most common malignancy for men and women, respectively. Although incidence increases with age, patients across the age spectrum may be affected, and MEL represents the third most common cancer for adolescents and young adults between the ages of 20 and 39.[52] Cutaneous melanomas on the head and neck account for 15% to 30% of all MEL, and are more common among older patients.[53–57] The primary etiology for cutaneous melanomas is UVR,[57,58] as evidenced by a mutational signature typified by frequent C>T transitions.[59] Other risk factors include fair skin, red hair, blue eye color, melanocytic nevi, older age, and immunosuppression.[60,61] Workup and diagnosis of a primary MEL tumor requires histopathologic confirmation.[62] Staging of melanoma according to the American Joint Committee on Cancer Tumor Node Metastasis (AJCC TNM) eighth edition entails assessment of primary tumor thickness and ulceration, as well as evaluation for regional nodal and distant metastases.[63]

Low-risk, pT1a tumors (smaller than 0.8 mm Breslow depth and nonulcerated) can be resected with 1-cm margins.[62] Patients with higher-risk lesions (thicker than 0.8 mm or ulcerated) require wide excision with up to 2-cm margins, and also lymphatic mapping with SLNB.[62,64,65] Compared with MEL at other anatomic sites, MELs of the head and neck are more aggressive, with thicker primary tumors, higher rates of ulceration and the nodular histology subtype.[53,54,56] Multiple studies indicate that SLNBs are less likely to be positive for primary head and neck MEL, despite having worse prognosis.[54,55] Two randomized, controlled trials (MSLT2 and DeCOG) did not demonstrate a survival advantage for immediate completion lymph node dissection among patients with positive SLNB.[66,67] However, only approximately 10% of the study population had head and neck primaries, and furthermore, completion lymph node dissections of the neck are not associated with lymphedema. Based on these results, patients with positive SLNB should receive close follow-up of the draining nodal basin with serial ultrasound imaging or undergo immediate complete lymph node dissection; this may vary by institutional practice. Meanwhile, patients with clinically detected lymph node metastases should directly undergo therapeutic lymphadenectomy.[68,69] Patients at very high risk of recurrence in the neck, may be carefully selected for adjuvant radiotherapy to prevent morbidity, although there is no survival benefit to this approach.[70] Following resection of stage III-IV disease, adjuvant therapy using either PD-1 inhibition, or MAPK inhibitors (MAPKi), should be offered to patients to reduce the risk of recurrence (approximately 60% vs 40% recurrence-free survival (RFS) compared with placebo at 3 years).[71-73] Adjuvant therapy using CTLA-4 inhibition is discouraged, given inferior efficacy and higher toxicity, as compared with PD-1 inhibitors.[71] For patients with unresectable or metastatic melanoma, systemic options include (1) immune checkpoint inhibitors (ICIs), or (2) targeted MAPKi. First-line ICI-based therapy for melanoma should include PD-1 blockade, either as monotherapy,[74,75] or in combination with CTLA-4.[76] Patients who achieve responses to treatment may have durable responses with median overall survival (mOS) ranging from 33 to 38 months with PD-1 alone, to as high as 60 months with combination therapy.[74-76] The decision between monotherapy versus combination therapy should take into consideration tumor burden and patient characteristics; single-agent therapy with PD-1 alone is better tolerated, whereas response rates are higher for the combination. To date, the use of combination ICI therapy in the first-line setting has resulted in the highest long-term survival rate for patients with advanced MEL, with as many as 50% of patients alive at 5 years.[76] Combination MAPKi therapy to target BRAF and MEK is an important option for patients with advanced MEL. Testing for the somatic BRAF V600 mutation is required to identify the approximately 50% of patients with MEL who will benefit from this therapy. MAPKi therapy leads to rapid responses with high disease control rates; however, MAPKi may have less durability compared with ICI (mOS 22–34), as acquired resistance is expected in most cases.[77-79] BRAF and MEK inhibitors should always be used in combination when possible; this not only leads to improved efficacy, but also prevents paradoxic MAPK activation, which can lead to development of secondary non-MEL skin cancers. There are 3 different combinations approved, each with differing toxicity profiles.[77-79] There are no published randomized controlled trials to compare ICI against MAPKi, nor how to sequence these therapies for patients with BRAF V600 mutations. Although ICIs offer durable responses and the potential for long-term survival, MAPKi may provide quicker palliation for patients with bulky disease. Recent efforts have investigated how to combine ICI with MAPKi. In the IMspire150 trial, combining the PD-L1 inhibitor, atezolizumab, with BRAF (vemurafenib) and MEK (cobimetinib) inhibition led to improved progression-free survival, when compared with BRAF and MEK inhibition alone.[80] This triplet regimen was subsequently approved by the FDA in July 2020. In-transit metastases and brain metastases are frequently seen in patients with advanced MEL and thus warrant special consideration. For patients with in-transit or superficial lymph node metastases, the oncolytic virus, talimogene laherparepvec, has single-agent activity as an intratumoral therapy, and may lead to durable responses for select patients without visceral disease, although no impact on survival has been demonstrated.[81] Brain metastases occur in up to 50% of patients with advanced MEL, and are frequently seen among patients with primary head and neck melanoma tumors.[82] Surgery and/or radiation are important mainstays of therapy, especially for symptomatic lesions. For small asymptomatic brain metastases, dual ICI therapy may provide adequate treatment and help forgo the need for local therapy.[83,84] In addition, combination MAPKi therapy has shown efficacy in treating MEL brain metastases, although outcomes are short-lived when compared with other extracranial tumors.[85]

MERKEL CELL CARCINOMA

MCC is an aggressive high-grade neuroendocrine malignancy of the skin that has the highest case fatality rate of any skin cancer. It often presents as a rapidly enlarging "cyst" or a pink or purple dome-shaped cutaneous lesion. Patients tend to be elderly, and approximately 8% of patients are immunosuppressed due to chronic lymphocytic leukemia, HIV, or a solid organ transplant.[86] The presence of a brisk T-cell infiltrate in primary tumors, measured by CD3+ cells or CD8+ cells, correlates with survival,[87] suggesting that the immune system plays an important role in this disease.

From an etiologic perspective, there are 2 distinct paths to carcinogenesis of MCC, UVR mutagenesis and the Merkel cell polyomavirus (MCPyV). In North America, 80% of MCC cases are caused by the oncogenic action of MCPyV.[88] The MCPyV was first described in 2008.[88] It is a small double-stranded DNA virus, which is normally a harmless component of the normal skin flora. However, in rare instances, the virus integrates into the DNA of a host cell and transforms the cell, resulting in expression of viral proteins, including the MCPyV T-antigen oncoprotein, which drives unregulated growth by inhibiting the retinoblastoma tumor suppressor.[89,90] MCPyV-specific T cells can be detected in tumor specimens, and their presence is associated with favorable survival. Most patients with virus-positive MCC (VP-MCC) mount a B-cell response against the T-antigen oncoproteins, and immunoglobulin G antibodies against the MCPyV small T antigen can be detected using a serology test.[91] Serology testing for an antibody to the MCPyV oncoprotein should be performed within 3 months of diagnosis to detect the antibody when it is at its highest, as it naturally decreases over time following successful treatment. The serology test has been prospectively validated as a surveillance tool for patients with VP-MCC who have been treated with curative intent. Although the TMB in VP-MCC tends to be very low, virus-negative MCC (VN-MCC) is characterized by a very high TMB. MCC is often found on sun-exposed skin.[86] UVR mutagenesis is thought to be the major cause of VN-MCC.

The primary MCC tumor is located in the head and neck region for approximately 30% of cases. More than 40% of patients present with metastases to the regional lymph nodes or distant metastases.[86] Other frequent sites of metastases are the liver, lung, bone, and bone marrow. Fluorine-18 fluorodeoxyglucose PET/computed tomography scans are useful to detect metastases, as the tumors tend to be highly avid.[92] In-transit and cutaneous metastases are common, and a full skin examination should be included in the initial workup. Because of the propensity for early spread, SLNB should be performed to complete staging on all patients without clinical evidence of lymph node metastases.

It is not uncommon for patients with MCC to present with a parotid mass or neck mass, and no evidence of a primary lesion.[86] Unknown primary patients are noted to have lower chance of recurrence than patients who have a primary lesion with in-transit and/or lymph node metastases (Stage IIIB).[93] The AJCC staging system was updated to reflect the more favorable prognosis of patients with unknown primary, who are now categorized as Stage IIIA instead of IIIB.[93] It is hypothesized that the patient's underlying immune system spontaneously rejected the primary tumor, eliminating it before it became clinically apparent.

The primary tumor is treated with wide local excision,[94] or definitive RT can substitute for surgery in cases in which resection is technically difficult (for example, on the eyelid).[95,96] MCC is exquisitely sensitive to low doses of RT. Doses of 50 to 55 Gy are recommended, and can be delivered in as few as 20 to 25 fractions,[95] but outcomes with radiation alone may be inferior to surgery, based on retrospective data.[94] Narrow excision with adjuvant RT has been reported with good disease control outcomes in a small series,[97] and is also an acceptable alternative when wide local excision is not feasible. Adjuvant RT may be recommended to the primary tumor site if the tumor has high-risk features, including size larger than 2 cm, close margins, or lymphovascular invasion. A recent study of 12 elderly patients with stage I and II MCC of the head and neck examined the use of a single 8-Gy fraction of RT following surgery, and found that there were no in-field local recurrences, suggesting that lower doses may minimize toxicity from RT without compromising efficacy.[98]

Adjuvant RT to the draining lymph node basin is recommended if the SLNB is positive.[99] Complete lymph node dissection is not necessary because the local control rates are excellent with adjuvant RT.[99,100] RT without complete lymph node dissection is also an acceptable treatment option for macroscopic lymph nodes at high-volume centers, where the in-field control rate with definitive RT is considered equivalent with surgery followed by RT.[100] The experience of the treatment center in this disease was associated with a significant survival advantage according to 3 analyses of the National Cancer Database[101–103]; thus, patients who are diagnosed at low-volume centers should be referred to a center that treats more than 3 cases per year.

Following adequate primary and adjuvant treatment, patients with Stage I to III MCC are at high risk of death from recurrent disease. A patient with stage IIIB disease has a 60% to 70% chance of death due to MCC in 5 years.[104] Eighty percent of occurrences will happen within the first 2 years; therefore, frequent imaging and physical examinations are critical during the first 24 months of follow-up. Monitoring serology test for an antibody against the Merkel cell polyomavirus oncoprotein can be useful in follow-up if the titer was detectable at baseline.[91]

For patients who present with widespread disease or patients who have a recurrence that is not salvageable by radiotherapy or surgery, palliative systemic therapy is indicated. Before immunotherapy, Merkel cell was treated like other high-grade small cell neuroendocrine cancers with chemotherapy, such as cisplatin and etoposide. Like small cell carcinoma of the lung, MCC has a high rate of response to chemotherapy (~65%), but the natural history is that the cancer tends to reoccur within a few months of stopping chemotherapy, and the average survival was approximately 9 months.[105–107] Now, the PD-L1 inhibitor avelumab and the PD-1 inhibitor pembrolizumab have replaced chemotherapy because they are more effective and less toxic.[108–111]

Avelumab was first studied in patients who had disease progression despite chemotherapy. The ORR to avelumab was 33%, and the 1-year OS was 52%.[108,109] Avelumab was then tested in treatment-naïve patients and 62% of them achieved a response.[110] The impressive therapeutic effect of inhibiting the PD-1 checkpoint axis in MCC was confirmed with pembrolizumab in a first-line trial conducted by the National Cancer Institute Cancer Immunotherapy Trial Network (NCI CITN).[111] The response rate was 56% (14 of 25), including 24% complete responders. The drugs pembrolizumab or avelumab have not been compared against each other. One notable difference between avelumab and pembrolizumab is that infusion reactions are more common with avelumab (23% vs 0%), but they are usually mild and do not preclude further therapy.

In patients in whom immunotherapy is not effective or is contraindicated (such as patients with a lung or heart transplant), second-line palliative therapy consists of

Table 1
Key trials using immune checkpoint inhibitors in the treatment of cutaneous malignancies

	Study	Population	Study Design	Sample Size	Endpoints
Melanoma	Ascierto et al (CheckMate 066)	First-line, advanced or metastatic melanoma	Phase 3, 1:1 randomization to nivolumab vs dacarbazine	n = 418	Median OS: 37.5 vs 11.2 mo, HR 0.46, P<.001 3-y OS: 51.2% vs 21.6%
	Robert et al (Keynote 006)	First-line, advanced or metastatic melanoma	Phase 3, 1:1:1 randomization to pembrolizumab (every 2 or 3 wk) vs ipilimumab	n = 834	Median OS: 32.7 vs 15.9 mo, HR 0.73, P = .0005 Median PFS 8.4 v 3.4 mo, HR 0.57, P < .0001
	Larkin et al (CheckMate 067)	First-line, advanced or metastatic melanoma	Phase 3, 1:1:1 randomization to nivolumab + ipilimumab vs nivolumab vs ipilimumab	n = 945	Median OS: >60 (NR) vs 36.9 vs 19.9 mo 5-y OS: 52% vs 44% vs 26% Median PFS 11.5 vs 6.9 vs 2.9 mo
	Ascierto et al (CheckMate 238)	Adjuvant melanoma, stage IIIB-IV	Phase 3, 1:1 randomization to nivolumab vs ipilimumab	n = 906	4-y RFS: 51.7% vs 41.2%, HR 0.71, P = .0003
	Eggermont et al (Keynote 054/EORTC 1325)	Adjuvant melanoma, stage IIIA-IIIC	Phase 3,1:1 randomization to pembrolizumab vs placebo	n = 1019	3-y RFS: 63.7% vs 44.1%, HR 0.56, P < .001
Cutaneous squamous cell carcinoma (CSCC)	Migden et al (RE6N2810)	Any line, locally advanced or metastatic CSCC	Phase 1/2, open-label cemiplimab	n = 163	Locally advanced: ORR 44%, 31% PR, 13% CR Metastatic: ORR 48%, 41% PR, 7% CR
	Maubec et al (CARSKIN)	First-line, locally advanced or metastatic CSCC	Phase 2, open-label pembrolizumab	n = 57	ORR (at week 15) 42%, 35% PR, 7% CR

(continued on next page)

Table 1
(continued)

	Study	Population	Study Design	Sample Size	Endpoints
Merkel cell carcinoma (MCC)	Kaufman et al (JAVELIN Merkel 200 Part A)	Second-line, metastatic MCC, after chemotherapy	Phase 2, open-label avelumab	n = 88	ORR 33.0%, 21.6% PR, 11.4% CR
	D'Angelo et al (JAVELIN Merkel 200 Part B)	First-line, metastatic MCC	Phase 2, open-label avelumab	n = 39	ORR 62.1%, 48.3% PR, 13.8% CR
	Nghiem et al,[111] (Keynote 017/NCI CITN-09)	First-line, advanced or metastatic MCC	Phase 2, open-label pembrolizumab	n = 50	ORR 56%, 32% PR, 24% CR
Basal cell carcinoma (BCC)	Stratigos et al,[50] (REGN2810)	Second-line, locally advanced BCC, after hedgehog inhibitors	Phase 2, open-label cemiplimab	n = 84	ORR 31%, 25% PR, 6% CR

Abbreviations: CR, complete remission; HR, hazard ratio; NR, not reached; ORR, overall odds ratio; OS, overall survival; PR, partial remission; RFS, recurrence-free survival.

off-label treatment regimens adapted from the treatment of other neuroendocrine malignancies, such as chemotherapy or octreotide, or participation in a clinical trial.

No systemic therapy has been demonstrated to improve outcomes in the adjuvant setting. Studies using adjuvant ICIs are currently enrolling. Adjuvant systemic therapy is not recommended outside of a clinical trial at this time.

SUMMARY

CMs arising on the head and neck regions are a common health problem. Most CMs are highly preventable through sun protection behaviors. Most KCs are easily cured with surgical excision. High-risk BCC and CSCC may recur or cause local destruction, but rarely metastasize. MEL and MCC have a high propensity to metastasize early on through the skin (in-transits), to lymph nodes, and/or distant organs, resulting in high mortality. In the head and neck area, anatomic and cosmetic factors make wide surgical margins impractical and a multidisciplinary management is important to tailor medical decision-making for each individual. ICI therapy is being used increasingly for metastatic CMs, and it is approved for adjuvant use in MEL (**Table 1**). The role of ICI and other systemic immunotherapies is likely to expand in the management of advanced CMs in the years to come.

CLINICS CARE POINTS

- Most of the cutaneous malignancies of the head and neck are UV-driven; hence, patients should have regular dermatologic examination and follow sun protection behaviors.
- Patients with underlying immune suppression are at greater risk of aggressive skin cancer.
- Melanoma and Merkel cell carcinoma have high mortality rates and should be managed in a multi-disciplinary setting.
- While uncommon, aggressive basal cell and cutaneous squamous cell carcinoma may result in local destruction of adjacent organs or metastatic disease, result in death.
- ICI therapy improves clinical outcomes for patients with advanced, cutaneous malignancies of the head and neck.
- Neither PD-L1 status or TMB has been demonstrated to be helpful for medical decision-making in any of the cutaneous malignancies.
- Patients with cutaneous malignancies refractory to ICI therapy should be referred for clinical trials.

DISCLOSURE

The authors have nothing to disclose.

REFERENCES

1. Zanetti R, Rosso S, Martinez C, et al. Comparison of risk patterns in carcinoma and melanoma of the skin in men: a multi-centre case-case-control study. Br J Cancer 2006;94:743–51.
2. Robsahm TE, Helsing P, Veierød MB. Cutaneous squamous cell carcinoma in Norway 1963-2011: increasing incidence and stable mortality. Cancer Med 2015;4:472–80.
3. Bavinck JN, Tieben LM, Van der Woude FJ, et al. Prevention of skin cancer and reduction of keratotic skin lesions during acitretin therapy in renal transplant

recipients: a double-blind, placebo-controlled study. J Clin Oncol 1995;13: 1933–8.

4. Moon TE, Levine N, Cartmel B, et al. Effect of retinol in preventing squamous cell skin cancer in moderate-risk subjects: a randomized, double-blind, controlled trial. Southwest Skin Cancer Prevention Study Group. Cancer Epidemiol Biomarkers Prev 1997;6:949–56.

5. Chen AC, Martin AJ, Choy B, et al. A Phase 3 randomized trial of nicotinamide for skin-cancer chemoprevention. N Engl J Med 2015;373:1618–26.

6. Howard RA, Dores GM, Curtis RE, et al. Merkel cell carcinoma and multiple primary cancers. Cancer Epidemiol Biomarkers Prev 2006;15:1545–9.

7. Kaae J, Hansen AV, Biggar RJ, et al. Merkel cell carcinoma: incidence, mortality, and risk of other cancers. J Natl Cancer Inst 2010;102:793–801.

8. Rogers HW, Weinstock MA, Feldman SR, et al. Incidence estimate of nonmelanoma skin cancer (keratinocyte carcinomas) in the U.S. population, 2012. JAMA Dermatol 2015;151:1081–6.

9. Criscione VD, Weinstock MA, Naylor MF, et al. Actinic keratoses: natural history and risk of malignant transformation in the Veterans Affairs Topical Tretinoin Chemoprevention Trial. Cancer 2009;115:2523–30.

10. Jansen MHE, Kessels J, Nelemans PJ, et al. Randomized trial of four treatment approaches for actinic keratosis. N Engl J Med 2019;380:935–46.

11. Senet P, Combemale P, Debure C, et al. Malignancy and chronic leg ulcers: the value of systematic wound biopsies: a prospective, multicenter, cross-sectional study. Arch Dermatol 2012;148:704–8.

12. Mullen JT, Feng L, Xing Y, et al. Invasive squamous cell carcinoma of the skin: defining a high-risk group. Ann Surg Oncol 2006;13:902–9.

13. Jensen AO, Svaerke C, Farkas D, et al. Skin cancer risk among solid organ recipients: a nationwide cohort study in Denmark. Acta Derm Venereol 2010;90: 474–9.

14. Rowe DE, Carroll RJ, Day CL. Prognostic factors for local recurrence, metastasis, and survival rates in squamous cell carcinoma of the skin, ear, and lip. Implications for treatment modality selection. J Am Acad Dermatol 1992;26: 976–90.

15. Silverman MK, Kopf AW, Grin CM, et al. Recurrence rates of treated basal cell carcinomas. Part 1: overview. J Dermatol Surg Oncol 1991;17:713–8.

16. Schmults CD, Karia PS, Carter JB, et al. Factors predictive of recurrence and death from cutaneous squamous cell carcinoma: a 10-year, single-institution cohort study. JAMA Dermatol 2013;149:541–7.

17. Gore SM, Shaw D, Martin RC, et al. Prospective study of sentinel node biopsy for high-risk cutaneous squamous cell carcinoma of the head and neck. Head Neck 2016;38(Suppl 1):E884–9.

18. Takahashi A, Imafuku S, Nakayama J, et al. Sentinel node biopsy for high-risk cutaneous squamous cell carcinoma. Eur J Surg Oncol 2014;40:1256–62.

19. Gurudutt VV, Genden EM. Cutaneous squamous cell carcinoma of the head and neck. J Skin Cancer 2011;2011:502723.

20. Sapir E, Tolpadi A, McHugh J, et al. Skin cancer of the head and neck with gross or microscopic perineural involvement: patterns of failure. Radiother Oncol 2016;120:81–6.

21. Balamucki CJ, Mancuso AA, Amdur RJ, et al. Skin carcinoma of the head and neck with perineural invasion. Am J Otolaryngol 2012;33:447–54.

22. Schulte KW, Lippold A, Auras C, et al. Soft x-ray therapy for cutaneous basal cell and squamous cell carcinomas. J Am Acad Dermatol 2005;53:993–1001.

23. Locke J, Karimpour S, Young G, et al. Radiotherapy for epithelial skin cancer. Int J Radiat Oncol Biol Phys 2001;51:748–55.
24. Porceddu SV, Bressel M, Poulsen MG, et al. Postoperative concurrent chemoradiotherapy versus postoperative radiotherapy in high-risk cutaneous squamous cell carcinoma of the head and neck: the randomized phase III TROG 05.01 trial. J Clin Oncol 2018;36:1275–83.
25. Bonner JA, Harari PM, Giralt J, et al. Radiotherapy plus cetuximab for squamous-cell carcinoma of the head and neck. N Engl J Med 2006;354:567–78.
26. Cognetta AB, Howard BM, Heaton HP, et al. Superficial x-ray in the treatment of basal and squamous cell carcinomas: a viable option in select patients. J Am Acad Dermatol 2012;67:1235–41.
27. Hernández-Machin B, Borrego L, Gil-García M, et al. Office-based radiation therapy for cutaneous carcinoma: evaluation of 710 treatments. Int J Dermatol 2007;46:453–9.
28. Migden MR, Rischin D, Schmults CD, et al. PD-1 blockade with cemiplimab in advanced cutaneous squamous-cell carcinoma. N Engl J Med 2018;379:341–51.
29. Migden MR, Khushalani NI, Chang ALS, et al. Cemiplimab in locally advanced cutaneous squamous cell carcinoma: results from an open-label, phase 2, single-arm trial. Lancet Oncol 2020;21:294–305.
30. Maubec E, Boubaya M, Petrow P, et al. Phase II study of pembrolizumab as first-line, single-drug therapy for patients with unresectable cutaneous squamous cell carcinomas. J Clin Oncol 2020;38:3051–61.
31. Maubec E, Petrow P, Scheer-Senyarich I, et al. Phase II study of cetuximab as first-line single-drug therapy in patients with unresectable squamous cell carcinoma of the skin. J Clin Oncol 2011;29:3419–26.
32. Jarkowski A, Hare R, Loud P, et al. Systemic therapy in advanced cutaneous squamous cell carcinoma (CSCC): the Roswell Park experience and a review of the literature. Am J Clin Oncol 2016;39:545–8.
33. van Dam RM, Huang Z, Rimm EB, et al. Risk factors for basal cell carcinoma of the skin in men: results from the health professionals follow-up study. Am J Epidemiol 1999;150:459–68.
34. Wang YJ, Tang TY, Wang JY, et al. Genital basal cell carcinoma, a different pathogenesis from sun-exposed basal cell carcinoma? A case-control study of 30 cases. J Cutan Pathol 2018;45:688–95.
35. Euvrard S, Kanitakis J, Claudy A. Skin cancers after organ transplantation. N Engl J Med 2003;348:1681–91.
36. Bøgelund FS, Philipsen PA, Gniadecki R. Factors affecting the recurrence rate of basal cell carcinoma. Acta Derm Venereol 2007;87:330–4.
37. Silverman MK, Kopf AW, Bart RS, et al. Recurrence rates of treated basal cell carcinomas. Part 3: surgical excision. J Dermatol Surg Oncol 1992;18:471–6.
38. Mosterd K, Krekels GA, Nieman FH, et al. Surgical excision versus Mohs' micrographic surgery for primary and recurrent basal-cell carcinoma of the face: a prospective randomised controlled trial with 5-years' follow-up. Lancet Oncol 2008;9:1149–56.
39. Smeets NW, Krekels GA, Ostertag JU, et al. Surgical excision vs Mohs' micrographic surgery for basal-cell carcinoma of the face: randomised controlled trial. Lancet 2004;364:1766–72.

40. McCusker M, Basset-Seguin N, Dummer R, et al. Metastatic basal cell carcinoma: prognosis dependent on anatomic site and spread of disease. Eur J Cancer 2014;50:774–83.

41. Mendenhall WM, Ferlito A, Takes RP, et al. Cutaneous head and neck basal and squamous cell carcinomas with perineural invasion. Oral Oncol 2012;48: 918–22.

42. Han A, Ratner D. What is the role of adjuvant radiotherapy in the treatment of cutaneous squamous cell carcinoma with perineural invasion? Cancer 2007; 109:1053–9.

43. Visch Marjolein Birgitte MB, Kreike Bas B, Gerritsen Marie-Jeanne Pieternel MJP. Long-term experience with radiotherapy for the treatment of non-melanoma skin cancer. J Dermatolog Treat 2020;31:290–5.

44. Avril MF, Auperin A, Margulis A, et al. Basal cell carcinoma of the face: surgery or radiotherapy? Results of a randomized study. Br J Cancer 1997;76:100–6.

45. Petit JY, Avril MF, Margulis A, et al. Evaluation of cosmetic results of a randomized trial comparing surgery and radiotherapy in the treatment of basal cell carcinoma of the face. Plast Reconstr Surg 2000;105:2544–51.

46. Basset-Séguin N, Hauschild A, Kunstfeld R, et al. Vismodegib in patients with advanced basal cell carcinoma: primary analysis of STEVIE, an international, open-label trial. Eur J Cancer 2017;86:334–48.

47. Dréno B, Kunstfeld R, Hauschild A, et al. Two intermittent vismodegib dosing regimens in patients with multiple basal-cell carcinomas (MIKIE): a randomised, regimen-controlled, double-blind, phase 2 trial. Lancet Oncol 2017;18:404–12.

48. Lear JT, Migden MR, Lewis KD, et al. Long-term efficacy and safety of sonidegib in patients with locally advanced and metastatic basal cell carcinoma: 30-month analysis of the randomized phase 2 BOLT study. J Eur Acad Dermatol Venereol 2018;32:372–81.

49. Xie P, Lefrançois P. Efficacy, safety, and comparison of sonic hedgehog inhibitors in basal cell carcinomas: a systematic review and meta-analysis. J Am Acad Dermatol 2018;79:1089–100.e17.

50. Stratigos A, Sekulic A, Peris K, et al. Primary analysis of phase II results for cemiplimab in patients (pts) with locally advanced basal cell carcinoma (laBCC) who progress on or are intolerant to hedgehog inhibitors (HHIs). Ann Oncol 2020;31:S1142–215.

51. Siegel RL, Miller KD, Jemal A. Cancer statistics, 2020. CA Cancer J Clin 2020; 70:7–30.

52. Miller KD, Fidler-Benaoudia M, Keegan TH, et al. Cancer statistics for adolescents and young adults, 2020. CA Cancer J Clin 2020;70:443–59.

53. Hoersch B, Leiter U, Garbe C. Is head and neck melanoma a distinct entity? A clinical registry-based comparative study in 5702 patients with melanoma. Br J Dermatol 2006;155:771–7.

54. Callender GG, Egger ME, Burton AL, et al. Prognostic implications of anatomic location of primary cutaneous melanoma of 1 mm or thicker. Am J Surg 2011; 202:659–64 [discussion 664-5].

55. Fadaki N, Li R, Parrett B, et al. Is head and neck melanoma different from trunk and extremity melanomas with respect to sentinel lymph node status and clinical outcome? Ann Surg Oncol 2013;20:3089–97.

56. Lachiewicz AM, Berwick M, Wiggins CL, et al. Survival differences between patients with scalp or neck melanoma and those with melanoma of other sites in the Surveillance, Epidemiology, and End Results (SEER) program. Arch Dermatol 2008;144:515–21.

57. Laskar R, Ferreiro-Iglesias A, Bishop DT, et al. Risk factors for melanoma by anatomical site: an evaluation of aetiological heterogeneity. Br J Dermatol 2020;184(6):1085–93.
58. Caini S, Gandini S, Sera F, et al. Meta-analysis of risk factors for cutaneous melanoma according to anatomical site and clinico-pathological variant. Eur J Cancer 2009;45:3054–63.
59. Lawrence MS, Stojanov P, Polak P, et al. Mutational heterogeneity in cancer and the search for new cancer-associated genes. Nature 2013;499:214–8.
60. Pampena R, Kyrgidis A, Lallas A, et al. A meta-analysis of nevus-associated melanoma: prevalence and practical implications. J Am Acad Dermatol 2017; 77(e4):938–45.
61. Gandini S, Sera F, Cattaruzza MS, et al. Meta-analysis of risk factors for cutaneous melanoma: III. Family history, actinic damage and phenotypic factors. Eur J Cancer 2005;41:2040–59.
62. Swetter SM, Tsao H, Bichakjian CK, et al. Guidelines of care for the management of primary cutaneous melanoma. J Am Acad Dermatol 2019;80:208–50.
63. Gershenwald J, Scolyer R, Hess K, et al. Melanoma of the skin. In: Amin MB, editor. AJCC cancer staging Manual. Eighth Edition. New York: Springer International Publishing; 2017. p. 563–85.
64. Hayes AJ, Maynard L, Coombes G, et al. Wide versus narrow excision margins for high-risk, primary cutaneous melanomas: long-term follow-up of survival in a randomised trial. Lancet Oncol 2016;17:184–92.
65. Morton DL, Thompson JF, Cochran AJ, et al. Final trial report of sentinel-node biopsy versus nodal observation in melanoma. N Engl J Med 2014;370: 599–609.
66. Faries MB, Thompson JF, Cochran AJ, et al. Completion dissection or observation for sentinel-node metastasis in melanoma. N Engl J Med 2017;376:2211–22.
67. Leiter U, Stadler R, Mauch C, et al. Final analysis of DeCOG-SLT trial: no survival benefit for complete lymph node dissection in patients with melanoma with positive sentinel node. J Clin Oncol 2019;37:3000–8.
68. Glover AR, Allan CP, Wilkinson MJ, et al. Outcomes of routine ilioinguinal lymph node dissection for palpable inguinal melanoma nodal metastasis. Br J Surg 2014;101:811–9.
69. van Akkooi AC, Bouwhuis MG, van Geel AN, et al. Morbidity and prognosis after therapeutic lymph node dissections for malignant melanoma. Eur J Surg Oncol 2007;33:102–8.
70. Henderson MA, Burmeister BH, Ainslie J, et al. Adjuvant lymph-node field radiotherapy versus observation only in patients with melanoma at high risk of further lymph-node field relapse after lymphadenectomy (ANZMTG 01.02/TROG 02.01): 6-year follow-up of a phase 3, randomised controlled trial. Lancet Oncol 2015;16:1049–60.
71. Ascierto PA, Del Vecchio M, Mandalá M, et al. Adjuvant nivolumab versus ipilimumab in resected stage IIIB-C and stage IV melanoma (CheckMate 238): 4-year results from a multicentre, double-blind, randomised, controlled, phase 3 trial. Lancet Oncol 2020;21:1465–77.
72. Eggermont AMM, Blank CU, Mandala M, et al. Longer follow-up confirms recurrence-free survival benefit of adjuvant pembrolizumab in high-risk stage III melanoma: updated results from the EORTC 1325-MG/KEYNOTE-054 trial. J Clin Oncol 2020;38:3925–36.
73. Dummer R, Hauschild A, Santinami M, et al. Five-year analysis of adjuvant dabrafenib plus trametinib in stage III melanoma. N Engl J Med 2020;383:1139–48.

74. Ascierto PA, Long GV, Robert C, et al. Survival outcomes in patients with previously untreated braf wild-type advanced melanoma treated with nivolumab therapy: three-year follow-up of a randomized phase 3 trial. JAMA Oncol 2019;5:187–94.

75. Robert C, Ribas A, Schachter J, et al. Pembrolizumab versus ipilimumab in advanced melanoma (KEYNOTE-006): post-hoc 5-year results from an open-label, multicentre, randomised, controlled, phase 3 study. Lancet Oncol 2019;20:1239–51.

76. Larkin J, Chiarion-Sileni V, Gonzalez R, et al. Five-year survival with combined nivolumab and ipilimumab in advanced melanoma. N Engl J Med 2019;381:1535–46.

77. Long GV, Flaherty KT, Stroyakovskiy D, et al. Dabrafenib plus trametinib versus dabrafenib monotherapy in patients with metastatic BRAF V600E/K-mutant melanoma: long-term survival and safety analysis of a phase 3 study. Ann Oncol 2017;28:1631–9.

78. Ascierto PA, McArthur GA, Dreno B, et al. Cobimetinib combined with vemurafenib in advanced BRAF(V600)-mutant melanoma (coBRIM): updated efficacy results from a randomised, double-blind, phase 3 trial. Lancet Oncol 2016;17:1248–60.

79. Ascierto PA, Dummer R, Gogas HJ, et al. Update on tolerability and overall survival in COLUMBUS: landmark analysis of a randomised phase 3 trial of encorafenib plus binimetinib vs vemurafenib or encorafenib in patients with BRAF V600-mutant melanoma. Eur J Cancer 2020;126:33–44.

80. Gutzmer R, Stroyakovskiy D, Gogas H, et al. Atezolizumab, vemurafenib, and cobimetinib as first-line treatment for unresectable advanced BRAF(V600) mutation-positive melanoma (IMspire150): primary analysis of the randomised, double-blind, placebo-controlled, phase 3 trial. Lancet 2020;395:1835–44.

81. Andtbacka RH, Kaufman HL, Collichio F, et al. Talimogene laherparepvec improves durable response rate in patients with advanced melanoma. J Clin Oncol 2015;33:2780–8.

82. Huismans AM, Haydu LE, Shannon KF, et al. Primary melanoma location on the scalp is an important risk factor for brain metastasis: a study of 1,687 patients with cutaneous head and neck melanomas. Ann Surg Oncol 2014;21:3985–91.

83. Long GV, Atkinson V, Lo S, et al. Combination nivolumab and ipilimumab or nivolumab alone in melanoma brain metastases: a multicentre randomised phase 2 study. Lancet Oncol 2018;19:672–81.

84. Tawbi HA, Forsyth PA, Algazi A, et al. Combined nivolumab and ipilimumab in melanoma metastatic to the brain. N Engl J Med 2018;379:722–30.

85. Davies MA, Saiag P, Robert C, et al. Dabrafenib plus trametinib in patients with BRAF(V600)-mutant melanoma brain metastases (COMBI-MB): a multicentre, multicohort, open-label, phase 2 trial. Lancet Oncol 2017;18:863–73.

86. Heath M, Jaimes N, Lemos B, et al. Clinical characteristics of Merkel cell carcinoma at diagnosis in 195 patients: the AEIOU features. J Am Acad Dermatol 2008;58:375–81.

87. Miller NJ, Church CD, Fling SP, et al. Merkel cell polyomavirus-specific immune responses in patients with Merkel cell carcinoma receiving anti-PD-1 therapy. J Immunother Cancer 2018;6:131.

88. Feng H, Shuda M, Chang Y, et al. Clonal integration of a polyomavirus in human merkel cell carcinoma. Science 2008;319:1096–100.

89. Dye KN, Welcker M, Clurman BE, et al. Merkel cell polyomavirus Tumor antigens expressed in Merkel cell carcinoma function independently of the ubiquitin ligases Fbw7 and β-TrCP. PLOS Pathog 2019;15:e1007543.

90. Houben R, Shuda M, Weinkam R, et al. Merkel cell polyomavirus-infected merkel cell carcinoma cells require expression of viral T antigens. J Virol 2010;84: 7064–72.

91. Paulson KG, Lewis CW, Redman MW, et al. Viral oncoprotein antibodies as a marker for recurrence of Merkel cell carcinoma: a prospective validation study. Cancer 2017;123:1464–74.

92. Akaike G, Akaike T, Fadl SA, et al. Imaging of merkel cell carcinoma: what imaging experts should know. Radiographics 2019;39:2069–84.

93. Harms KL, Healy MA, Nghiem P, et al. Analysis of prognostic factors from 9387 merkel cell carcinoma cases forms the basis for the new 8th edition AJCC staging system. Ann Surg Oncol 2016;23:3564–71.

94. Wright GP, Holtzman MP. Surgical resection improves median overall survival with marginal improvement in long-term survival when compared with definitive radiotherapy in Merkel cell carcinoma: a propensity score matched analysis of the National Cancer Database. Am J Surg 2018;215:384–7.

95. Veness M, Foote M, Gebski V, et al. The role of radiotherapy alone in patients with merkel cell carcinoma: reporting the Australian experience of 43 patients. Int J Radiat Oncol Biol Phys 2010;78:703–9.

96. Pape E, Rezvoy N, Penel N, et al. Radiotherapy alone for Merkel cell carcinoma: a comparative and retrospective study of 25 patients. J Am Acad Dermatol 2011;65:983–90.

97. Tarabadkar ES, Fu T, Lachance K, et al. Narrow excision margins are appropriate for Merkel cell carcinoma when combined with adjuvant radiation: analysis of 188 cases of localized disease and proposed management algorithm. J Am Acad Dermatol 2021;84:340–7.

98. Cook MM, Schaub SK, Goff PH, et al. Postoperative, single-fraction radiation therapy in Merkel cell carcinoma of the head and neck. Adv Radiat Oncol 2020;5:1248–54.

99. Perez MC, Oliver DE, Weitman ES, et al. Management of sentinel lymph node metastasis in merkel cell carcinoma: completion lymphadenectomy, radiation, or both? Ann Surg Oncol 2019;26:379–85.

100. Fang LC, Lemos B, Douglas J, et al. Radiation monotherapy as regional treatment for lymph node-positive Merkel cell carcinoma. Cancer 2010;116:1783–90.

101. Chipidza FE, Thakuria M, Schoenfeld JD, et al. Association between treatment center experience and survival after diagnosis of stage I to III Merkel cell carcinoma treated with surgery with or without postoperative radiation therapy. J Am Acad Dermatol 2020;84(3):875–7.

102. Yoshida EJ, Luu M, Freeman M, et al. The association between facility volume and overall survival in patients with Merkel cell carcinoma. J Surg Oncol 2020;122:254–62.

103. Cheraghlou S, Agogo GO, Girardi M. The impact of facility characteristics on Merkel cell carcinoma outcomes: a retrospective cohort study. J Am Acad Dermatol 2019;S0190-9622(19)32664-7.

104. Fields RC, Busam KJ, Chou JF, et al. Five hundred patients with Merkel cell carcinoma evaluated at a single institution. Ann Surg 2011;254:465–73 [discussion 473-5].

105. Tai PTH, Yu E, Winquist E, et al. Chemotherapy in neuroendocrine/Merkel cell carcinoma of the skin: case series and review of 204 cases. J Clin Oncol 2000;18:2493–9.
106. Allen PJ, Bowne WB, Jaques DP, et al. Merkel cell carcinoma: prognosis and treatment of patients from a single institution. J Clin Oncol 2005;23:2300–9.
107. Iyer JG, Blom A, Doumani R, et al. Response rates and durability of chemotherapy among 62 patients with metastatic Merkel cell carcinoma. Cancer Med 2016;5:2294–301.
108. Kaufman HL, Russell J, Hamid O, et al. Avelumab in patients with chemotherapy-refractory metastatic Merkel cell carcinoma: a multicentre, single-group, open-label, phase 2 trial. Lancet Oncol 2016;17:1374–85.
109. Kaufman HL, Russell JS, Hamid O, et al. Updated efficacy of avelumab in patients with previously treated metastatic Merkel cell carcinoma after ≥1 year of follow-up: JAVELIN Merkel 200, a phase 2 clinical trial. J ImmunoTherapy Cancer 2018;6(1):7.
110. D'Angelo SP, Russell J, Lebbé C, et al. Efficacy and safety of first-line avelumab treatment in patients with stage IV metastatic Merke cell carcinoma: a pre-planned interim analysis of a clinical trial. JAMA Oncol 2018;4:e180077.
111. Nghiem P, Bhatia S, Lipson EJ, et al. Durable tumor regression and overall survival in patients with advanced Merkel cell carcinoma receiving pembrolizumab as first-line therapy. J Clin Oncol 2019;37:693–702.

Managing Recurrent Metastatic Head and Neck Cancer

Hira Shaikh, MD[a], Vidhya Karivedu, MD[b],
Trisha M. Wise-Draper, MD, PhD[a],*

KEYWORDS

- Head and neck cancer • Recurrent • Metastatic • Systemic therapy
- Chemotherapy • Targeted therapy • Immunotherapy

KEY POINTS

- Surgery and/or reirradiation may provide long-term disease control or cure in some locally recurrent/oligometastatic HNSCC.
- Pembrolizumab plus chemotherapy as well as pembrolizumab monotherapy (PD-L1 CPS≥1) has been approved as a frontline treatment of R/M HNSCC.
- Cetuximab either in combination with platinum-based doublet or as a single agent after the failure of platinum-based chemotherapy is a reasonable treatment option.

BACKGROUND

Head and neck squamous cell carcinoma (HNSCC) is the sixth most common cancer worldwide.[1] More than half of the patients with advanced stage disease (stage III or IV) develop local and/or regional recurrence with or without distant metastases within 3 years of definitive treatment.[2] Treatment of locally recurrent disease often includes combined modality approaches (surgery, radiotherapy [RT], with or without chemotherapy). If deemed operable, salvage surgery alone is considered the standard of care, providing durable disease control in ~15% of patients,[3] whereas reirradiation with or without chemotherapy is usually considered in select unresectable tumors.[4] Reirradiation after salvage surgery has shown to improve locoregional control and

Funding: Dr T.M. Wise-Draper is supported by a National Center for Advancing Translational Sciences of the National Institutes of Health 2UL1TR001425-05A1 Research Scholars Grant, RSG-19-111-01-CCE from the American Cancer Society, Brandon C. Gromada Head and Neck Cancer Foundation pilot grant, and start-up funds provided by the University of Cincinnati.
[a] Division of Hematology/Oncology, University of Cincinnati, 3125 Eden Avenue, Cincinnati, OH 45267-0562, USA; [b] Division of Medical Oncology, The Ohio State University, 1335 Lincoln Tower, 1800 Cannon Drive, Columbus, OH 43210, USA
* Corresponding author. 3125 Eden Avenue, ML 0562, Cincinnati, OH 45267.
E-mail address: wiseth@ucmail.uc.edu

Hematol Oncol Clin N Am 35 (2021) 1009–1020
https://doi.org/10.1016/j.hoc.2021.05.009
hemonc.theclinics.com

disease-free survival (DFS) but not overall survival (OS) albeit with increased toxicity.[4] However, most recurrent and/or metastatic (R/M) HNSCCs are not amenable to curative therapy because of significant treatment-related morbidity and toxicity. In those with locoregionally recurrent disease not amenable to surgery or radiation, the treatment approach is similar to that for patients with metastatic disease including palliative systemic treatment.

Historically, chemotherapy, most frequently a combination of platinum-based therapy with or without cetuximab, was favored.[5] In recent years, immunotherapy, particularly immune checkpoint inhibitors (ICIs), has become the "4th modality" for cancer treatment. Inhibitors of programmed death-1 (PD-1) or its corresponding ligand, PD-L1, have been approved by the US Food and Drug Administration (FDA) in multiple lines of therapy for various cancers.[6–8]

In 2016, treatment with PD-1-inhibiting antibodies, pembrolizumab and nivolumab, were approved by the FDA for the treatment of platinum-refractory R/M HNSCC.[6,7] In 2019, further approval allowed for pembrolizumab alone or in combination with chemotherapy depending on the PD-L1 combined positive score (CPS) as frontline treatment of R/M HNSCC.[8] However, less than 20% of patients elicit a response to immunotherapy, necessitating development of novel treatment to overcome resistance and biomarkers to better guide the use of immunotherapy in the appropriate patients.

ROLE OF SURGERY IN RECURRENT HEAD AND NECK CANCER

Locoregional failure occurs in approximately 33% of patients with locally advanced, human papillomavirus (HPV)-negative and 17% of HPV-positive HNSCC treated with cisplatin-based chemoradiation (CRT).[9] In locoregional failure or recurrence, treatment with curative-intent surgical salvage is not always technically feasible and carries a high risk of postoperative morbidity and mortality. However, surgery continues to offer the best chance of long-term survival in medically operable patients with limited-volume disease.[10] Importantly, patients with factors such as high disease volume, short time to recurrence, hypopharyngeal cancer, and multiple patient comorbidities have particularly poor outcomes.[11,12]

According to a meta-analysis of 16 studies, surgical resection in patients with locoregional recurrence following primary RT or CRT can yield a 5-year OS of 37%.[13] Major reported complications included fistulas (33%), followed by wound infections (24%) and flap failure (3%).[14] Despite the high rate of complications, if feasible and patients are appropriately selected, salvage surgery continues to be a preferred treatment option.

ROLE OF RADIATION IN RECURRENT HEAD AND NECK CANCER

There are 3 main roles for reirradiation for recurrent locoregional disease: curative intent for patients who are not surgical candidates, adjuvant treatment following salvage surgery, and palliative treatment for symptom control.[10,15] Reirradiation in locoregional recurrence is often a viable option, albeit with a higher rate of complications.[4] However, feasibility is a concern in most cases due to recurrent tumor proximity to the site of prior irradiation. Complications of reirradiation include osteoradionecrosis, fistulas, skin/wound breakdown, stroke, and major vessel necrosis or rupture.[16] Brands and colleagues[17] reported a 40% incidence of severe late toxicities, with 10% treatment-related mortality and 2-year survival of 10% to 30% in patients with unresectable disease who received definitive reirradiation with or without chemotherapy.

The role of adjuvant therapy following salvage surgery was also studied in a randomized study, in which patients were randomized to adjuvant CRT versus observation after primary resection. Adjuvant therapy resulted in improved DFS but not OS. In addition, there was an increase in both acute and late toxicity.[4] Palliative RT historically has been used for symptom control including bleeding or pain. With the emergence of stereotactic body radiation therapy, palliative RT produces comparable survival and toxicity profiles compared with palliative chemotherapy.[18]

Recently, intraoperative radiation therapy (IORT) has gained attention given its advantages, including greater accuracy, avoidance of tumor cell proliferation by rapid delivery, and reduction in hospital visits. Emami and colleagues[19] demonstrated a response rate (RR) of 86% in patients with recurrent HNSCC receiving IORT during salvage surgery. Another study showed 5-year recurrence-free survival and OS of 49% and 26%, respectively, in a similar setting.[20] Outcomes were better in those who achieved negative margins compared with those with positive margins (1-year in-field control, 82% vs 56% respectively).[21] However, the use of IORT in recurrent HNSCC is limited to few centers given the paucity of required equipment and the need for multidisciplinary effort. In addition, the results need to be verified in randomized phase 3 trials.

OLIGOMETASTATIC HEAD AND NECK CANCER

In oligometastatic HNSCC (1–5 metastases), outcomes have been reported with surgery (5-year OS, ~30%), which remains the gold standard whenever feasible.[22,23] Young and colleagues[22] demonstrated efficacy of pulmonary metastasectomy for pulmonary metastases from HNSCC in a meta-analysis, with a 5-year survival rate of 29%. Poor prognostic factors included cervical lymph node metastases at diagnosis (5-year survival rates 24% [N+] versus 60% [N0]),[24] oral cavity as primary site (5-year survival rates 15.4% vs 45.2%, $P = .01$),[24] multiple pulmonary nodules, and incomplete pulmonary resection. Importantly, HPV-positive patients have a high rate of long-term disease control with single metastasis-directed local therapy, with a median OS reported to be 41 months.[25]

Radiation alone for oligometastatic disease has been reported to yield outcomes similar to surgical resection and can serve as an alternative to invasive surgery.[26] In the cases of solitary metastases, both surgery and RT showed good outcomes with a 5-year survival rate of up to 56% ($P = .001$).[27] Florescu and Thariat[23] reported 5-year survival rates of greater than 20% after pulmonary/liver metastasectomy in selected patients. Corry and colleagues[28] reported RR of 50% to 70% with a "Quad Shot regimen," consisting of 3 courses of twice-daily 3.7-Gy fractions for 2 consecutive days, given over 8 to 9 weeks. Thus, multimodality treatment involving surgery and radiation can play an important role in oligometastatic disease and potentially provide a cure for some relapsed HNSCC.

ROLE OF SYSTEMIC THERAPY
Chemotherapy and Targeted Agents

Single-agent cytotoxic chemotherapy is often preferred over combination treatment for patients with a poor performance status. Commonly used drugs include platinum, 5-fluorouracil (5-FU), taxanes, and methotrexate; none of these options have shown superiority over the other.[29–32] When used alone, these agents result in response in only 15% to 30% of cases; have a short duration of response (DoR), ~3 to 5 months; and only rarely a complete response is observed.[29] Although combination chemotherapy increases the RR, it does not translate into an OS benefit and has greater toxicity.[33] Hence, combination chemotherapy is usually reserved for patients with good functional status requiring quicker and deeper tumor response. However, cytotoxic agents are now often reserved for later lines of treatment given the development of targeted agents and immunotherapy.

About 80% to 90% of patients with HNSCC overexpress the epidermal growth factor receptor (EGFR), which has been linked to tumorigenesis.[34] Cetuximab is a human-murine chimeric immunoglobulin G1 (IgG1) monoclonal antibody, which competitively binds to the extracellular domain of EGFR. Single-agent activity of cetuximab is minimal in the platinum-refractory R/M HNSCC setting, with an RR of 13%, median progression-free survival (PFS) of 70 days, and median OS of approximately 6 months.[35] However, cetuximab, when combined with platinum and 5-FU (EXTREME regimen) in the first-line metastatic setting, improved RR (36% vs 20%), PFS (5.6 vs 3.3 months; $P<.001$), and OS (10.1 vs 7.4 months; $P = .04$), compared with chemotherapy alone in the EXTREME trial (results detailed in **Table 1**).[5]

However, the EXTREME regimen is associated with grade 3 to 4 toxicities of 82% and a treatment discontinuation rate of 20%.[5] Thus it is mostly reserved for the fittest patients. In clinical practice, a taxane is frequently substituted for 5-FU.[36] In the TPExtreme randomized phase 3 trial, 539 patients with R/M HNSCC were randomly assigned to either 6 cycles of the EXTREME regimen or 4 cycles of cetuximab plus cisplatin and docetaxel (TPEx).[36] Noninferiority was demonstrated between the 2 arms in regard to OS at a median follow-up of 30 months (14.5 [TPEx] vs 13.4 months [EXTREME]; $P = .15$), with decreased toxicity (grade ≥ 4 events 36% [TPEx] vs 51% [EXTREME]; $P = .001$). Owing to the manageable toxicity profile and the convenience of same-day administration, docetaxel is viewed as a reasonable replacement for 5-FU.

Afatinib, an irreversible pan-ErbB inhibitor (EGFR, HER2, and HER4), showed superior PFS over methotrexate (2.6 months vs 1.7 months, respectively; $P = .03$) but no significant difference in OS (6.8 months vs 6 months, respectively, hazard ratio [HR] 0.96; $P = .70$).[37] RR was 10% and 6% ($P = 0.10$) in afatinib and methotrexate arms, respectively. A phase 2 trial comparing afatinib to cetuximab in platinum-refractory R/M HNSCC (n = 121) showed comparable RRs between the 2 agents. Sustained clinical responses were observed with sequential EGFR/ErbB treatment, thus indicating an absence of cross-resistance between the 2 drugs.[38] Given the promising outcomes, afatinib may be another potential option in R/M HNSCC. However, longer follow-up of these trials is required. Recently, impressive responses were observed with tipifarnib, a selective inhibitor of farnesyltransferase, the enzyme responsible for HRAS function, in HRAS mutant R/M HNSCC in a phase 2 trial, with an RR 56% and PFS of 6.1 months.[39]

Advent of Immunotherapy in the Management of Recurrent and/or Metastatic Head and Neck Squamous Cell Carcinoma

Previously, patients with R/M HNSCC who progressed on platinum-based therapy had a median OS reported to be around 1.8 months with best supportive care.[40] However, a phase 1b study, KEYNOTE-012, in platinum-refractory R/M HNSCC showed promise for novel immunotherapy.[7] Patients were heavily pretreated with chemotherapy, many having received 4 previous lines of systemic therapy. RR was ~18%, but responses were durable and median DoR was not reached (see **Table 1**). One-year OS rate was 38% with PFS of 17%. Treatment-related adverse events (TRAEs) of grade 3 to 4 occurred in 13% patients. Results of KEYNOTE-012 were further supported by a phase 2 trial, KEYNOTE-055, that investigated

Table 1
Published studies of major treatment options in R/M HNSCC

Study Name	Phase	Line of Therapy	Agent	Comparator	PD-L1 Expression (%)	Patients Randomized (n)	Response Rate (%)	Median Overall Survival (mo)	Median Duration of Response (mo)	Treatment-Related Adverse Events
Checkpoint inhibitors										
KEYNOTE-012 (Mehra et al,[7] 2018)	1b	Second line or beyond	Pembrolizumab	None	PD-L1 ≥1 (initial cohort); any (expansion cohort)	192	Overall: 18 TPS ≥1: 21 TPS<1: 6	8	NR (range 2+ to 30+)	Gr. 3-4: 13%
KEYNOTE-055 (Bauml et al,[41] 2017)	2	Second line or beyond	Pembrolizumab	IC chemotherapy	Any (substratified into CPS≥1 [82%] and CPS<1)	171	Overall: 16 CPS≥1: 18 CPS<1: 12	8	8	Gr. 3-4: 15%
KEYNOTE-040 (Cohen et al,[42] 2019)	3	Second line	Pembrolizumab	IC chemotherapy	Any (substratified into CPS ≥1 [79%] and TPS ≥50 [26%])	495	14.6 vs 10·1	Overall: 8.4 vs 6.9 TPS ≥50: 11.6 vs 6.6 CPS≥1: 8.7 vs 7.1	18.4 vs 5	Gr. 3-5: 13% vs 36%
Checkmate 141 (Ferris et al,[6] 2018)	3	Second line	Nivolumab	IC chemotherapy	Any (substratified into TPS ≥1 [57%] and <1)	361	13.3 vs 5.8	7.5 vs 5.1 PD-L1 ≥1: 8.7 vs 4.6 PD-L1 <1: 5.7 vs 5.8	2 vs 2.3 (P = .32)	Gr. 3-4: 13% vs 35%

(continued on next page)

Table 1
(continued)

Study Name	Phase	Line of Therapy	Agent	Comparator	PD-L1 Expression (%)	Patients Randomized (n)	Response Rate (%)	Median Overall Survival (mo)	Median Duration of Response (mo)	Treatment-Related Adverse Events
KEYNOTE-048 (Burtness et al,[8] 2019; Greil et al,[46] 2020)	3	First line	Pembrolizumab + chemotherapy	EXTREME	Any (substratified into CPS ≥1 [85%] and ≥20 [43%])	882	Overall: 36 vs 36; CPS ≥20: 44 vs 38; CPS ≥1: 37 vs 36	13 vs 10.7; CPS ≥20: 14.7 vs 11; CPS ≥1: 13.6 vs 10.6	6·7 vs 4·3	Gr. 3–5: 85% vs 83%
			Pembrolizumab	EXTREME			Overall: 17 vs 36; CPS ≥20: 23 vs 36; CPS ≥1: 19 vs 35	11.5 vs 10.7 (P = .199); CPS ≥20: 14.9 vs 10.8; CPS ≥1: 12.3 vs 10.4	23.4 vs 4.5	Gr. 3–5: 55% vs 83%
Targeted agents										
LUX-Head & Neck 1 (Machiels et al,[37] 2015)	3	Second line	Afatinib	Methotrexate	N/A	483	10 vs 6	6.8 vs 6 (P = .70)	N/A	Gr. 3–5 40% vs 36%
EXTEME (Vermorken et al,[5] 2008)	3	First line	Cetuximab/ platinum/5-FU	Platinum/5-FU	N/A	442	36 vs 20	10 vs 7.4	5.6 vs 4.7 (P = .2)	Gr. 3–4: 82% vs 76%

Abbreviations: DCR, disease control rate (RR + stable disease); EXTREME, platinum + 5-florouracil + cetuximab; Gr., grade; IC, investigator's choice; N/A, not applicable/available; NR, not reached; TPS, tumor-positive score.

pembrolizumab in 171 patients with HNSCC who had progressed on both platinum and cetuximab treatment.[41] The RR was 16%, and the mean DoR was 8 months.

The phase 3 KEYNOTE-040 investigated pembrolizumab over standard treatment (methotrexate, docetaxel, or cetuximab) in 495 patients with R/M HNSCC leading to the first approval of immunotherapy in second line and beyond.[42] Beside demonstrating improved median OS (8.4 months vs 6.9 months; HR, 0.80; $P = .016$), the study confirmed the significance of the predictive biomarker, PD-L1. On subgroup analysis, patients with PD-L1 expression with CPS $\geq$1 (79% of all patients) had greater benefit with pembrolizumab (median OS 8.7 months vs 7.1 months, HR 0.74, $P<.01$). Fewer grade $\geq$3 TRAEs were noted with pembrolizumab (13% and 36% for pembrolizumab vs chemotherapy, respectively).

At the same time, nivolumab, another PD-1 inhibitor, was investigated in the CheckMate 141 trial when compared with investigator's choice of chemotherapy (single-agent cetuximab, methotrexate, or docetaxel) in 361 patients with platinum-refractory R/M HNSCC.[6] Both RR (13.3% vs 5.8%, $P<.01$) and median OS (7.5 months vs 5 months, $P<.01$) were improved. Consequently, both pembrolizumab and nivolumab were approved by the FDA for platinum-refractory R/M SCCHN in 2016.

The pembrolizumab/lenvatinib combination has also shown promise in a phase 1b/2 trial involving multiple solid tumors (n = 137). The trial included 22 patients with HNSCC, with a 24-week RR of 36%, median DoR of 8.2 months (95% confidence interval [CI], 2.2–12.6 months), and a median PFS of 4.7 months (95% CI, 4.0–9.8 months).[43] At present, a phase 3 trial, LEAP-010, is underway studying pembrolizumab with or without lenvatinib in a similar cohort of patients who are PD-L1 positive (CPS $\geq$1).[44] In addition, LEAP-009 is investigating pembrolizumab in combination with lenvatinib versus chemotherapy in patients with R/M HNSCC who have previously received platinum therapy and ICI.[45] These studies indicate lenvatinib as a potential viable target in future combinations with ICIs or targeted agents.

Chemoimmunotherapy and Immunotherapy as the Frontline Treatment for Recurrent and/or Metastatic Head and Neck Squamous Cell Carcinoma

Given the success of pembrolizumab in the second-line setting, KEYNOTE-048 evaluated immunotherapy for front-line treatment of R/M HNSCC in 882 patients.[8] Three arms were compared: pembrolizumab as a single agent, combination of pembrolizumab and platinum-doublet chemotherapy (platinum and 5-FU), and cetuximab with platinum-doublet chemotherapy (EXTREME regimen).

During the annual European Society for Medical Oncology conference 2020,[46] updated results were reported with a median study follow-up of 46.2 months for pembrolizumab versus EXTREME and 45.6 months for pembrolizumab/chemotherapy versus EXTREME. Pembrolizumab and pembrolizumab/chemotherapy improved OS versus EXTREME in the CPS $\geq$20 and CPS $\geq$1 groups, whereas pembrolizumab/chemotherapy also improved OS in the total population (see **Table 1**). Grade 3 to 5 TRAEs were noted in 17% of the pembrolizumab arm, 72% of the pembrolizumab/chemotherapy arm, and 69% of the EXTREME arm. Detailed results are available in **Table 1**. For patients without PD-L1 expression (CPS<1), ICI combined with platinum-based chemotherapy or combination chemotherapy is preferred.

Pembrolizumab plus chemotherapy was approved by the FDA in June 2019 as frontline treatment of R/M HNSCC in all patients, whereas pembrolizumab monotherapy was approved as a frontline treatment of R/M HNSCC with PD-L1 CPS$\geq$1 or $\geq$20, changing the standard of care for these patients. When using pembrolizumab plus chemotherapy combination, 5-FU is often substituted with a taxane due to better tolerability, extrapolating results from the TPEx trial, and the widespread use of the combination in lung cancer based on KEYNOTE-407 trial.[47] This regimen is currently being studied in the trial NCT04030455.[48]

BIOMARKERS OF RESPONSE TO IMMUNOTHERAPY

Immune approaches are believed to be effective in HNSCC because of multiple methods of immune evasion, including presence of CD8[+] T cells in the tumor microenvironment, viral etiology associated with HPV-positive tumors, and high mutational burden associated with smoking.[49] P16 with a standard cutoff of positivity being 70% staining of tumor cells remains a surrogate for HPV. Increased tumor PD-L1 expression (ranging 42%–68%)[50] and PD-L2 (>50%) expression has been reported in HNSCC.[51]

In practice, only a minority of patients with R/M HNSCC will gain benefit from immunotherapy demonstrating the need of novel biomarkers to guide treatment options.[46] In addition, although PD-L1 is used as a predictive biomarker for response to ICIs in HNSCC, multiple trials have demonstrated their benefit in PD-L1-negative patients, including KEYNOTE-012, KEYNOTE-055, and CHECKMATE 141.[6,7,41] Tumor mutational burden, interferon-γ signature, HPV status, and the host microbiome have emerged as potential predictors of immune response and are currently under investigation in clinical trials.[49,52]

CLINICAL RELEVANCE
Previously Untreated Recurrent and/or Metastatic Head and Neck Squamous Cell Carcinoma

The results of KEYNOTE-048 changed the treatment paradigm for R/M HNSCC in the frontline setting. Single-agent pembrolizumab gained favor in those with PD-L1 CPS≥1. In patients with rapidly progressive tumors, pembrolizumab alone might not be the best option given longer time to response, whereas the addition of chemotherapy increases RR. For those negative (CPS<1) for PD-L1, pembrolizumab with platinum plus 5-FU (or taxane) chemotherapy, or combination chemotherapy is preferred, depending on patient performance status and potential ICI ineligibility (high levels of steroid use, autoimmune disease or transplant requiring immunosuppression, etc.).

Immunotherapy after Failure of Chemotherapy or Targeted Treatment in Recurrent and/or Metastatic Head and Neck Squamous Cell Carcinoma

Given most patients with R/M HNSCC will receive ICIs in the frontline, few will qualify for ICIs as a subsequent treatment option. However, in those receiving non-ICI regimens in the frontline, both pembrolizumab and nivolumab are approved by the FDA for platinum-refractory R/M HNSCC. As monotherapy, anti-PD-1 therapies induce responses in 13% to 15% of patients and double the survival rate at 1-year[6,42]

Systemic Treatment after Failure of Immunotherapy

In patients who are platinum-refractory and are either ineligible for or fail immunotherapy, clinical trials are preferred. However, cetuximab may also be considered if clinical condition and performance status allow. Cetuximab has shown activity as a single agent in R/M HNSCC as detailed earlier.[35] Single-agent taxane,[30] platinum,[31] or methotrexate,[32] can serve as other options for second-line treatment and beyond in R/M HNSCC. Taxanes have shown efficacy following nivolumab in a retrospective study in 13 patients with R/M HNSCC, with median PFS 3.8 months and median OS 10 months indicating that sequencing taxanes after immunotherapy failure may be a viable option.[30] Platinum-based chemotherapy has also shown favorable outcomes in patients with R/M HNSCC who have previously received ICIs, with an RR of 50% and median OS of 15 months.[53]

CLINICS CARE POINTS

- Surgery and/or reirradiation can potentially provide a cure in some locally recurrent/oligometastatic HNSCC.
- Pembrolizumab plus chemotherapy has been approved as a frontline treatment of R/M HNSCC. Pembrolizumab monotherapy is also approved as a frontline option for patients with R/M HNSCC with PD-L1 CPS $\geq$ 1.
- Both pembrolizumab and nivolumab are preferred options for platinum-refractory R/M HNSCC. As monotherapy, anti-PD-1 therapies induce responses in 13% to 18% of patients and double the survival rate at 1 year.
- Cetuximab either in combination with platinum-based doublet or as a single agent after the failure of platinum-based chemotherapy is a reasonable treatment option. The former is usually reserved for the fittest patients due to higher rate of toxicities.

SUMMARY

Checkpoint inhibitors have transformed the treatment paradigm of R/M HNSCC. Nevertheless, the overcoming resistance and enhancing treatment response is under active investigation. In addition, better predictive and prognostic biomarkers to guide treatment become imperative to serve the purpose of personalized medicine.

DISCLOSURE

Dr H. Shaikh and Dr V. Karivedu have no disclosures. Dr T.M. Wise-Draper discloses ownership interest in High Enroll, LLC, Honoraria from Physician Education Resources and research funding from Merck & Co, AstraZeneca/Medimmune, GlaxoSmithKline/Tesaro, Caris Life Sciences, and Bristol-Myers Squibb; he also serves on advisory boards for Shattuck Labs, Exicure, and Rakuten.

REFERENCES

1. Hunter KD, Parkinson EK, Harrison PR. Profiling early head and neck cancer. Nat Rev Cancer 2005;5(2):127–35.
2. Lydiatt WM, Patel SG, O'Sullivan B, et al. Head and Neck cancers-major changes in the American Joint Committee on cancer eighth edition cancer staging manual. CA Cancer J Clin 2017;67(2):122–37.
3. Gilbert H, Kagan AR. Recurrence patterns in squamous cell carcinoma of the oral cavity, pharynx, and larynx. J Surg Oncol 1974;6(5):357–80.
4. Janot F, de Raucourt D, Benhamou E, et al. Randomized trial of postoperative re-irradiation combined with chemotherapy after salvage surgery compared with salvage surgery alone in head and neck carcinoma. J Clin Oncol 2008;26(34):5518–23.
5. Vermorken JB, Mesia R, Rivera F, et al. Platinum-based chemotherapy plus cetuximab in head and neck cancer. N Engl J Med 2008;359(11):1116–27.
6. Ferris RL, Blumenschein G Jr, Fayette J, et al. Nivolumab vs investigator's choice in recurrent or metastatic squamous cell carcinoma of the head and neck: 2-year

long-term survival update of CheckMate 141 with analyses by tumor PD-L1 expression. Oral Oncol 2018;81:45–51.

7. Mehra R, Seiwert TY, Gupta S, et al. Efficacy and safety of pembrolizumab in recurrent/metastatic head and neck squamous cell carcinoma: pooled analyses after long-term follow-up in KEYNOTE-012. Br J Cancer 2018;119(2):153–9.

8. Burtness B, Harrington KJ, Greil R, et al. Pembrolizumab alone or with chemotherapy versus cetuximab with chemotherapy for recurrent or metastatic squamous cell carcinoma of the head and neck (KEYNOTE-048): a randomised, open-label, phase 3 study. Lancet 2019;394(10212):1915–28.

9. Ang KK, Zhang Q, Rosenthal DI, et al. Randomized phase III trial of concurrent accelerated radiation plus cisplatin with or without cetuximab for stage III to IV head and neck carcinoma: RTOG 0522. J Clin Oncol 2014;32(27):2940–50.

10. Goodwin WJ Jr. Salvage surgery for patients with recurrent squamous cell carcinoma of the upper aerodigestive tract: when do the ends justify the means? Laryngoscope 2000;110(3 Pt 2 Suppl 93):1–18.

11. Zafereo M. Surgical salvage of recurrent cancer of the head and neck. Curr Oncol Rep 2014;16(5):386.

12. Lim JY, Lim YC, Kim SH, et al. Factors predictive of successful outcome following salvage treatment of isolated neck recurrences. Otolaryngol Head Neck Surg 2010;142(6):832–7.

13. Elbers JBW, Veldhuis LI, Bhairosing PA, et al. Salvage surgery for advanced stage head and neck squamous cell carcinoma following radiotherapy or chemoradiation. Eur Arch Otorhinolaryngol 2019;276(3):647–55.

14. Hasan Z, Dwivedi RC, Gunaratne DA, et al. Systematic review and meta-analysis of the complications of salvage total laryngectomy. Eur J Surg Oncol 2017;43(1): 42–51.

15. Kasperts N, Slotman BJ, Leemans CR, et al. Results of postoperative reirradiation for recurrent or second primary head and neck carcinoma. Cancer 2006;106(7): 1536–47.

16. Machtay M, Rosenthal DI, Chalian AA, et al. Pilot study of postoperative reirradiation, chemotherapy, and amifostine after surgical salvage for recurrent head-and-neck cancer. Int J Radiat Oncol Biol Phys 2004;59(1):72–7.

17. Brands MT, Smeekens EAJ, Takes RP, et al. Time patterns of recurrence and second primary tumors in a large cohort of patients treated for oral cavity cancer. Cancer Med 2019;8(12):5810–9.

18. Strom T, Wishka C, Caudell JJ. Stereotactic body radiotherapy for recurrent unresectable head and neck cancers. Cancer Control 2016;23(1):6–11.

19. Emami B, Borrowdale RW, Sethi A, et al. Intraoperative radiation therapy in head and neck cancers. Int J Radiat Oncol Biol Phys 2017;99(2 Supplement):E335–6.

20. Zeidan YH, Yeh A, Weed D, et al. Intraoperative radiation therapy for advanced cervical metastasis: a single institution experience. Radiat Oncol 2011;6:72.

21. Scala LM, Hu K, Urken ML, et al. Intraoperative high-dose-rate radiotherapy in the management of locoregionally recurrent head and neck cancer. Head Neck 2013;35(4):485–92.

22. Young ER, Diakos E, Khalid-Raja M, et al. Resection of subsequent pulmonary metastases from treated head and neck squamous cell carcinoma: systematic review and meta-analysis. Clin Otolaryngol 2015;40(3):208–18.

23. Florescu C, Thariat J. Local ablative treatments of oligometastases from head and neck carcinomas. Crit Rev Oncol Hematol 2014;91(1):47–63.

24. Nibu K, Nakagawa K, Kamata S, et al. Surgical treatment for pulmonary metastases of squamous cell carcinoma of the head and neck. Am J Otolaryngol 1997; 18(6):391–5.
25. Fleming CW, Ward MC, Woody NM, et al. Identifying an oligometastatic phenotype in HPV-associated oropharyngeal squamous cell cancer: Implications for clinical trial design. Oral Oncol 2021;112:105046.
26. Sutera P, Clump DA, Kalash R, et al. Initial results of a multicenter phase 2 trial of stereotactic ablative radiation therapy for oligometastatic cancer. Int J Radiat Oncol Biol Phys 2019;103(1):116–22.
27. Leeman JE, Patel SH, Anderson ES, et al. Long-term survival in oligometastatic head and neck cancer patients. J Clin Oncol 2017;35(15_suppl):6029.
28. Corry J, Peters LJ, Costa ID, et al. The 'QUAD SHOT'–a phase II study of palliative radiotherapy for incurable head and neck cancer. Radiother Oncol 2005; 77(2):137–42.
29. Molin Y, Fayette J. Current chemotherapies for recurrent/metastatic head and neck cancer. Anticancer Drugs 2011;22(7):621–5.
30. moloney c, Sukor S, McCarthy MT, et al. A review of head and neck squamous cell carcinoma response to taxane chemotherapy treatment in the pre versus post nivolumab era. J Clin Oncol 2020;38(15_suppl):e18504.
31. Al-Sarraf M, Metch B, Kish J, et al. Platinum analogs in recurrent and advanced head and neck cancer: a Southwest Oncology Group and Wayne State University Study. Cancer Treat Rep 1987;71(7–8):723–6.
32. Stewart JS, Cohen EE, Licitra L, et al. Phase III study of gefitinib compared with intravenous methotrexate for recurrent squamous cell carcinoma of the head and neck [corrected]. J Clin Oncol 2009;27(11):1864–71.
33. Gibson MK, Li Y, Murphy B, et al. Randomized phase III evaluation of cisplatin plus fluorouracil versus cisplatin plus paclitaxel in advanced head and neck cancer (E1395): an intergroup trial of the Eastern Cooperative Oncology Group. J Clin Oncol 2005;23(15):3562–7.
34. Denaro N, Russi EG, Adamo V, et al. State-of-the-art and emerging treatment options in the management of head and neck cancer: news from 2013. Oncology 2014;86(4):212–29.
35. Vermorken JB, Trigo J, Hitt R, et al. Open-label, uncontrolled, multicenter phase II study to evaluate the efficacy and toxicity of cetuximab as a single agent in patients with recurrent and/or metastatic squamous cell carcinoma of the head and neck who failed to respond to platinum-based therapy. J Clin Oncol 2007;25(16): 2171–7.
36. Guigay J, Fayette J, Mesia R, et al. TPExtreme randomized trial: TPEx versus Extreme regimen in 1st line recurrent/metastatic head and neck squamous cell carcinoma (R/M HNSCC). J Clin Oncol 2019;37(15_suppl):6002.
37. Machiels JP, Haddad RI, Fayette J, et al. Afatinib versus methotrexate as second-line treatment in patients with recurrent or metastatic squamous-cell carcinoma of the head and neck progressing on or after platinum-based therapy (LUX-Head & Neck 1): an open-label, randomised phase 3 trial. Lancet Oncol 2015;16(5): 583–94.
38. Seiwert TY, Fayette J, Cupissol D, et al. A randomized, phase II study of afatinib versus cetuximab in metastatic or recurrent squamous cell carcinoma of the head and neck. Ann Oncol 2014;25(9):1813–20.
39. Ho AL, Hanna GJ, Scholz CR, et al. Preliminary activity of tipifarnib in tumors of the head and neck, salivary gland and urothelial tract with HRAS mutations. J Clin Oncol 2020;38(15_suppl):6504.

40. León X, Hitt R, Constenla M, et al. A retrospective analysis of the outcome of patients with recurrent and/or metastatic squamous cell carcinoma of the head and neck refractory to a platinum-based chemotherapy. Clin Oncol 2005;17(6):418–24.
41. Bauml J, Seiwert TY, Pfister DG, et al. Pembrolizumab for platinum- and cetuximab-refractory head and neck cancer: results from a single-arm, phase II study. J Clin Oncol 2017;35(14):1542–9.
42. Cohen EEW, Soulieres D, Le Tourneau C, et al. Pembrolizumab versus methotrexate, docetaxel, or cetuximab for recurrent or metastatic head-and-neck squamous cell carcinoma (KEYNOTE-040): a randomised, open-label, phase 3 study. Lancet 2019;393(10167):156–67.
43. Taylor MH, Lee C-H, Makker V, et al. Phase IB/II Trial of lenvatinib plus pembrolizumab in patients with advanced renal cell carcinoma, endometrial cancer, and other selected advanced solid tumors. J Clin Oncol 2020;38(11):1154–63.
44. Siu LL, Burtness B, Cohen EEW, et al. Phase III LEAP-010 study: first-line pembrolizumab with or without lenvatinib in recurrent/metastatic (R/M) head and neck squamous cell carcinoma (HNSCC). J Clin Oncol 2020;38(15_suppl):TPS6589.
45. Harrington K, Cohen E, Siu L, et al. 351Pembrolizumab plus lenvatinib vs chemotherapy and lenvatinib monotherapy for recurrent/metastatic head and neck squamous cell carcinoma that progressed on platinum therapy and immunotherapy: LEAP-009. J ImmunoTherapy Cancer 2020;8(Suppl 3):A214.
46. Greil R, Rischin D, Harrington KJ, et al. 915MO Long-term outcomes from KEYNOTE-048: Pembrolizumab (pembro) alone or with chemotherapy (pembro+C) vs EXTREME (E) as first-line (1L) therapy for recurrent/metastatic (R/M) head and neck squamous cell carcinoma (HNSCC). Ann Oncol 2020;31:S660–1.
47. Paz-Ares L, Luft A, Vicente D, et al. Pembrolizumab plus chemotherapy for squamous non–small-cell lung cancer. N Engl J Med 2018;379(21):2040–51.
48. Center MDAC, National Cancer I. Cisplatin, docetaxel, and pembrolizumab in treating patients with stage II-III Laryngeal cancer. Available at: https://ClinicalTrials.gov/show/NCT04030455.
49. Mandal R, Şenbabaoğlu Y, Desrichard A, et al. The head and neck cancer immune landscape and its immunotherapeutic implications. JCI Insight 2016;1(17):e89829.
50. Qiao X-w, Jiang J, Pang X, et al. The evolving landscape of PD-1/PD-L1 pathway in head and neck cancer. 10.3389/fimmu.2020.01721. Front Immunol 2020;11:1721.
51. Yearley JH, Gibson C, Yu N, et al. PD-L2 expression in human tumors: relevance to anti-PD-1 therapy in cancer. Clin Cancer Res 2017;23(12):3158.
52. Wang J, Sun H, Zeng Q, et al. HPV-positive status associated with inflamed immune microenvironment and improved response to anti-PD-1 therapy in head and neck squamous cell carcinoma. Scientific Rep 2019;9(1):13404.
53. Kacew AJ, Harris EJ, Lorch JH, et al. Chemotherapy after immune checkpoint blockade in patients with recurrent, metastatic squamous cell carcinoma of the head and neck. Oral Oncol 2020;105:104676.

Immunotherapy for Head and Neck Cancer

Sumita Trivedi, MD[1], Lova Sun, MD[1], Charu Aggarwal, MD, MPH*

KEYWORDS

- Head and neck cancers • Immunotherapy • Immune checkpoint inhibitors • PD-L1
- Human papillomavirus

KEY POINTS

- Anti-PD-1 therapy is now standard first-line therapy for metastatic and unresectable head and neck cancers.
- Immune-related adverse events can affect any organ system.
- There is a need for improved biomarkers to inform patient selection for use of immunotherapy as well as novel treatment combination strategies to overcome resistance and improve outcomes.
- Combination immune checkpoint inhibition, therapeutic vaccines, and adoptive T-cell therapy are currently being investigated in head and neck cancer.

INTRODUCTION

Head and neck cancer, the seventh most common cancer worldwide, is diagnosed in more than 800,000 patients per year, and is responsible for more than 400,000 deaths.[1–3] Most patients with head and neck squamous cell carcinoma (HNSCC), which comprises more than 90% of head and neck cancers, present with locally advanced disease and are managed with multimodality therapy, including surgical resection, radiotherapy, and/or chemotherapy. However, despite advances in local and systemic therapy, the risk for local or distant recurrence is high, and overall survival remains poor (5-year overall survival <50%).[4]

As with many other tumor types, the immune system plays an important role in the progression of HNSCC, which has a relatively high tumor mutation burden[5] and is often associated with impaired immune cell function.[6] In particular, human papilloma virus (HPV)-mediated cancers, which have been increasing in incidence over the past several decades, are more likely to exhibit an immunologically active tumor microenvironment,[7,8]

Department of Medicine, Division of Hematology-Oncology, University of Pennsylvania, Perelman Center for Advanced Medicine, 3400 Civic Center Boulevard, Philadelphia, PA 19104, USA
[1] First authors contributed equally to this article.
* Corresponding author.
E-mail address: Charu.aggarwal@pennmedicine.upenn.edu

Hematol Oncol Clin N Am 35 (2021) 1021–1037
https://doi.org/10.1016/j.hoc.2021.05.010

and present an attractive target for various novel immune-targeted approaches. In addition, smoking, a known driver of HNSCC carcinogenesis, has been associated with poor immune cell infiltration and higher mutation numbers; and tumors harboring genetic smoking signatures may respond particularly well to immune therapy.[8] In this review, we summarize recent and ongoing developments in incorporating immunotherapy into the treatment of recurrent/metastatic HNSCC, and discuss emerging strategies for incorporation of immunotherapy in the locally advanced setting.

IMMUNE CHECKPOINT INHIBITORS IN RECURRENT/METASTATIC HEAD AND NECK SQUAMOUS CELL CARCINOMA

The historical standard of care for recurrent or metastatic (R/M) HNSCC in the first-line setting was platinum-based chemotherapy with cetuximab.

In the past few years, immune checkpoint inhibitors have significantly expanded and improved treatment options for R/M HNSCC. Many cancers take advantage of the body's normal downregulatory immune checkpoint pathways to evade immune recognition and killing of tumor cells. Immunotherapy agents, including immune checkpoint inhibitors, enhance immune surveillance and tumor cell killing, and have been shown to lead to durable, long-term responses and survival in many cancers, including HNSCC. The anti-programmed death 1 (PD-1) immune checkpoint inhibitors pembrolizumab and nivolumab first showed improved survival and durable responses in the second-line setting after progression on chemotherapy; pembrolizumab has now become incorporated into standard first-line therapy as well (**Table 1**).

Immunotherapy in the Second-Line Setting

KEYNOTE-012 was a phase Ib basket trial of pembrolizumab, a humanized monoclonal antibody against PD-1. In 192 patients with pretreated recurrent or metastatic HNSCC, 74% of whom had received at least 2 prior lines of systemic therapy, an objective response rate (ORR) of 18% was observed, including 8 patients with complete response,[9,10] and overall survival at 12 months was 38%. Whereas the initial cohort of 60 patients enrolled in this study were required to have evidence of PD-L1–positive tumors (tumor cells or stroma with $\geq$1% PD-L1 expression), the remaining 132 enrolled patients were not required to have PD-L1 positivity. Based on these results, pembrolizumab was granted accelerated approval in patients with platinum-refractory R/M HNSCC. The phase II KEYNOTE-055 trial also showed treatment efficacy (ORR 16%) with good response duration and acceptable toxicity profile in 171 heavily pretreated patients with disease progression within 6 months of platinum and cetuximab therapy.[11] The subsequent randomized phase III KEYNOTE-040 trial compared pembrolizumab to investigator's choice chemotherapy in a cohort of 495 patients with R/M HNSCC, and Food and Drug Administration (FDA) approval was maintained based on prolongation of survival (median overall survival [mOS] 8.4 vs 6.9 months, hazard ratio [HR] 0.80, 95% confidence interval [CI] 0.65–0.98), as well as improved side-effect profile, with pembrolizumab.[12] Notably, patients with higher PD-L1 expression derived more pronounced benefit with pembrolizumab.[12]

Nivolumab, another PD-1 inhibitor, was also approved in the second-line setting based on the randomized phase III CheckMate 141 study, which enrolled 361 patients with disease progression within 6 of months of platinum-based chemotherapy. Patients were randomized 2:1 to either nivolumab 3 mg/kg every 2 weeks or investigator's choice systemic therapy. The nivolumab group had improved overall survival (mOS 7.5 vs 5.1 months, HR 0.7, 95% CI 0.51–0.96) and ORR (13.3% vs 5.8%), as well as lower incidence of severe adverse events (13.1% vs 35.1%), compared with

Table 1
Trials of immune checkpoint inhibitors in recurrent/metastatic head and neck squamous cell carcinoma

Trial	Agent	Phase	Response Rate/Effect	HPV/PDL1 Subgroup Differentiation
Second or later line setting				
KEYNOTE-012[9,10]	Pembrolizumab	Ib	ORR 18% mPFS 2.1 mo mOS 8 mo	Higher ORR in HPV+ (24% vs 16%); Higher ORR in PD-L1 CPS≥1 (21% vs 6%)
KEYNOTE-055[11]	Pembrolizumab	II	ORR 16% mPFS 2 mo	Similar ORR in PD-L1+ (18%) and PD-L1- (12%)
KEYNOTE-040[12]	Pembrolizumab (vs chemo)	III	mOS 8.4 mo vs 6.9 mo with chemo (HR 0.80)	Longer mOS in PD-L1+ CPS≥1: HR 0.75, mOS 8.7 mo CPS≥50: HR 0.64, mOS 11.6 mo
CheckMate 141[13,14]	Nivolumab (vs chemo)	III	mOS 7.5 vs 5.1 mo with chemo (HR 0.7) ORR 13.3%	PD-L1 CPS≥1: HR 0.55 (mOS 8.7 mo) Benefit regardless of HPV status
HAWK[16]	Durvalumab	II	ORR 16.2%	Restricted enrollment to PD-L1 TPS ≥25% HPV+: ORR 16.2% HPV-: ORR 10.9%
EAGLE[17,21]	Durvalumab Tremelimumab (vs chemo)	III	12-mo OS 37% (D), 30.4% (D + T), 30.5% (chemo)	Survival advantage with D ± T over chemo in TMB-high subgroup (≥16 mut/Mb)
First line				
KEYNOTE-048[18]	Pembrolizumab Monotherapy (vs chemotherapy)	III	mOS 11.6 vs 10.7 mo, HR 0.85 (noninferior) ORR 16.9%	CPS ≥ 20: mOS 14.9 vs 10.7 mo, HR 0.61 CPS ≥ 1: mOS 12.3 vs 10.3 mo, HR 0.78
	Pembrolizumab with platinum doublet (vs chemotherapy)	III	mOS 13.0 vs 10.7 mo, HR 0.77 ORR 42.9% (CPS≥20), 36.4 (CPS ≥1)	CPS ≥ 20: mOS 14.7 vs 11.0 mo, HR 0.70 CPS ≥ 1: 13.6 vs 10.4 mo, HR 0.65

Abbreviations: CPS, combined positive score; D, Durvalumab; HPV, human papilloma virus; HR, hazard ratio; mOS, median overall survival; mPFS, median progression-free survival; ORR, overall response rate; PD-L1, programmed death-L1; T, Tremelimumab; TMB, tumor mutation burden; TPS, tumor proportional score.

the chemotherapy group.[13] Two-year results confirmed OS benefit of nivolumab irrespective of PD-L1 expression and HPV status.[14]

In 2016, both pembrolizumab and nivolumab were FDA approved for patients with advanced R/M HNSCC who have progressed after platinum-based chemotherapy, regardless of PD-L1 expression.[15] Other checkpoint inhibitors, including durvalumab, a PD-1 inhibitor, and tremelimumab, a CTLA-4 inhibitor, have been also investigated in the second-line setting. Although the phase II HAWK trial showed encouraging antitumor activity of durvalumab, with an ORR of 16.2%,[16] the phase III EAGLE trial did not demonstrate statistically significant survival benefit of durvalumab with or without tremelimumab over chemotherapy in the overall population.[17]

Immunotherapy in the First-Line Setting

KEYNOTE-048 was a randomized phase III trial conducted in patients with treatment-naïve metastatic HNSCC, or recurrent disease incurable by local therapies. In this 3-arm trial, 882 patients were randomized to pembrolizumab monotherapy, pembrolizumab in combination with platinum doublet chemotherapy (cisplatin or carboplatin and 5-FU), or standard of care chemotherapy with the EXTREME regimen.[18] Pembrolizumab monotherapy demonstrated superior OS in the PD-L1 combined positive score (CPS) $\geq$20 (mOS 14.9 vs 10.7 months, HR 0.61, P = .0007) and CPS$\geq$1 populations (mOS 12.3 vs 10.3 months HR 0.78, P = .0086) compared with the EXTREME arm, and was noninferior in the total population (mOS 11.6 vs 10.7 months, HR 0.85). Pembrolizumab with chemotherapy demonstrated improved OS compared with EXTREME chemotherapy in the total population (mOS 13.0 vs 10.7 months, HR 0.77, P = .0034) as well as the CPS $\geq$20 (14.7 vs 11.0 months, HR 0.70, P = .0004) and CPS $\geq$1 (13.6 vs 10.4 months, HR 0.65, P < .0001) subpopulations.[18]

Based on results from KEYNOTE-048, in June 2019, the FDA approved pembrolizumab for first-line treatment of patients with metastatic or unresectable recurrent HNSCC. Whereas pembrolizumab in combination with platinum and fluorouracil was approved for all patients, the approval for single-agent pembrolizumab was limited to patients whose tumors express PD-L1 (CPS $\geq$1). Although pembrolizumab monotherapy produced deep and durable responses in some patients, the ORR of pembrolizumab monotherapy in the total population (16%) was markedly lower than chemotherapy (36%), and pembrolizumab monotherapy did not improve survival compared with the EXTREME regimen in the total PD-L1-unselected population. Thus, pembrolizumab monotherapy may be most appropriate in patients with PD-L1 CPS $\geq$20 with less bulky or asymptomatic disease, such as lung metastases only, whereas pembrolizumab plus chemotherapy may be preferred when rapid response rate is critical, such as in bulky locoregional disease at risk of airway or bleeding complications.

BIOMARKERS TO PREDICT RESPONSE TO IMMUNE CHECKPOINT INHIBITION

Despite these advances in systemic treatment options, approximately 85% to 95% of patients with R/M HNSCC do not respond to immunotherapy alone, or have a nondurable response followed by disease progression. Thus, there is a clear need for improved biomarkers to inform patient selection, as well as for improved treatment combinations and strategies to overcome resistance and improve outcomes.

Programmed Death-L1

Currently, the FDA approval for single-agent pembrolizumab in the first-line setting is limited to patients whose tumors express PD-L1 CPS $\geq$1. Approximately half of

HNSCCs express PD-L1 on tumor cells (ie, tumor proportion score), but up to 85% have PD-L1 expression when considering both tumor and immune cells (ie, CPS). PD-L1 expression has shown utility as a predictive biomarker of response to PD-1 blockade in multiple cancer types; however, important limitations of PD-L1, including dynamic expression over time and intratumor heterogeneity,[19] as well as nonstandardized assays corresponding to different PD-1/PD-L1 inhibitors, have led to inconsistent findings across trials. Several of the studies discussed previously, including the phase 3 KEYNOTE-040 and CheckMate 141 trials, showed that PD-L1 expression on tumor cells (tumor proportional score [TPS]) predicted improved clinical benefit and survival with anti-PD-1 therapy,[12,14] although higher expression levels did not correlate with improved survival in longer-term follow-up in the CheckMate 141 trial.[14] In KEYNOTE 012, CPS, which assesses PD-L1 expression on both tumor and tumor-infiltrating immune cells, was more predictive of outcomes than TPS alone[9]; accordingly, subsequent trials including KEYNOTE-048 have assessed PD-L1 expression via CPS. Consensus guidelines also recommend PD-L1 testing with CPS.[15] Although PD-L1 expression may predict clinical benefit with immune checkpoint inhibitor therapy, patients with PD-L1–negative HNSCC can also derive benefit and should not be excluded from anti-PD-1 agents. Combining PD-L1 expression with other biomarkers has the potential to enhance the ability to predict benefit from immunotherapy; investigation into these approaches is ongoing.

Other Biomarkers

Tumor mutation burden (TMB) has been extensively investigated as a predictor of immunotherapy response, based on the rationale that a greater number of mutations corresponds to an increased range of neoepitopes that can be targeted by an activated immune system. Within the HNSCC cohort of a cancer genomics dataset of pembrolizumab-treated patients, higher TMB predicted a greater frequency of clinical response, particularly among HPV-negative patients.[20] In the phase III EAGLE study, which investigated durvalumab with or without tremelimumab in patients who had progressed on platinum-based chemotherapy, patients with high tumor mutational burden ($\geq$16 mutations/megabase, assessed via circulating tumor DNA) treated with immunotherapy had improved survival compared with those treated with chemotherapy, with hazard ratios for overall survival improved by at least 60%.[21] In addition to being independently predictive, joint use of TMB with other biomarkers including PD-L1 and T-cell activated gene expression profile (GEP) may also have utility in characterizing and predicting clinical responses to immunotherapy.[22]

Similar factors as discussed with PD-L1, including tumor heterogeneity, change over time, and assay standardization, have limited the value of TMB and its incorporation into clinical decision making.[23] In addition, as discussed in the following, the impact of HPV status on predictive utility of TMB has yet to be definitively established. Finally, other biomarkers including PD-L2, immune infiltration, inflammatory GEP, and microbiota have been investigated, but not yet validated in HNSCC.[22,24]

OTHER CONSIDERATIONS IN THE USE OF IMMUNOTHERAPY FOR HEAD AND NECK SQUAMOUS CELL CARCINOMA
Human Papilloma Virus Status

Though HNSCC has historically been associated with tobacco and alcohol use, HPV-driven cancers, particularly of the oropharynx, have been increasing in incidence over the past few decades.[25,26] HPV-associated oropharyngeal cancer represents a distinct entity that affects younger individuals and carries a more favorable prognosis.

The impact of HPV status on outcomes with immune checkpoint inhibition (ICI) remains unclear. HPV infection has been hypothesized to induce an inflamed immune microenvironment and GEP, leading to increased T-cell infiltration and heightened efficacy of ICI.[7] In both the KEYNOTE-012 and HAWK trials, patients with HPV+ disease had higher response rates than patients with HPV− disease when treated with ICI therapy.[9,10,16] In the CheckMate 141 study, the benefit of nivolumab compared with chemotherapy was initially more pronounced in patients with HPV+ cancers (HR 0.56, 95% CI 0.32–0.99) than HPV− cancers (HR 0.73, 95% CI 0.42–1.25); however, on updated results, benefit of nivolumab was seen regardless of HPV status.[13,14] Conversely, in KEYNOTE-040, HPV− cancers appeared to have greater benefit from pembrolizumab than HPV + cancers.[12] Overall, patients with both HPV+ and HPV− HNSCC can derive benefit from ICIs; and current guidelines recommend that HPV status should not influence the decision to treat patients with R/M HNSCC with standard of care immunotherapy.[15]

Other immunotherapeutic approaches targeting HPV as well as Epstein Barr Virus (EBV), a key player in the pathogenesis of many nasopharynx cancers, include therapeutic vaccines and adoptive T-cell therapy; these are discussed later in this article.

Monitoring for Response to Treatment

Patterns of response and progression to immunotherapy often differ in kinetics from response to conventional cytotoxic chemotherapy. For instance, radiographic tumor shrinkage may occur in a delayed fashion after initial disease progression on therapy, a phenomenon called pseudoprogression initially described in patients with advanced melanoma.[27,28] Larger trials in other tumor types have also described pseudoprogression, although generally occurring at rates lower than 10%.[29] In a subgroup analysis of CheckMate 141, treatment with nivolumab beyond RECIST 1.1-defined disease progression led to clinical benefit, including tumor reduction, in some patients.[30] Generally, however, radiographically documented pseudoprogression in HNSCC is a relatively rare phenomenon.[31]

Conversely, hyperprogression refers to rapid disease progression defined as an increase in tumor growth rate by a factor or 2 after checkpoint inhibitor initiation,[32] and has been reported with checkpoint inhibitor therapy in HNSCC.[33] Although it remains controversial whether this observation represents true immunotherapy-induced acceleration of tumor growth or natural biology of tumor growth, hyperprogression has been shown to correlate with poorer outcomes.[32] In HNSCC, this pattern can be particularly dangerous when rapid tumor growth of locoregionally advanced disease causes compromise of adjacent anatomic structures.

To more accurately assess responses to immunotherapy and capture additional response patterns beyond those described by Response Evaluation in Solid Tumors (RECIST) and World Health Organization criteria, newer response criteria including immune-specific related response criteria (irRC),[27] immune-related RECIST (irRECIST), and immunotherapy RECIST (iRECIST),[34] have been developed to standardize and harmonize response evaluation for both clinical practice and immunotherapy trials.[35] These criteria incorporate features such as confirmation of disease progression and allowance of new metastases, allow patients with atypical responses to continue therapy without being labeled as disease progression and having premature cessation of treatment,[36] and facilitate improved trial endpoints in immunotherapy trials.

Immune-Related Adverse Events and Contraindications to Immunotherapy

Although checkpoint inhibitors are generally better tolerated than standard chemotherapy, immune-related adverse events (irAEs), including pneumonitis, colitis, and endocrinopathies, are a known risk of immunotherapy. These complications can affect any organ system, can be life threatening, and often require management with treatment cessation and/or corticosteroids and other immunomodulatory medications, depending on grade and severity.[37] Monitoring for and management of irAE in patients with HNSCC on immunotherapy largely mirrors that of other cancer types. However, patients with bulky disease may be at additional risk for bleeding/vascular blowout, airway compromise, and facial edema with immune infiltration or inflammation from immunotherapy. Patients with progressive symptoms, concern for airway compromise, or vascular encasement should have surgical consultation early in their treatment course and consideration of cessation of immunotherapy.[15]

Exclusion criteria for enrollment on nivolumab and pembrolizumab clinical trials in HNSCC included autoimmune disease, organ transplantation, immunosuppressive therapy, chronic viral infections (human immunodeficiency virus [HIV], hepatitis B virus [HBV], hepatitis C virus [HCV]), poor performance status, and brain metastases.[10,13] An accumulating body of literature suggests that immunotherapy can be safe and effective in patients with HIV, HBV, and HCV[38,39]; and efforts are ongoing to increase inclusion rates of patients with chronic viral infections in immunotherapy trials.[40] Current FDA approvals for checkpoint inhibitors in HNSCC do not carry specific eligibility restrictions; thus, clinical judgment is paramount in weighing risks and benefits for individual patients with relative contraindications to immunotherapy.

IMMUNOTHERAPY IN THE LOCALLY ADVANCED SETTING

Current standard of care for locally advanced HNSCC consists of definitive chemoradiotherapy or surgery followed by adjuvant radiation therapy with or without chemotherapy depending on pathologic risk stratification. Despite aggressive management resulting in significant morbidity, there continues to be up to a 50% rate of recurrence in HPV-unrelated HNSCC.[41] The addition of immunotherapy is currently being explored to improve disease-free survival while reducing toxicity in this subset of patients (**Table 2**). JAVELIN head and neck 100 sought to determine whether the anti-PD-L1 monoclonal antibody, avelumab, with concurrent chemoradiation followed by maintenance avelumab could delay disease progression in locally advanced HNSCC (NCT02952586). No improvement in survival was demonstrated with the addition of avelumab to chemoradiation, and the trial was terminated prematurely. Interestingly, the addition of pembrolizumab to concurrent cisplatin-sensitized radiation showed promising results in a phase IB trial (NCT02586207). Treatment included neoadjuvant pembrolizumab administered 7 days before concurrent chemoradiation, as well as in combination with chemoradiation. Complete response rates were 85.3% in HPV+ and 78.3% in HPV− HNSCC.[42] Neoadjuvant pembrolizumab in patients with high-risk, locally advanced HNSCC was additionally found to be safe and feasible in a single-arm phase II trial (NCT02296684), with 43% of the 21 patients demonstrating pathologic treatment to a single dose of pembrolizumab. The randomized, open-label phase III study KEYNOTE-689 evaluated the addition of neoadjuvant and adjuvant pembrolizumab in combination with cisplatin-sensitized radiation (NCT03765918). Pembrolizumab was found to be safe, with pathologic response noted in 44% of patients.[43] Although pembrolizumab appears to be biologically active in locally active HNSCC, the optimal sequencing in the current treatment paradigm is currently under investigation with several ongoing trials. GORTEC 2015 to 01 is an ongoing phase II study comparing pembrolizumab and radiation with standard of care cetuximab and radiation in patients with locally advanced HNSCC (NCT02707588). No difference was noted in the primary endpoint of locoregional

Table 2
Trials of immune checkpoint inhibitors in locally advanced head and neck squamous cell carcinoma

Trial	Agent	Phase	Trial Design	Response Rate/Effect	Clinicaltrials.gov Identifier
JAVELIN 100 head and neck	Avelumab	III	Avelumab plus concurrent CRT vs placebo plus CRT	mPFS HR 1.21 (95% CI 0.93–1.57, $P = .92$) mOS HR 1.31 (95% CI 0.93–1.85, $P = .937$)	NCT02952586
KEYNOTE-412	Pembrolizumab	III	Pembrolizumab plus concurrent CRT vs placebo plus CRT		NCT03040999
RTOG 3504	Nivolumab	I	Nivolumab plus weekly cisplatin CRT vs Nivolumab plus 3 weekly cisplatin CRT vs Nivolumab plus cetuximab CRT vs RT alone		NCT02764593
GORTEC 2015–01	Pembrolizumab	II	Pembrolizumab with RT vs cetuximab with RT	Locoregional control at 15 mo 60% vs 59% with cetux-RT 2-y PFS 42% vs 40% with cetux-RT (HR 0.83) 2-y OS 62% vs 55% with cetux-RT (HR 0.83)	NCT02707588
KEYNOTE-689	Pembrolizumab	III	Neoadjuvant pembrolizumab followed by surgical resection then SOC plus adjuvant pembrolizumab vs surgical resection followed by adjuvant SOC		NCT03765918

Abbreviations: CI, confidence interval; CRT, Chemoradiotherapy; HR, hazard ratio; mOS, median overall survival; mPFS, median progression-free survival; RT, Radiotherapy; SOC, Standard of care.

control at 15 months (60% vs 59% with cetuximab-RT) or secondary endpoints of 2-year progression-free survival (42% vs 40% with cetux-RT HR = 0.83, 95% CI 0.53–1.29, P = .41) or OS (62% vs 55% with cetuximab-RT HR 0.83, 95% CI 0.49–1.40, P = .49). KEYNOTE-412 is a phase III study to determine the safety and efficacy of concomitant cisplatin-sensitized radiation with pembrolizumab compared with placebo with cisplatin-radiation (NCT03040999). The addition of another anti-PD-1 monoclonal antibody, nivolumab, to either cisplatin or cetuximab-sensitized radiation or radiation alone was the subject of a phase I trial of patients with intermediate or high-risk locally advanced HNSCC (NCT02764593). Early safety data for the cohort of patients receiving nivolumab with weekly cisplatin-sensitized radiation showed nivolumab to be safe and feasible.

COMBINATION IMMUNE CHECKPOINT INHIBITION
Dual-Checkpoint Blockade

Inhibition of the PD-1/PD-L1 axis may result in adaptive resistance with upregulation of expression of other immune checkpoints.[44] Combined checkpoint inhibition may improve tumor immune responses and multiple checkpoint inhibitor combinations are targeting costimulatory pathways. Cytotoxic T lymphocyte antigen (CTLA-4) is expressed by several immune cells in the tumor microenvironment, including regulatory T cells (Tregs), which produce the immunosuppressive molecule transforming growth factor-β (TGF-β) when activated with CD28.[45] CTLA-4 induces T-cell dysfunction and downregulation of the immune response necessary under normal conditions to prevent immune overactivity; however, tumor cell secretion of TGF-β can in turn stimulate CTLA-4 expression, leading to T-cell exhaustion.[46] Anti-CTLA-4 agents could potentially complement anti-PD-1effects on T cells and the immunosuppressive tumor microenvironment. Two trials, EAGLE and CONDOR, studied the combination of durvalumab and tremelimumab. Results of the phase III EAGLE trial demonstrated that the combination durvalumab and tremelimumab did not improve overall survival (HR 1.04, CI 0.85–1.26) compared with chemotherapy. ORR with durvalumab and tremelimumab was 18%, similar to durvalumab monotherapy with increased toxicity seen in the combination arm.[17] Similarly, CheckMate 714, a randomized phase II trial using a combination anti-CTLA-4 and anti-PD-1 versus anti-PD-1 monotherapy did not meet its primary endpoint in the platinum-refractory population (NCT02823574). CheckMate 358, a phase I/II trial to investigate the safety and effectiveness of nivolumab alone or in combination with ipilimumab or relatlimab (an anti-LAG-3 monoclonal antibody) in HPV and EBV-associated cancers was recently completed (NCT02488759). Ongoing trials continue to investigate alternative combinations of anti-CTLA-4 and anti-PD-1 therapy (NCT02741570, NCT02551159).

Immunotherapy in Combination with Small Molecule Drugs

Signaling inhibitors block pathways necessary for tumor growth and proliferation and have been the target of therapeutic intervention for many tumors. Bintrafusp alfa (M7824) is a bifunctional fusion protein composed of 2 extracellular domains of TGF-βRII fused to an anti-PD-1 monoclonal antibody. Bintrafusp alfa was evaluated in a phase II (NCT03427411) trial that included patients with advanced, pretreated HPV-associated solid tumors. Preliminary results demonstrated ORRs of 30.5%.[47] Vascular endothelial growth factor receptor pathway inhibition has shown efficacy in combination with immune checkpoint blockade in multiple solid tumors and is under evaluation in HNSCC. Lenvatinib is a multikinase inhibitor that was evaluated for safety and efficacy in an open-label phase Ib/II trial of patients with advanced solid tumors including HNSCC and the combination of lenvatinib and pembrolizumab (NCT02501096). ORRs at 24 weeks was reported as 36% in 22 patients with HNSCC.[48] Based on these data, an ongoing phase III trial, LEAP 010, which compares the combination of lenvatinib and pembrolizumab with pembrolizumab and placebo is under way (NCT04199104).

VACCINE THERAPY

Over recent decades, increasing rates of HPV infection have generated interest in prophylactic vaccination strategies, initially targeting HPV-related cervical cancers, the 9-valent vaccine received expanded approval by the FDA for use in the prevention of HPV-related HNSCC in 2020. Prophylactic vaccinations induce an immune response resulting in antibodies against HPV major capsid protein L1, effectively neutralizing the presenting HPV virus and preventing infection.[49] L1 expression is lost after established HPV infection and, therefore, prophylactic vaccines do not exert therapeutic effects on existing HPV-associated malignancies.[50]

HPV viral oncoproteins E6 and E7 are continuously expressed by HPV-related cancer cells and are essential to maintain transformation of HPV+ HNSCC and therefore form the target of several therapeutic vaccines.[51,52] These are 2 of 8 genes encoded by the HPV genome that are expressed early in the virus life cycle and are the first viral proteins expressed following infection.[53] E6 and E7 perform multifunctional roles in oncogenesis, promoting p53 degradation and inactivating pRb respectively, resulting in uncontrolled host DNA synthesis and cell division and initiating the cascade that results in malignant cell transformation.[54] Tumor-specific antigens such as E6/E7 are ideal targets for therapeutic vaccines, as they often generate robust cytolytic T-cell responses. HPV vaccines, either alone or in combination with chemotherapy or immunotherapy have gained enthusiasm, with several clinical trials under way in this arena. The optimal vaccine strategy is yet to be identified; the possibilities include vector-based, peptide-based, DNA or mRNA vaccines, and dendritic vaccines. DNA vaccines produce antigens that can induce cytotoxic T-cell and B-cell immunity without eliciting antivector immune responses.[55] The antigen is produced in the body and the DNA backbone serves as an immunologic adjuvant.[56] Although DNA vaccines have been shown to be safe and easily scalable, they demonstrated low immunogenicity in early clinical trials.[57] Methods to increase DNA uptake include electroporation, liposomes, tattooing, and cationic polymers. A recently completed phase I/IIa trial assessed the safety, tolerability, and immunogenicity of 2 DNA plasmids encoding E6 and E7 proteins of HPV 16 and 18 in combination with a DNA vaccine encoding interleukin-2 (MEDI0457) delivered intramuscularly followed by electroporation (NCT02163057). A total of 22 patients were enrolled in the trial with promising initial results and was followed by a phase I/II trial to assess the vaccine in combination with a PD-L1 blocking monoclonal antibody, durvalumab (NCT03162224). At interim data cutoff, an ORR of 22% was shown in all patients who received MEDI0457 in combination with durvalumab and was found to be safe and well tolerated.

mRNA vaccines produce high antigen expression, as they can accumulate at high concentrations in the cytoplasm. They may additionally benefit from enhanced vaccine efficacy by inducing innate immune responses.[58] A phase I/II clinical trial using an intradermal, mRNA vaccine targeting HPV-16 E6 and E7 is currently under way (NCT03418480).

Peptide vaccines contain amino acid sequences that form immunogenic peptides corresponding to CD8 epitopes on tumor antigens that bind to a particular HLA allele. The peptide vaccine activates cytotoxic T lymphocytes, which in turn recognize peptide-major histocompatibility complex (MHC) I complexes on the surface of tumor cells.[59] These vaccines are restricted to bind only the specific HLA subclass for which they were designed. Peptide vaccines that contain long, single, or overlapping peptides containing both CD8 and CD4 epitopes overcome the HLA restriction issues. Although safe, peptide vaccines are poorly immunogenic and often combined with adjuvants to enhance their immunogenicity.[60] In a phase I/II trial, patients with advanced HPV-associated cancers received a vaccine of a synthetic long peptide derived from p16 in combination with an oil-in-water adjuvant (Monatanide). Cellular and humoral responses were induced by the peptide without unexpected serious adverse events (NCT01462838). Results of a recently completed phase I trial of subcutaneous MAGE-A3 or HPV-16 Trojan Peptide vaccine in patients with recurrent or metastatic HNSCC (NCT00257738) as well as a phase I trial with HPV-16 E6 and E7 peptides in HPV-related cancers including HNSCC (NCT00019110) are anticipated. The combination of peptide vaccines with immunotherapy is an additional area of interest and a phase II trial of nivolumab in combination with a synthetic long peptide HPV-16 vaccine (ISA101) demonstrated promising results. ISA101, consists 9 overlapping E6 peptides and 4 overlapping E7 peptides covering the complete sequence of the E6 and E7 oncoproteins. Patients who received the combination of nivolumab with ISA101 demonstrated an ORR of 33% (90% CI 19%–50%) with an mOS of 17.5 months (95% CI 17.5 to inestimable).[61] and 2 phase II clinical trials using HPV-16 E6/E7 overlapping peptides in combination with either anti-PD-1 antibody (Nivolumab) or an anti-CD137 immune stimulatory antibody (Utomilumab) are ongoing (NCT02426892, NCT03258008).

Viral and bacterial vector-based vaccines deliver tumor antigen packaged in attenuated viruses and function as immune adjuvants by triggering an immune response to a perceived infection.[62] A well-characterized, attenuated, facultative intracellular bacterium, *Listeria monocytogenes* has been used in a phase I trial and a phase II window of opportunity trial as an adjuvant in combination with an HPV-16 E7 vaccine with or without an anti-PD-L1 monoclonal antibody, Durvalumab (NCT02002182 and NCT02291055). A phase I trial of a modified vaccinia vector (Ankara) to encode a functionally inactive fusion protein of EBV recently demonstrated EBV-specific T-cell responses in eight of 14 patients.[63]

ADOPTIVE T-CELL THERAPY

Adoptive T-cell transfer (ACT) is a promising immunotherapy strategy that involves isolating T cells from a patient, modifying them to enhance their activity, then reintroducing them into the patient with a goal to improve the immune system's anticancer response.[64] Virally mediated cancers such as HPV-associated and EBV-associated HNSCC represent a potentially attractive system, as they contain specific tumor targets at which T cells can be directed. A phase I study of an intradermal vaccine of irradiated tumor cells followed by infusion of in vitro expanded T cells derived from resected inguinal lymph nodes, demonstrated disease control in 6 of 17 patients.[65] Two recently completed trials in R/M HPV-related cancers, including HNSCC, explored the use of T-cell receptor–engineered T cells and tumor-infiltrating lymphocytes (NCT02280811 and NCT01585428). The use of ACT in nasopharyngeal cancers has been studied in multiple trials, including a phase I study of ex vivo expanded autologous T cells in R/M EBV-associated nasopharyngeal cancers and another phase I study in which patients received EBV-transformed peripheral blood mononuclear cells.[66,67] With the successful application of chimeric antigen receptor (CAR) T cells in hematological malignancies, there has been enthusiasm for their application to other solid tumors, including HNSCC. CAR T cells are composed of 4 structural components, an extracellular antigen recognition region with a single-chain antibody fragment derived from a monoclonal antibody that can recognize specific tumor-related antigens without MHC, a transmembrane domain, an intracellular signaling domain, and an extracellular hinge domain.[68] A benefit of CAR T cells is their ability to function in an MHC independent manner. Several tumor-related antigens are currently being evaluated for use as HNSCC-specific CAR T therapy. Mucin 1, cell surface associated protein (MUC1) targeting CAR T cells are currently being studied in advanced refractory solid tumors, including pancreatic, breast, and non–small-cell lung cancer (NCT02587689). MUC1 has been shown to be overexpressed in HNSCC and demonstrated antitumor effects in preclinical studies.[69,70] A phase I/II trial in locoregional HNSCC using a second-generation panErbB-specific CAR T, which has been shown to be overexpressed in HNSCC,[71,72] is currently under way (NCT01818323). Combining CAR T cells with other therapies could increase their efficacy, and there is a phase I trial under way to study the effect of a HER2-specific CAR T in combination with an oncolytic adenovirus (NCT03740256).

SUMMARY

Immunotherapy has changed the therapeutic landscape of many cancers, including HNSCC, by improving survival and reducing toxicity over previous strategies. The addition of immune checkpoint inhibitors in the first-line setting offers a novel therapeutic option for patients with recurrent and metastatic disease. PD-L1 immunohistochemistry has shown utility in guiding patient selection for treatment options with other biomarkers that are currently under investigation. Studies evaluating the role for immunotherapy in locally advanced disease will provide useful information on this potential strategy to reduce toxicity while improving recurrence-free survival in this subset of patients. Much effort is now focused on identifying combinations to overcome adaptive resistance induced by immune checkpoint monotherapy while increasing response rates and duration in patients. Dual-checkpoint inhibitors as well as small molecule drugs in combination with standard of therapy or immune therapies are under investigation in multiple trials. New approaches including therapeutic vaccines and adoptive T-cell therapy have been developed in both solid and hematological malignancies and are now being studied in HNSCC.

As our understanding of the tumor microenvironment and its relationship to the immune system continues to expand, we expect the field of immunotherapy for HNSCC to evolve and ultimately improve outcomes for patients with this disease.

CLINICS CARE POINTS

- Despite advances in local and systemic therapies for head and neck cancer, the risk for recurrence is high and overall survival remains poor.
- In recent years, immune checkpoint inhibitors have expanded and improved the treatment options for recurrent and metastatic head and neck cancer.
- Anti-PD-1 therapy has now been approved in the first-line and second-line setting for recurrent and metastatic head and neck cancers.
- PD-L1 CPS is currently the most useful predictive biomarker of response to PD-1 blockade.
- Trials evaluating combination immune checkpoint blockade, therapeutic cancer vaccines, and adoptive T-cell therapy are currently under way in head and neck cancer.

DISCLOSURE

Dr C. Aggarwal has served as a consultant or advisor to AstraZeneca, BluPrint, Daichii Sankyo, Celgene, Genentech, Lilly, Merck, and Roche; and has received institutional research funding from AstraZeneca/MedImmune, Genentech/Roche, Incyte, Macro-Genics, and Merck Sharp & Dohme. Dr L. Sun has served as a consultant to Targeted Therapy.

REFERENCES

1. Gupta B, Johnson NW, Kumar N. Global epidemiology of head and neck cancers: a continuing challenge. Oncology 2016;91:13–23.
2. Fitzmaurice C, Allen C, Barber RM, et al. Global, regional, and national cancer incidence, mortality, years of life lost, years lived with disability, and disability-adjusted life-years for 32 cancer groups, 1990 to 2015: a systematic analysis for the Global Burden of Disease Study. JAMA Oncol 2017;3:524–48.
3. Bray F, Ferlay J, Soerjomataram I, et al. Global cancer statistics 2018: GLOBO-CAN estimates of incidence and mortality worldwide for 36 cancers in 185 countries. CA Cancer J Clin 2018;68:394–424.
4. Vermorken JB, Mesia R, Rivera F, et al. Platinum-based chemotherapy plus cetuximab in head and neck cancer. N Engl J Med 2008;359:1116–27.
5. Lawrence MS, Stojanov P, Polak P, et al. Mutational heterogeneity in cancer and the search for new cancer-associated genes. Nature 2013;499:214–8.
6. Ferris RL, Whiteside TL, Ferrone S. Immune escape associated with functional defects in antigen-processing machinery in head and neck cancer. Clin Cancer Res 2006;12:3890–5.
7. Wang J, Sun H, Zeng Q, et al. HPV-positive status associated with inflamed immune microenvironment and improved response to anti-PD-1 therapy in head and neck squamous cell carcinoma. Scientific Rep 2019;9:13404.
8. Mandal R, Şenbabaoğlu Y, Desrichard A, et al. The head and neck cancer immune landscape and its immunotherapeutic implications. JCI Insight 2016;1.
9. Mehra R, Seiwert TY, Gupta S, et al. Efficacy and safety of pembrolizumab in recurrent/metastatic head and neck squamous cell carcinoma: pooled analyses after long-term follow-up in KEYNOTE-012. Br J Cancer 2018;119:153–9.
10. Seiwert TY, Burtness B, Mehra R, et al. Safety and clinical activity of pembrolizumab for treatment of recurrent or metastatic squamous cell carcinoma of the head and neck (KEYNOTE-012): an open-label, multicentre, phase 1b trial. Lancet Oncol 2016;17:956–65.
11. Bauml J, Seiwert TY, Pfister DG, et al. Pembrolizumab for platinum- and cetuximab-refractory head and neck cancer: results from a single-arm, phase II study. J Clin Oncol 2017;35:1542–9.
12. Cohen EEW, Soulières D, Le Tourneau C, et al. Pembrolizumab versus methotrexate, docetaxel, or cetuximab for recurrent or metastatic head-and-neck squamous cell carcinoma (KEYNOTE-040): a randomised, open-label, phase 3 study. Lancet 2019;393:156–67.
13. Ferris RL, Blumenschein G, Fayette J, et al. Nivolumab for recurrent squamous-cell carcinoma of the head and neck. N Engl J Med 2016;375:1856–67.
14. Ferris RL, Blumenschein G Jr, Fayette J, et al. Nivolumab vs investigator's choice in recurrent or metastatic squamous cell carcinoma of the head and neck: 2-year long-term survival update of CheckMate 141 with analyses by tumor PD-L1 expression. Oral Oncol 2018;81:45–51.

15. Cohen EEW, Bell RB, Bifulco CB, et al. The Society for Immunotherapy of Cancer consensus statement on immunotherapy for the treatment of squamous cell carcinoma of the head and neck (HNSCC). J Immunother Cancer 2019;7:184.

16. Zandberg DP, Algazi AP, Jimeno A, et al. Durvalumab for recurrent or metastatic head and neck squamous cell carcinoma: Results from a single-arm, phase II study in patients with ≥25% tumour cell PD-L1 expression who have progressed on platinum-based chemotherapy. Eur J Cancer 2019;107:142–52.

17. Ferris RL, Haddad R, Even C, et al. Durvalumab with or without tremelimumab in patients with recurrent or metastatic head and neck squamous cell carcinoma: EAGLE, a randomized, open-label phase III study. Ann Oncol 2020;31:942–50.

18. Burtness B, Harrington KJ, Greil R, et al. Pembrolizumab alone or with chemotherapy versus cetuximab with chemotherapy for recurrent or metastatic squamous cell carcinoma of the head and neck (KEYNOTE-048): a randomised, open-label, phase 3 study. Lancet 2019;394:1915–28.

19. Taube JM, Klein A, Brahmer JR, et al. Association of PD-1, PD-1 ligands, and other features of the tumor immune microenvironment with response to anti-PD-1 therapy. Clin Cancer Res 2014;20:5064–74.

20. Cristescu R, Mogg R, Ayers M, et al. Pan-tumor genomic biomarkers for PD-1 checkpoint blockade–based immunotherapy. Science 2018;362:eaar3593.

21. Li W, Wildsmith S, Ye J, et al. Plasma-based tumor mutational burden (bTMB) as predictor for survival in phase III EAGLE study: Durvalumab (D) ± tremelimumab (T) versus chemotherapy (CT) in recurrent/metastatic head and neck squamous cell carcinoma (R/M HNSCC) after platinum failure. J Clin Oncol 2020;38:6511.

22. Seiwert TY, Haddad R, Bauml J, et al. Abstract LB-339: Biomarkers predictive of response to pembrolizumab in head and neck cancer (HNSCC). Cancer Res 2018;78:LB-339.

23. Riaz N, Havel JJ, Makarov V, et al. Tumor and microenvironment evolution during immunotherapy with nivolumab. Cell 2017;171:934–49.e916.

24. Oliva M, Spreafico A, Taberna M, et al. Immune biomarkers of response to immune-checkpoint inhibitors in head and neck squamous cell carcinoma. Ann Oncol 2019;30:57–67.

25. Chaturvedi AK, Engels EA, Pfeiffer RM, et al. Human papillomavirus and rising oropharyngeal cancer incidence in the United States. J Clin Oncol 2011;29:4294–301.

26. Gillison ML, Chaturvedi AK, Anderson WF, et al. Epidemiology of human papillomavirus-positive head and neck squamous cell carcinoma. J Clin Oncol : official J Am Soc Clin Oncol 2015;33:3235–42.

27. Wolchok JD, Hoos A, O'Day S, et al. Guidelines for the evaluation of immune therapy activity in solid tumors: immune-related response criteria. Clin Cancer Res 2009;15:7412–20.

28. Wolchok JD, Hamid O, Ribas A, et al. Atypical patterns of response in patients (pts) with metastatic melanoma treated with pembrolizumab (MK-3475) in KEYNOTE-001. J Clin Oncol 2015;33:3000.

29. Borcoman E, Nandikolla A, Long G, et al. Patterns of response and progression to immunotherapy. Am Soc Clin Oncol Educ Book 2018;169–78.

30. Haddad R, Ferris RL, Blumenschein G, et al. Abstract CT157: Treatment beyond progression with nivolumab in patients with recurrent or metastatic squamous cell carcinoma of the head and neck in the phase 3 Checkmate 141 study. Cancer Res 2017;77:CT157.

31. Baxi SS, Dunn LA, Burtness BA. Amidst the excitement: a cautionary tale of immunotherapy, pseudoprogression and head and neck squamous cell carcinoma. Oral Oncol 2016;62:147–8.
32. Champiat S, Dercle L, Ammari S, et al. Hyperprogressive disease is a new pattern of progression in cancer patients treated by anti-PD-1/PD-L1. Clin Cancer Res 2017;23:1920–8.
33. Saâda-Bouzid E, Defaucheux C, Karabajakian A, et al. Hyperprogression during anti-PD-1/PD-L1 therapy in patients with recurrent and/or metastatic head and neck squamous cell carcinoma. Ann Oncol 2017;28:1605–11.
34. Hoos A, Eggermont AM, Janetzki S, et al. Improved endpoints for cancer immunotherapy trials. J Natl Cancer Inst 2010;102:1388–97.
35. Seymour L, Bogaerts J, Perrone A, et al. iRECIST: guidelines for response criteria for use in trials testing immunotherapeutics. The Lancet Oncol 2017;18:e143–52.
36. Hodi FS, Hwu W-J, Kefford R, et al. Evaluation of immune-related response criteria and RECIST v1.1 in patients with advanced melanoma treated with pembrolizumab. J Clin Oncol 2016;34:1510–7.
37. John AT, Bryan JS, Julie B, et al. Management of immunotherapy-related toxicities, version 1.2019, NCCN clinical practice guidelines in oncology. J Natl Compr Cancer Netw 2019;17:255–89.
38. Shah NJ, Al-Shbool G, Blackburn M, et al. Safety and efficacy of immune checkpoint inhibitors (ICIs) in cancer patients with HIV, hepatitis B, or hepatitis C viral infection. J ImmunoTherapy Cancer 2019;7:353.
39. Cook MR, Kim C. Safety and efficacy of immune checkpoint inhibitor therapy in patients with HIV infection and advanced-stage cancer: a systematic review. JAMA Oncol 2019;5:1049–54.
40. Reuss JE, Stern D, Foster JC, et al. Assessment of cancer therapy evaluation program advocacy and inclusion rates of people living with HIV in anti–PD1/PDL1 clinical trials. JAMA Netw Open 2020;3:e2027110.
41. Stafford M, Kaczmar J. The neoadjuvant paradigm reinvigorated: a review of pre-surgical immunotherapy in HNSCC. Cancers Head Neck 2020;5:4.
42. Powell SF, Gold KA, Gitau MM, et al. Safety and efficacy of pembrolizumab with chemoradiotherapy in locally advanced head and neck squamous cell carcinoma: a phase IB study. J Clin Oncol 2020;38:2427–37.
43. Uppaluri R, Campbell KM, Egloff AM, et al. Neoadjuvant and adjuvant pembrolizumab in resectable locally advanced, human papillomavirus-unrelated head and neck cancer: a multicenter, phase II trial. Clin Cancer Res 2020;26:5140–52.
44. Koyama S, Akbay EA, Li YY, et al. Adaptive resistance to therapeutic PD-1 blockade is associated with upregulation of alternative immune checkpoints. Nat Commun 2016;7:10501.
45. Wang CJ, Schmidt EM, Attridge K, et al. Immune regulation by CTLA-4–relevance to autoimmune diabetes in a transgenic mouse model. Diabetes Metab Res Rev 2011;27:946–50.
46. Sullivan TJ, Letterio JJ, van Elsas A, et al. Lack of a role for transforming growth factor-beta in cytotoxic T lymphocyte antigen-4-mediated inhibition of T cell activation. Proc Natl Acad Sci U S A 2001;98:2587–92.
47. Strauss J, Gatti-Mays ME, Cho BC, et al. Bintrafusp alfa, a bifunctional fusion protein targeting TGF-beta and PD-L1, in patients with human papillomavirus-associated malignancies. J Immunother Cancer 2020;8.
48. Taylor MH, Lee CH, Makker V, et al. Phase IB/II trial of lenvatinib plus pembrolizumab in patients with advanced renal cell carcinoma, endometrial cancer, and other selected advanced solid tumors. J Clin Oncol 2020;38:1154–63.

49. Lowy DR, Schiller JT. Prophylactic human papillomavirus vaccines. J Clin Invest 2006;116:1167–73.
50. Schiller JT, Castellsague X, Garland SM. A review of clinical trials of human papillomavirus prophylactic vaccines. Vaccine 2012;30(Suppl 5):F123–38.
51. Rampias T, Sasaki C, Weinberger P, et al. E6 and e7 gene silencing and transformed phenotype of human papillomavirus 16-positive oropharyngeal cancer cells. J Natl Cancer Inst 2009;101:412–23.
52. Bagarazzi ML, Yan J, Morrow MP, et al. Immunotherapy against HPV16/18 generates potent TH1 and cytotoxic cellular immune responses. Sci Transl Med 2012;4:155ra138.
53. Schiffman M, Doorbar J, Wentzensen N, et al. Carcinogenic human papillomavirus infection. Nat Rev Dis Primers 2016;2:16086.
54. Munoz N, Castellsague X, de Gonzalez AB, et al. Chapter 1: HPV in the etiology of human cancer. Vaccine 2006;24(Suppl 3). S3/1-10.
55. Gildener-Leapman N, Lee J, Ferris RL. Tailored immunotherapy for HPV positive head and neck squamous cell cancer. Oral Oncol 2014;50:780–4.
56. Krieg AM. CpG motifs in bacterial DNA and their immune effects. Annu Rev Immunol 2002;20:709–60.
57. Low L, Mander A, McCann K, et al. DNA vaccination with electroporation induces increased antibody responses in patients with prostate cancer. Hum Gene Ther 2009;20:1269–78.
58. Grunwitz C, Kranz LM. mRNA cancer vaccines-messages that prevail. Curr Top Microbiol Immunol 2017;405:145–64.
59. Huppa JB, Davis MM. T-cell-antigen recognition and the immunological synapse. Nat Rev Immunol 2003;3:973–83.
60. Melief CJ, van Hall T, Arens R, et al. Therapeutic cancer vaccines. J Clin Invest 2015;125:3401–12.
61. Massarelli E, William W, Johnson F, et al. Combining immune checkpoint blockade and tumor-specific vaccine for patients with incurable human papillomavirus 16-related cancer: a phase 2 clinical trial. JAMA Oncol 2019;5:67–73.
62. Ryman KD, Klimstra WB. Host responses to alphavirus infection. Immunol Rev 2008;225:27–45.
63. Taylor GS, Jia H, Harrington K, et al. A recombinant modified vaccinia ankara vaccine encoding Epstein-Barr Virus (EBV) target antigens: a phase I trial in UK patients with EBV-positive cancer. Clin Cancer Res 2014;20:5009–22.
64. June CH. Adoptive T cell therapy for cancer in the clinic. J Clin Invest 2007;117:1466–76.
65. To WC, Wood BG, Krauss JC, et al. Systemic adoptive T-cell immunotherapy in recurrent and metastatic carcinoma of the head and neck: a phase 1 study. Arch Otolaryngol Head Neck Surg 2000;126:1225–31.
66. Chia WK, Teo M, Wang WW, et al. Adoptive T-cell transfer and chemotherapy in the first-line treatment of metastatic and/or locally recurrent nasopharyngeal carcinoma. Mol Ther 2014;22:132–9.
67. Smith C, Tsang J, Beagley L, et al. Effective treatment of metastatic forms of Epstein-Barr virus-associated nasopharyngeal carcinoma with a novel adenovirus-based adoptive immunotherapy. Cancer Res 2012;72:1116–25.
68. Srivastava S, Riddell SR. Chimeric antigen receptor T cell therapy: challenges to bench-to-bedside efficacy. J Immunol 2018;200:459–68.
69. Rabassa ME, Croce MV, Pereyra A, et al. MUC1 expression and anti-MUC1 serum immune response in head and neck squamous cell carcinoma (HNSCC): a multivariate analysis. BMC Cancer 2006;6:253.

70. Mei Z, Zhang K, Lam AK, et al. MUC1 as a target for CAR-T therapy in head and neck squamous cell carinoma. Cancer Med 2020;9:640–52.
71. Pollock NI, Grandis JR. HER2 as a therapeutic target in head and neck squamous cell carcinoma. Clin Cancer Res 2015;21:526–33.
72. Pollock NI, Wang L, Wallweber G, et al. Increased Expression of HER2, HER3, and HER2:HER3 Heterodimers in HPV-positive HNSCC using a novel proximity-based assay: implications for targeted therapies. Clin Cancer Res 2015;21: 4597–606.

UNITED STATES POSTAL SERVICE®

Statement of Ownership, Management, and Circulation
(All Periodicals Publications Except Requester Publications)

1. Publication Title	2. Publication Number	3. Filing Date
HEMATOLOGY/ONCOLOGY CLINICS OF NORTH AMERICA	002 – 473	9/18/2021

4. Issue Frequency	5. Number of Issues Published Annually	6. Annual Subscription Price
FEB, APR, JUN, AUG, OCT, DEC	6	$456.00

7. Complete Mailing Address of Known Office of Publication (Not printer) (Street, city, county, state, and ZIP+4®)

ELSEVIER INC.
230 Park Avenue, Suite 800
New York, NY 10169

Contact Person
Malathi Samayan

Telephone (Include area code)
91-44-4299-4507

8. Complete Mailing Address of Headquarters or General Business Office of Publisher (Not printer)

ELSEVIER INC.
230 Park Avenue, Suite 800
New York, NY 10169

9. Full Names and Complete Mailing Addresses of Publisher, Editor, and Managing Editor (Do not leave blank)

Publisher (Name and complete mailing address)

Dolores Meloni, ELSEVIER INC.
1600 JOHN F KENNEDY BLVD. SUITE 1800
PHILADELPHIA, PA 19103-2899

Editor (Name and complete mailing address)

STACY EASTMAN, ELSEVIER INC.
1600 JOHN F KENNEDY BLVD. SUITE 1800
PHILADELPHIA, PA 19103-2899

Managing Editor (Name and complete mailing address)

PATRICK MANLEY, ELSEVIER INC.
1600 JOHN F KENNEDY BLVD. SUITE 1800
PHILADELPHIA, PA 19103-2899

10. Owner (Do not leave blank. If the publication is owned by a corporation, give the name and address of the corporation immediately followed by the names and addresses of all stockholders owning or holding 1 percent or more of the total amount of stock. If not owned by a corporation, give the names and addresses of the individual owners. If owned by a partnership or other unincorporated firm, give its name and address as well as those of each individual owner. If the publication is published by a nonprofit organization, give its name and address.)

Full Name	Complete Mailing Address
WHOLLY OWNED SUBSIDIARY OF REED/ELSEVIER, US HOLDINGS	1600 JOHN F KENNEDY BLVD. SUITE 1800 PHILADELPHIA, PA 19103-2899

11. Known Bondholders, Mortgagees, and Other Security Holders Owning or Holding 1 Percent or More of Total Amount of Bonds, Mortgages, or Other Securities. If none, check box ▶ ☐ None

Full Name	Complete Mailing Address
N/A	

12. Tax Status (For completion by nonprofit organizations authorized to mail at nonprofit rates) (Check one)
The purpose, function, and nonprofit status of this organization and the exempt status for federal income tax purposes:
☒ Has Not Changed During Preceding 12 Months
☐ Has Changed During Preceding 12 Months (Publisher must submit explanation of change with this statement)

PS Form 3526, July 2014 [Page 1 of 4 (see instructions page 4)] PSN: 7530-01-000-9931 PRIVACY NOTICE: See our privacy policy on www.usps.com

13. Publication Title	14. Issue Date for Circulation Data Below
HEMATOLOGY/ONCOLOGY CLINICS OF NORTH AMERICA	JUNE 2021

15. Extent and Nature of Circulation			Average No. Copies Each Issue During Preceding 12 Months	No. Copies of Single Issue Published Nearest to Filing Date
a. Total Number of Copies (Net press run)			157	137
b. Paid Circulation (By Mail and Outside the Mail)	(1)	Mailed Outside-County Paid Subscriptions Stated on PS Form 3541 (Include paid distribution above nominal rate, advertiser's proof copies, and exchange copies)	62	49
	(2)	Mailed In-County Paid Subscriptions Stated on PS Form 3541 (Include paid distribution above nominal rate, advertiser's proof copies, and exchange copies)	0	0
	(3)	Paid Distribution Outside the Mails Including Sales Through Dealers and Carriers, Street Vendors, Counter Sales, and Other Paid Distribution Outside USPS®	48	40
	(4)	Paid Distribution by Other Classes of Mail Through the USPS (e.g. First-Class Mail®)	0	0
c. Total Paid Distribution (Sum of 15b (1), (2), (3), and (4))		▶	110	89
d. Free or Nominal Rate Distribution (By Mail and Outside the Mail)	(1)	Free or Nominal Rate Outside-County Copies included on PS Form 3541	31	29
	(2)	Free or Nominal Rate In-County Copies Included on PS Form 3541	0	0
	(3)	Free or Nominal Rate Copies Mailed at Other Classes Through the USPS (e.g. First-Class Mail)	0	0
	(4)	Free or Nominal Rate Distribution Outside the Mail (Carriers or other means)	0	0
e. Total Free or Nominal Rate Distribution (Sum of 15d (1), (2), (3) and (4))		▶	31	29
f. Total Distribution (Sum of 15c and 15e)		▶	141	118
g. Copies not Distributed (See Instructions to Publishers #4 (page #3))		▶	16	19
h. Total (Sum of 15f and g)		▶	157	137
i. Percent Paid (15c divided by 15f times 100)		▶	78.01%	75.42%

* If you are claiming electronic copies, go to line 16 on page 3. If you are not claiming electronic copies, skip to line 17 on page 3.

16. Electronic Copy Circulation		Average No. Copies Each Issue During Preceding 12 Months	No. Copies of Single Issue Published Nearest to Filing Date
a. Paid Electronic Copies	▶		
b. Total Paid Print Copies (Line 15c) + Paid Electronic Copies (Line 16a)	▶		
c. Total Print Distribution (Line 15f) + Paid Electronic Copies (Line 16a)	▶		
d. Percent Paid (Both Print & Electronic Copies) (16b divided by 16c × 100)	▶		

☒ I certify that 50% of all my distributed copies (electronic and print) are paid above a nominal price.

17. Publication of Statement of Ownership

☒ If the publication is a general publication, publication of this statement is required. Will be printed
in the OCTOBER 2021 issue of this publication.

☐ Publication not required.

18. Signature and Title of Editor, Publisher, Business Manager, or Owner

Malathi Samayan *(signature)*

Malathi Samayan - Distribution Controller

Date
9/18/2021

I certify that all information furnished on this form is true and complete. I understand that anyone who furnishes false or misleading information on this form or who omits material or information requested on the form may be subject to criminal sanctions (including fines and imprisonment) and/or civil sanctions (including civil penalties).

PS Form 3526, July 2014 (Page 3 of 4) PRIVACY NOTICE: See our privacy policy on www.usps.com